PET/CT and PET/MRI for Assessment of Structural and Functional Relationships in Disease Conditions

Guest Editors

DREW A. TORIGIAN, MD, MA
ABASS ALAVI, MD, PhD (Hon), DSc (Hon)

PET CLINICS

www.pet.theclinics.com

Consulting Editor
ABASS ALAVI, MD, PhD (Hon), DSc (Hon)

July 2008 • Volume 3 • Number 3

SAUNDERS an imprint of ELSEVIER, Inc.

W.B. SAUNDERS COMPANY
A Division of Elsevier Inc.

1600 John F. Kennedy Boulevard • Suite 1800 • Philadelphia, Pennsylvania 19103-2899

http://www.theclinics.com

PET CLINICS Volume 3, Number 3
July 2008 ISSN 1556-8598, ISBN 10: 1-4160-6646-2, ISBN-13: 978-1-4160-6646-0

Editor: Barton Dudlick
Developmental Editor: Theresa Collier

PET Clinics (ISSN 1556-8598) is published quarterly by W.B. Saunders, 360 Park Avenue South, New York, NY 10010-1710. Months of publication are January, April, July, and October. Business and Editorial Offices: 1600 John F. Kennedy Blvd., Suite 1800, Philadelphia, PA 19103-2899. Accounting and Circulation Offices: 11830 Westline Industrial Drive, St. Louis, MO 63146. Periodicals postage paid at New York, NY, and additional mailing offices. Subscription prices per year are $196.00 (US individuals), $274.00 (US institutions), $97.00 (US students), $223.00 (Canadian individuals), $306.00 (Canadian institutions), $118.00 (Canadian students), $237.00 (foreign individuals), $306.00 (foreign institutions), and $118.00 (foreign students). To receive student and resident rate, orders must be accompanied by name of affiliated institution, date of term, and the signature of program/residency coordinator on institution letterhead. Orders will be billed at individual rate until proof of status is received. Foreign air speed delivery is included in all Clinics subscription prices. All prices are subject to change without notice. POSTMASTER: Send address changes to PET Clinics, Elsevier Periodicals Customer Service, 11830 Westline Industrial Drive, St. Louis, MO 63146. **Customer service: 1-800-654-2452 (US). From outside of the United States, call 314-453-7041. Fax: 314-453-5170. E-mail: JournalsCustomerService-usa@elsevier.com (for print support); JournalsOnlineSupport-usa@elsevier.com (for online support).**

Reprints. For copies of 100 or more of articles in this publication, please contact the Commercial Reprints Department, Elsevier Inc., 360 Park Avenue South, New York, NY 10010-1710. Tel.: 212-633-3812; Fax: 212-462-1935; E-mail: reprints@elsevier.com.

Printed in the United States of America.

Contributors

CONSULTING EDITOR

ABASS ALAVI, MD, PhD (Hon), DSc (Hon)
Professor of Radiology, Division of Nuclear
Medicine, Hospital of the University of
Pennsylvania, Philadelphia, Pennsylvania

GUEST EDITORS

DREW A. TORIGIAN, MD, MA
Assistant Professor, Department of Radiology,
University of Pennsylvania School of Medicine,
Philadelphia, Pennsylvania

ABASS ALAVI, MD, PhD (Hon), DSc (Hon)
Professor of Radiology, Division of Nuclear
Medicine, Hospital of the University of
Pennsylvania, Philadelphia, Pennsylvania

AUTHORS

ABASS ALAVI, MD, PhD (Hon), DSc (Hon)
Professor of Radiology, Division of Nuclear
Medicine, Hospital of the University of
Pennsylvania, Philadelphia, Pennsylvania

VALENTINA AMBROSINI, MD, PhD
Department of Nuclear Medicine and Centre
for PET/CT, Zentralklinik Bad Berka, Germany

RICHARD P. BAUM, MD, PhD
Department of Nuclear Medicine and Centre
for PET/CT, Zentralklinik Bad Berka, Germany

JUDY BLEBEA, MD
Pending Visiting Associate Professor, Cleveland
Clinic Lerner School of Medicine; Staff Radiologist at
Imaging Institute, Cleveland Clinic, Cleveland, Ohio

SANJEEV CHAWLA, PhD
Research Associate, Department of Radiology,
Hospital of the University of Pennsylvania,
Philadelphia, Pennsylvania

KAREN CHEN, MD
Musculoskeletal Radiology Fellow, Department
of Radiology, Hospital of the University of
Pennsylvania, Philadelphia, Pennsylvania

WENGEN CHEN, MD, PhD
Resident in Nuclear Medicine, Department of
Radiology, University of Pennsylvania School
of Medicine, Philadelphia, Pennsylvania

BENOIT DESJARDINS, MD, PhD
Assistant Professor, Department of Radiology,
University of Pennsylvania School of Medicine,
Philadelphia, Pennsylvania

STEFANO FANTI, MD
Professor, Department of Nuclear Medicine,
S. Orsola-Malpighi Polyclinic, University
of Bologna, Bologna, Italy

THOMAS FERRARA, BS
Department of Radiology, Hospital of the
University of Pennsylvania School of Medicine,
Philadelphia, Pennsylvania

MICHAEL F. GOLDBERG, MD, MPH
Neuroradiology Fellow, Department of Radiology,
Hospital of the University of Pennsylvania,
Philadelphia, Pennsylvania

ROLAND HUSTINX, MD, PhD
Division of Nuclear Medicine, University Hospital
of Liège, Campus Universitaire du Sart Tilman,
Liège, Belgium

SHARYN KATZ, MD
Department of Radiology, Hospital of the
University of Pennsylvania School of Medicine,
Philadelphia, Pennsylvania

ANN K. KIM, MD
Department of Radiology, Division
of Neuroradiology, Hospital of the University
of Pennsylvania, Philadelphia, Pennsylvania

RAKESH KUMAR, MD
Department of Nuclear Medicine, All India Institute
of Medical Sciences, New Delhi, India

JEAN-DENIS LAREDO, MD
Professor, Department of Radiology, Hospital
of the University of Pennsylvania, Philadelphia,
Pennsylvania

LAURIE A. LOEVNER, MD
Professor of Radiology, Otorhinolaryngology,
Head and Neck Surgery, Neurosurgery,
Department of Radiology, Division of
Neuroradiology, Hospital of the University
of Pennsylvania, Philadelphia, Pennsylvania

ELIAS R. MELHEM, MD, PhD
Professor, Department of Radiology, Hospital
of the University of Pennsylvania, Philadelphia,
Pennsylvania

IGOR MIKITYANSKY, MD
Department of Radiology, Division
of Neuroradiology, Hospital of the University
of Pennsylvania, Philadelphia, Pennsylvania

MARIE-LOUISE MONTANDON, PhD
Division of Nuclear Medicine, Geneva University
Hospital, Geneva, Switzerland

ERIK S. MUSIEK, MD, PhD
Department of Neurology, University
of Pennsylvania Medical Center, Philadelphia,
Pennsylvania

GAUTHIER NAMUR, MD
Division of Nuclear Medicine, University Hospital
of Liège, Campus Universitaire du Sart Tilman,
Liège, Belgium

CRISTINA NANNI, MD
UO Medicina Nucleare, Azienda
Ospedaliero-Universitaria di Bologna Policlinico
S. Orsola-Malpighi, Bologna, Italy

ANDREW B. NEWBERG, MD
Division of Nuclear Medicine, Department
of Radiology, University of Pennsylvania Medical
Center, Philadelphia, Pennsylvania

VIKAS PRASAD, MD
Department of Nuclear Medicine and Centre for
PET/CT, Zentralklinik Bad Berka, Germany

SHAMIM AHMED SHAMIM, MD
Department of Nuclear Medicine, All India Institute
of Medical Sciences, New Delhi, India

DAVID B. STOUT, PhD
Department of Molecular and Medical
Pharmacology, Crump Institute for Molecular
Imaging, The David Geffen School of Medicine at
University of California Los Angeles, Los Angeles,
California

AMOL TAKALKAR, MD
Associate Medical Director, PET Imaging Center,
Biomedical Research Foundation of Northwest
Louisiana; Assistant Professor of Clinical
Radiology, Department of Radiology, LSUHSC-S,
Shreveport, Louisiana

DREW A. TORIGIAN, MD, MA
Assistant Professor, Department of Radiology,
University of Pennsylvania School of Medicine,
Philadelphia, Pennsylvania

HABIB ZAIDI, PhD, PD
Division of Nuclear Medicine, Geneva University
Hospital, Geneva, Switzerland

Contents

Applications of Small Animal Imaging with PET, PET/CT, and PET/MR Imaging   243

Cristina Nanni and Drew A. Torigian

> Small animal techniques of PET, MR imaging, and CT are most frequently applied in preclinical oncology research, but cardiovascular and neurologic research protocols can also take advantage of these innovative approaches. PET is used to provide functional information about disease activity. Using small animal PET and MR imaging, one can observe the response of a disease condition to a new therapeutic agent or the development of disease, significantly reducing the number of animals employed and increasing the reliability of the results. By employing the same technology (PET, MR imaging, or CT) in the experimental setting and in clinical practice, the step between preclinical science and clinical applications in human patients is shortened.

Preclinical Multimodality Imaging in Vivo   251

David B. Stout and Habib Zaidi

> Multimodality small-animal molecular imaging has become increasingly important as transgenic and knockout mice are produced to model human diseases. With the ever-increasing number and importance of human disease models, particularly in rodents (mice and rats), the ability of high-resolution multimodality molecular imaging instrumentation to contribute unique information is becoming more common and necessary. Multimodality imaging with high spatial resolution and good sensitivity, which combines modalities and records sequentially or simultaneously complementary information, offers many advantages in certain research experiments. This article discusses the current trends and new horizons in preclinical multimodality imaging in-vivo and its role in biomedical research.

The Clinical Role of Fusion Imaging Using PET, CT, and MR Imaging   275

Habib Zaidi, Marie-Louise Montandon, and Abass Alavi

> Multimodality image registration and fusion have a key role in routine diagnosis, staging, restaging, and the assessment of response to treatment, surgery, and radiotherapy planning of malignant disease. The complementarity between anatomic (CT and MR imaging) and molecular (SPECT and PET) imaging modalities is well established and the role of fusion imaging widely recognized as a central piece of the general tree of clinical decision making. Moreover, dual modality imaging technologies including SPECT/CT, PET/CT, and, in the future, PET/MR imaging, now represent the leading component of contemporary health care institutions. This article discusses recent advances in clinical multimodality imaging, the role of correlative fusion imaging in a clinical setting, and future opportunities and challenges facing the adoption of multimodality imaging.

PET and MR Imaging of Brain Tumors   293

Michael F. Goldberg, Sanjeev Chawla, Abass Alavi, Drew A. Torigian, and Elias R. Melhem

> A better understanding of tumorigenesis is crucial for the development of specific molecular therapies that specifically target the neoplasm and reduce patient

morbidity and mortality. PET measures a wide range of physiologic processes critical for understanding the pathophysiology of brain neoplasms with high sensitivity. Continuous developments in PET provide new insights into the diagnosis, classification, and pathophysiology of brain neoplasms. As such, PET has played an increasingly important role in the staging of brain neoplasms, image-guided therapy planning, and treatment monitoring. This article addresses the most commonly used agents in PET imaging of brain tumors.

Neuroimaging with positron emission tomography (PET) provides metabolic and molecular information that cannot be obtained from other imaging modalities and provides novel insights into the pathogenesis and diagnosis of a diverse array of neurologic diseases. As the library of novel PET ligands expands, so does the potential role for PET in the study of neurologic disease. The emergence of PET amyloid imaging reveals the incredible potential for PET neuroimaging. Recent technical advances in our ability to combine structural MR imaging data with functional and molecular PET data have enhanced the power of PET for the study of the brain. Thus, PET and MR imaging should continue to play an expanding role in the diagnosis and investigation of neurologic disease conditions.

This article emphasizes the strengths and potential pitfalls of functional and anatomic imaging in patients who have head and neck cancer with an emphasis on the treated neck, including patients who have undergone surgery and/or radiation therapy. Anatomic and molecular imaging together allow optimal evaluation and interpretation of a patient who has cancer. Effective assessment of patients who have head and neck cancer can be achieved through a careful review of pertinent anatomy, with awareness of the physiologic variations (especially those in the treated head and neck) seen in PET imaging, and analysis of both the PET and cross-sectional images.

In-111 Octreoscan is considered the gold standard for imaging of neuroendocrine tumors (NET). However, in the absence of morphologic imaging correlation, the exact localization of the tumor is often difficult. Also the sensitivity of PET imaging is more than Gamma camera (SPECT) imaging. Ga-68 labeled somatostatin analogs (SMS-R) are interesting radiopharmaceuticals for PET receptor imaging of NET. Some other radiopharmaceuticals e.g. F-18 DOPA can also be used to assess metabolism and functional status of NET. The importance of these radiopharmaceuticals, especially SMS-R increases in the absence of any specific biochemical marker or clinical parameter for follow-up of patients after therapy (eg. peptide receptor radionuclide therapy, surgery, chemoembolisation, etc). New criteria based on molecular, metabolic and morphologic imaging needs to be developed for correct assessment of response to therapy for these slow-growing, solid tumors.

This review focuses mainly on clinical applications of PET/CT in patients with breast cancer. It discusses the role of 2-[18F]-fluoro-2-deoxy-D-glucose (FDG) PET/CT (and FDG PET) in the diagnosis and initial staging of breast cancer, in monitoring the response of disease to chemotherapy, and in identifying metastatic and recurrent disease. In addition, it discusses the role of MR imaging and potential future hybrid modalities such as PET/MR imaging.

Imaging of patients with thoracic malignancy usually requires a multimodality approach. Each of these modalities has its own strengths and weaknesses. CT remains central to the staging and restaging of thoracic malignancies, but has recently been complemented with [18F]-2-fluoro-2-deoxy-D-glucose(FDG)–positron emission tomography (PET) imaging to maximize its potential. Furthermore, because FDG-PET/CT is useful at all stages of the workup and treatment of these patients, this modality has taken hold in the clinical realm for evaluation of patients with thoracic malignancy and is rapidly replacing PET-only imaging. MR imaging is also occasionally used in some patients with thoracic malignancies to improve disease staging or lesion characterization. PET/MR imaging may come to be used to evaluate patients with thoracic malignancies as well.

PET provides high-resolution images of radiopharmaceutical biodistribution in vivo. Fluorine-18–labeled fluorodeoxyglucose (FDG)–PET is an established entity in the work-up of several oncologic disorders and is making forays in the diagnosis of inflammatory diseases, leading to increased use for cardiac and neurologic applications. Combined myocardial perfusion and metabolism imaging using FDG-PET is the gold standard for noninvasive assessment of myocardial viability. Advances in imaging instrumentation (including CT and MR imaging technology) facilitate noninvasive assessment of cardiovascular pathologies. MR imaging is best placed to provide the most comprehensive cardiac evaluation. This article addresses evaluation of the cardiovascular system by PET, CT, and MR imaging.

This article reviews the current performance and status of PET/CT and MR imaging in four different abdominopelvic malignancies: cervical, pancreatic, and rectal cancers and liver metastases, as well as in Crohn's disease. The authors discuss the complementary aspects of these imaging techniques to evaluate the nature of the lesion, its local extent, and distant spread. These disease conditions represent pertinent clinical models in which PET/MRI may, if and when available, constitute a powerful tool in the management of patients.

18F-2-fluoro-2-deoxy-D-glucose–PET has an established role in the evaluation of hip periprosthetic infection and musculoskeletal malignancies. Determination of its role in the management of inflammatory arthritis and diabetic foot complications is ongoing. The reintroduction of fluorine F 18 sodium fluoride as a PET radiotracer may advantageously replace technetium Tc 99 m methylene diphosphonate for some non-oncologic applications, including treatment monitoring of Paget's disease and fibrous dysplasia. The combination of CT or MR imaging with PET imaging synergistically maximizes the diagnostic potential of a combined structural-functional imaging approach for the detection, characterization, and monitoring of myriad musculoskeletal disorders.

PET Clinics

THE CLINICS ARE NOW AVAILABLE ONLINE!

Access your subscription at:
www.theclinics.com

GOAL STATEMENT

The goal of the *PET Clinics* is to keep practicing radiologists and radiology residents up to date with current clinical practice in positron emission tomography by providing timely articles reviewing the state of the art in patient care.

ACCREDITATION

PET Clinics is planned and implemented in accordance with the Essential Areas and Policies of the Accreditation Council for Continuing Medical Education (ACCME) through the joint sponsorship of the University of Virginia School of Medicine and Elsevier. The University of Virginia School of Medicine is accredited by the ACCME to provide continuing medical education for physicians.

The University of Virginia School of Medicine designates this educational activity for a maximum of 15 *AMA PRA Category 1 Credits*™ for each issue, 60 credits per year. Physicians should only claim credit commensurate with the extent of their participation in the activity.

The American Medical Association has determined that physicians not licensed in the US who participate in this CME activity are eligible for a maximum of 15 *AMA PRA Category 1 Credits*™ for each issue, 60 credits per year.

Category 1 credit can be earned by reading the text material, taking the CME examination online at http://www.theclinics.com/home/cme, and completing the evaluation. After taking the test, you will be required to review any and all incorrect answers. Following completion of the test and evaluation, your credit will be awarded and you may print your certificate.

FACULTY DISCLOSURE/CONFLICT OF INTEREST

The University of Virginia School of Medicine, as an ACCME accredited provider, endorses and strives to comply with the Accreditation Council for Continuing Medical Education (ACCME) Standards of Commercial Support, Commonwealth of Virginia statutes, University of Virginia policies and procedures, and associated federal and private regulations and guidelines on the need for disclosure and monitoring of proprietary and financial interests that may affect the scientific integrity and balance of content delivered in continuing medical education activities under our auspices.

The University of Virginia School of Medicine requires that all CME activities accredited through this institution be developed independently and be scientifically rigorous, balanced and objective in the presentation/discussion of its content, theories and practices.

All authors/editors participating in an accredited CME activity are expected to disclose to the readers relevant financial relationships with commercial entities occurring within the past 12 months (such as grants or research support, employee, consultant, stock holder, member of speakers bureau, etc.). The University of Virginia School of Medicine will employ appropriate mechanisms to resolve potential conflicts of interest to maintain the standards of fair and balanced education to the reader. Questions about specific strategies can be directed to the Office of Continuing Medical Education, University of Virginia School of Medicine, Charlottesville, Virginia.

The faculty and staff of the University of Virginia Office of Continuing Medical Education have no financial affiliations to disclose.

The authors/editors listed below have identified no professional or financial affiliations for themselves or their spouse/partner:

Abass Alavi, MD, PhD (Hon), DSc (Hon) (Guest and Consulting Editor); Valentina Ambrosini, MD, PhD; Richard P. Baum, MD, PhD; Judy S. Blebea, MD; Sanjeev Chawla, PhD; Karen Chen, MD: Wengen Chen, MD, PhD; Benoit Desjardins, MD, PhD; Barton Dudlick (Acquisitions Editor); Stefano Fanti, MD; Thomas Ferrara, BS; Michael F. Goldberg, MD, MPH; Roland Hustinx, MD, PhD; Sharyn I. Katz, MD; Ann K. Kim, MD; Rakesh Kumar, MD; Jean-Denis Laredo, MD; Laurie A. Loevner, MD; Elias R. Melhem, MD, PhD; Igor Mikityansky, MD; Marie-Louise Montandon, PhD; Erik S. Musiek, MD, PhD; Gauthier Namur, MD; Cristina Nanni, MD; Andrew B. Newberg, MD; Vikas Prasad, MD; Patrice Rehm, MD (Test Author); Shamim Ahmed Shamim, MD; Amol M. Takalkar, MD; Drew A. Torigian, MD, MA (Guest Editor); and Habib Zaidi, PhD, PD.

The authors/editors listed below identified the following professional or financial affiliations for themselves or their spouse/partner:

David B. Stout, PhD owns stock in Molecular Imaging Products, is a consultant for Siemens Preclinical Solutions, and owns a patent with M2M Imaging.

Disclosure of Discussion of Non-FDA Approved Uses for Pharmaceutical Products and/or Medical Devices.
The University of Virginia School of Medicine, as an ACCME provider, requires that all faculty presenters identify and disclose any off-label uses for pharmaceutical and medical device products. The University of Virginia School of Medicine recommends that each physician fully review all the available data on new products or procedures prior to clinical use.

TO ENROLL

To enroll in the PET Clinics Continuing Medical Education program, call customer service at 1-800-654-2452 or visit us online at www.theclinics.com/home/cme. The CME program is available to subscribers for an additional fee of $175.00.

Preface

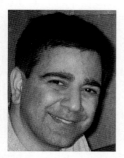

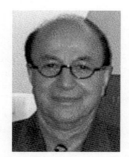

Drew A. Torigian, MD, MA   Abass Alavi, MD, PhD (Hon), DSc (Hon)

Guest Editors

For those individuals who were in the medical and scientific fields during the early 1970s, it was an exciting time to be alive. In 1973, the first clinically available computed tomography (CT) scanner was introduced due to the groundbreaking efforts of Drs. Godfrey Hounsfield and Allan Cormack in years prior.[1,2] The first magnetic resonance (MR) image was published by Dr. Paul Lauterbur in 1973 following the introduction of the use of gradients in the magnetic field to create images, and in 1977 the first human magnetic resonance imaging (MRI) scan was performed. CT and MRI have revolutionized structural tomographic imaging. Also in 1973, the concept of ^{18}F-fluorodeoxyglucose (FDG) for purposes of in vivo positron emission tomography (PET) imaging was born via the combined efforts of Drs. Abass Alavi, David Kuhl, and Martin Reivich at the University of Pennsylvania, which has revolutionized nuclear medicine and molecular imaging.[3] Simultaneously, Drs. Michael Ter-Pogossian, Michael Phelps, and Edward Hoffman at Washington University and Dr. Gerd Muehllehner at Searle Radiographics successfully assembled instrumentation for optimal in vivo PET imaging of positron-emitting radionuclides in humans.[4,5] In 1976, the first human brain and whole body FDG scintigraphic images were acquired on a single photon emission CT instrument at the University of Pennsylvania.

Subsequently, in 1998, PET/CT was introduced by Drs. Townsend and co-workers at the University of Pittsburgh, which allowed for the optimal combination of structural and functional assessment of human patients in vivo.[6,7] As a result, PET instrument sales have markedly decreased whereas PET/CT instrument sales have markedly increased. PET/MRI prototype instruments have recently been assembled in recent years and offer many advantages compared with PET/CT.[8] These include a lack of additional ionizing radiation, superior soft tissue contrast resolution, and an ability to provide additional gross functional imaging data using diffusion-weighted imaging, dynamic perfusion imaging, MR elastography, or MR spectroscopy.[9] However, CT generally remains superior to MRI for evaluation of the lungs, tracheobronchial tree, bowel, and cortical bone, and challenges still remain with regards to attenuation correction using MR images. It is conceivable that hybrid PET/CT/MRI instruments may therefore be assembled to become the standard imaging platform in the future for optimal structural and functional evaluation of all parts of the body.

It is now clear in retrospect how the natural evolution of these originally separate and now frequently combined imaging modalities progressed over the years. There is a natural synergy between PET and CT/MRI, allowing one to obtain the maximal amount of information per imaging session. Hybrid structural and functional imaging provides for partial volume correction of standardized uptake values from PET images via volumetric measurements on CT/MRI examinations, improved anatomical localization of radiotracer uptake seen on PET via coregistration with CT/MRI images, improved sensitivity, specificity, and accuracy of disease assessment, and combination of quantitative structural data from CT/MRI with quantitative molecular data from PET into single integrated quantitative parameters of global disease assessment that are easy to use and take into account structural and functional components of a disease process.[10,11] As such, the future of standalone CT, MRI, or PET

PET Clin 3 (2009) xiii–xiv

doi:10.1016/j.cpet.2009.05.007

pet.theclinics.com

instrumentation may be in question except for use in particular niche applications.

In this issue of *PET Clinics*, we provide a series of articles regarding the application of combined PET, CT, and MRI to small animal preclinical imaging and clinical imaging, brain tumors, non-neoplastic neurologic disorders, the head and neck, breast cancer, thoracic malignancy, the cardiovascular system, abdominopelvic disorders, musculoskeletal disorders, and the endocrine system. It is our hope that the readers of these articles will learn much and therefore apply much to the future practice of combined structural-functional quantitative PET/CT/MR imaging in the 21st century.

Drew A. Torigian, MD, MA

Abass Alavi, MD, PhD (Hon), DSc (Hon)
Department of Radiology
Hospital of the University of Pennsylvania
3400 Spruce Street
Philadelphia, PA 19104, USA

E-mail addresses:
Drew.Torigian@uphs.upenn.edu (D.A. Torigian)
Abass.Alavi@uphs.upenn.edu (A. Alavi)

REFERENCES

1. Hounsfield GN. Computerized transverse axial scanning (tomography). 1. Description of system. Br J Radiol 1973;46(552):1016–22.
2. Cormack AM. Reconstruction of densities from their projections, with applications in radiological physics. Phys Med Biol 1973;18(2):195–207.
3. Alavi A, Reivich M. Guest editorial: the conception of FDG-PET imaging. Semin Nucl Med 2002;32(1):2–5.
4. Ter-Pogossian MM, Phelps ME, Hoffman EJ, et al. A positron-emission transaxial tomograph for nuclear imaging (PETT). Radiology 1975;114(1):89–98.
5. Muehllehner G. Positron camera with extended counting rate capability. J Nucl Med 1975;16(7):653–7.
6. Beyer T, Townsend DW, Brun T, et al. A combined PET/CT scanner for clinical oncology. J Nucl Med 2000;41(8):1369–79.
7. Townsend DW. Positron emission tomography/computed tomography. Semin Nucl Med 2008;38(3):152–66.
8. Pichler BJ, Judenhofer MS. Wehrl HF. PET/MRI hybrid imaging: devices and initial results. Eur Radiol 2008;18(6):1077–86.
9. Zaidi H, Mawlawi O, Orton CG. Point/counterpoint. Simultaneous PET/MR will replace PET/CT as the molecular multimodality imaging platform of choice. Med Phys 2007;34(5):1525–8.
10. Torigian DA, Huang SS, Houseni M, et al. Functional imaging of cancer with emphasis on molecular techniques. CA Cancer J Clin 2007;57(4):206–24.
11. Basu S, Zaidi H, Houseni M, et al. Novel quantitative techniques for assessing regional and global function and structure based on modern imaging modalities: implications for normal variation, aging and diseased states. Semin Nucl Med 2007;37(3):223–39.

Applications of Small Animal Imaging with PET, PET/CT, and PET/MR Imaging

Cristina Nanni, MD[a],*, Drew A. Torigian, MD, MA[b]

KEYWORDS

- Small animal imaging • Molecular imaging
- Positron emission tomography (PET)
- Computed tomography (CT)
- Magnetic resonance imaging (MRI) • PET/CT • PET/MRI

Molecular imaging includes a range of techniques meant to visualize molecular events at the cellular level in living organisms in a noninvasive fashion. In the preclinical setting, the most interesting molecular imaging techniques are PET[1] and MR imaging with molecular contrast agents that allow in vivo accurate quantitation or semiquantitation of many molecular phenomena. Another important technique is CT with or without vascular or liver contrast agents. CT does not provide molecular information but is useful for observing the morphology of tissues and lesions (eg, to accurately measure a tumoral mass over time) because it is very fast and complements the data obtained by PET and MR imaging.

It is now possible for one to purchase small animal PET, MR imaging, and CT scanners, but the future includes the production of hybrid scanners. Currently, small animal PET/CT scanners are available, whereas only prototypes of PET/MR imaging scanners are available. The most common way to combine data from these methods consists of post acquisition image coregistration.

Oncology is by far the field of preclinical research in which all of these imaging techniques are most frequently applied, but cardiovascular and neurologic research protocols can also take advantage of these innovative approaches. For example, PET is used to provide information about tumoral metabolic activity[2,3] and allows for the exploration of different metabolic pathways in physiologic and pathologic tissues. The main advantage of small animal PET and MR imaging over standard methods of preclinical experimentation requiring ex vivo examination is the possibility to analyze the same animal more than once over time, allowing one to observe the response of a disease condition to a new therapeutic agent or the development of disease, thereby significantly reducing the number of animals employed and increasing the reliability of the results.

Furthermore, the use of small animal PET technology allows for the detection of very low (picomolar) concentrations of radiotracers with great sensitivity even with very small uptake variations.[1] Although less sensitive than PET, MR imaging produces high resolution imaging.

Another interesting characteristic of preclinical molecular imaging is summarized in the word "translational." By employing the same technology (PET, MR imaging, or CT) in the experimental setting and in clinical practice, the step between preclinical science and clinical applications in human patients is shortened, reducing the overall time required to effectively verify the

[a] UO Medicina Nucleare, Azienda Ospedaliero-Universitaria di Bologna Policlinico S.Orsola-Malpighi, Via Massarenti 9, 40138 Bologna, Italy
[b] Department of Radiology, Hospital of the University of Pennsylvania, 3400 Spruce Street, Philadelphia, PA 19104, USA
* Corresponding author.
E-mail address: cristina.nanni@aosp.bo.it (C. Nanni).

PET Clin 3 (2009) 243–250
doi:10.1016/j.cpet.2009.01.002

clinical utility of a new approach. One significant example in this field is the in vivo testing of new radiolabeled compounds designed to increase the specificity of PET imaging for a specific disease. The creation of animal models of human disease for in vivo testing of new compounds avoids the human translation of compounds that do not bind to the disease site or are not specific for the disease process of interest.

The translational applicability of these techniques, the possibility of accurate quantitation,[3] the high spatial resolution (1 mm for PET and <1 mm for MR imaging and CT) which is very important when studying small animals such as rodents in vivo, the high sensitivity, and the possibility of using targeted probes to increase the specificity of disease characterization are features that make these procedures desirable in the preclinical scenario despite their relatively high cost when compared with standard ex vivo studies.

APPLICATIONS OF SMALL ANIMAL PET

In the literature, the vast majority of studies employing a small animal PET scanner have not compared the results of PET with those of other preclinical imaging procedures but instead taken into consideration histochemical analyses or autoradiography to verify imaging results. This approach is mainly due to the high costs of the scanners, which makes it difficult to access the multiple modality technology. In the future, more complementary imaging techniques will be employed for evaluation of the same animal models.

Oncology

Small animal PET allows one to noninvasively measure a range of tumor-relevant parameters at the cellular and molecular level, which can be observed longitudinally over time. Studies to evaluate tumor response to a therapeutic intervention can achieve statistical significance using smaller groups of animals, because tumor cell physiology and tumor burden can be accurately determined before and after therapeutic intervention.

The most widely employed PET imaging probe is [18F]-2-fluoro-2-deoxy-D-glucose (FDG), which achieves tumor-specific accumulation because tumor cells have a higher rate of glucose uptake and metabolism (glycolysis) than normal tissues. FDG is generally used in oncology to predict cancer cell engraftment[4] and to measure the response to therapy. [18F]-3'-fluoro-3'-deoxy-L-thymidine (FLT) and its analogues (eg, [18F]-1-(2'-deoxy-2'-fluoro-β-D-arabinofuranosyl)thymine) are another family of compounds that are widely used in preclinical PET because they demonstrate the proliferative index of tumor masses with an accuracy that is far higher for animal models of cancer than for human patients.[5]

Many other PET probes have either been developed or are under development to obtain tumor specificity via a variety of tumor-specific mechanisms. The development of targeted radiolabeled ligands has enabled PET to image many aspects of in vivo tumor biology. Radiolabeled annexin-V, arginine-glycine-aspartic acid (RGD) peptide, vascular endothelial growth factor (VEGF), and $\alpha_v\beta_3$ integrin have been successfully tested in tumor models as well as models of cardiac infarction. The pharmacokinetics and pharmacodynamics of radiolabeled anticancer therapeutics can, in principle, also be monitored by these methods, leading to rapid improvements in drug dose scheduling or design.

The effects of receptor therapies (eg, inhibitors of androgen receptors, estrogen receptors, and epithelial growth factor receptor) can theoretically be predicted owing to the in vivo demonstration of the receptor after injection of a particular radiolabeled ligand.[3]

The literature includes studies on a wide number of PET radiolabeled compounds for preclinical evaluation of specific molecular events. It would be difficult to provide a complete list of all proposed compounds for oncological studies from the past decade in this article.

Cardiology

The applications of small animal PET imaging in preclinical cardiology can basically be divided into measurement of myocardial viability, measurement of myocardial perfusion, measurement of cardiac function, and targeting of specific processes (eg, angiogenesis, apoptosis, and injected stem cells following myocardial infarction).

The imaging of myocardial viability is based on the use of FDG. This approach relies on the concept that all viable myocardial cells (especially under conditions of hyperinsulinism) have increased glucose uptake. The signal obtained from the heart resembles the distribution of viability. Fibrotic and infracted areas are obviously hypometabolic.[6,7] Regarding the evaluation of myocardial perfusion, [13N]-NH$_3$ and [15O]-H$_2$O are suitable radiotracers for this application, and their use is already standard for human studies. Another possible way of assessing myocardial perfusion is to use [11C]-acetate with dynamic image acquisition, because the myocardial blood flow measured with [15O]-H$_2$O and [11C]-acetate is directly correlated. Acetate has several advantages over other tracers, including easy synthesis and a longer half-life.[8]

Besides studying myocardial viability and perfusion, it is possible to visualize other more specific cardiac processes. Angiogenesis consists of the formation of new capillaries by cellular outgrowth from existing microvessels. It occurs as part of the natural healing process after ischemic injury and involves local proliferation and migration of vascular smooth muscle and endothelial cells to form new capillaries. Many factors can stimulate angiogenesis, including tissue ischemia and hypoxia, inflammation, and shear stress via circulating angiogenic factors such as VEGF, angiopoietins, basic fibroblast growth factor, transforming growth factor, extracellular matrix, and integrins (the most important being $\alpha_v\beta_3$). Approaches for the targeted imaging of angiogenesis include evaluation of the altered expression of VEGF receptors and $\alpha_v\beta_3$ integrins.[9]

VEGF receptors can be considered as targets for imaging the mediators of ischemia-induced angiogenesis, such as through use of VEGF121 as the targeting ligand. [64Cu]-DOTA-VEGF121 for small animal PET studies was recently synthesized and tested in vivo with successful results in murine tumor models. Another way to image angiogenesis is based on integrins. The $\alpha_v\beta_3$ integrin is a protein expressed in angiogenic vessels that mediates intercellular adhesion for all proteins with an exposed RGD tripeptide sequence. Haubner and coworkers reported the synthesis of cyclic RGD peptides that can be labeled with [18F]-galacto and [64Cu]-DOTA for PET studies.[10] The value of the $\alpha_v\beta_3$ targeted imaging approach for assessment of myocardial angiogenesis was recently confirmed, even though most studies are based on single photon emitter labeled compounds. It was demonstrated that these radiotracers bind to myocardial ischemic areas that have reduced [99mTc]-sestamibi uptake.

Apoptosis, or programmed cell death, occurs in association with many cardiovascular diseases. Cells undergoing apoptosis express phosphatidylserine on their cell membranes, which is a favorable target for imaging.[6,7] Annexin-V is a medium-sized physiologic human protein with a high Ca^{2+}-dependent affinity toward the phosphatidylserine on the outer leaflet of the cell membrane. Annexin-V can be labeled with a radionuclide and used for apoptosis imaging. Although [99mTc]-labeled annexin-V is now available for imaging cardiac apoptosis in vivo in clinical practice (to detect small infarctions undetectable with [99mTc]-sestamibi and to monitor rejection in cardiac transplants), the positron emitter labeled compound [124I]-annexin-V has to date only been tested in an animal model of hepatic apoptosis and not in the setting of cardiac infarction.[11]

In recent years, the use of reporter genes to monitor gene expression has helped in advancing the understanding of many biologic processes. The introduction of a reporter gene within the DNA of a specific cell that must be tracked in vivo leads to the production of a specific reporter protein that becomes the specific target for a PET probe. In this way, according to the stability of the reporter gene, it is possible to detect the viability and location of the genetically marked cells over a long period of time (up to months). The most common approach for PET studies involves the use of 9-[4-[18F]-fluoro-3-(hydroxymethyl)butyl]-guanine as a reporter probe for imaging the enzyme-based reporter gene herpes simplex virus type 1 thymidine kinase (HSV1-tk) and its mutant derivative, HSV1-sr39tk.[12]

For cardiac applications, the importance of the reporter gene–reporter probe technique derives from the idea of treating cardiac infarction with stem cells to prevent the left ventricle from remodeling. After initial disappointment, it was found that the association of stem cells with specific growth factors inducing their differentiation into myocytes gives good results in terms of viability and contractility recovery; however, for definitive assessment it would be necessary to ascertain in vivo cell survival, final location, and function.

Neurology

Owing to the small size of the brains and brain structures of rodents, small animal PET is less employed in this field than in cardiology and oncology. Furthermore, anesthesia, which is essential for correct intravenous injection and image acquisition, tends to modify the brain and body metabolism and neurotransmitter distribution and is a cause of alteration in PET tracer biodistribution.[13] To obtain meaningful images of tiny structures (eg, the basal ganglia and striatonigral region), it is important to use high-sensitivity and high-resolution scanners, the correct anesthesia procedure, radiotracers with high specific activities (especially for receptor studies), and long image acquisition times. In view of all of the issues connected with small animal PET scanning of the brain, the preclinical evaluation of neurologic diseases in animal models is mainly based on well-established compounds, most of which are routinely employed in clinical practice. FDG is a metabolic tracer that is used in animal models of Alzheimer's disease or epilepsy (for the evaluation of response to new therapies), highlighting the activity of cellular hexokinase. 6-[18F]-fluoro-L-dopa detects aromatic amino acid decarboxylase activity related to movement disorders, [11C]-raclopride and [18F]-fluoroethylspiperone are receptor tracers for dopamine D2 receptors, [11C]-flumazenil binds to benzodiazepine receptors, and [11C]-methionine is an indicator of amino acid transporters mainly used for the evaluation of brain tumors.[14]

APPLICATIONS OF SMALL ANIMAL PET/CT

Small animal CT can be used as a supporting modality for small animal PET for three main reasons. First, as in the clinical setting, it allows the correct anatomic localization of PET findings. This localization is of particular interest in the field of small animal imaging because the use of experimental and specific radiotracers prevents the delineation of the animal shape from PET images alone. In particular, the PET image sometimes demonstrates one or more foci of radiotracer uptake whose anatomic localization is impossible in the absence of an anatomic reference. Second, the CT image can be used as an attenuation correction map for PET images, as in the clinical setting for humans. Because the animal body is very small, highly energetic photons are subjected to negligible attenuation by tissues, although it can be important to achieve accurate quantitation of PET radiotracer uptake when one is studying larger animals such as primates. Third, CT images can be useful to integrate the metabolic results obtained by PET. The CT images can be used to exactly measure the sizes or volumes of organs or tumors, with these measurements noninvasively monitored over time. CT also provides an attenuation map that can be very useful to diagnose entities such as the onset of lesional necrosis, small hepatic lesions, ascites, and so on. Small animal CT is especially useful for the evaluation of osseous structures and the lungs, even in the absence of intravenous contrast material.[15]

Recently, a technological development has led to the possibility of acquiring CT images with cardiac or respiratory gating. Respiratory gating is used to improve the spatial resolution predominantly at the lung bases by compensating for respiratory motion artifacts. Cardiac gating has much more scientific utility. In fact, it can be used as an alternative method to measure the ejection fraction for cardiac studies, because it is possible to intravenously inject contrast agents to allow one to differentiate the ventricular wall from the ventricular cavity. Such structural data can be combined with any of the PET functional imaging results described previously.

Most of the published studies regarding small animal PET/CT imaging have been performed using two separate scanners. This technique is possible owing to the introduction of multimodality gantry beds which can be shifted from one scanner to the other with the same animal located upon it. In this way, the change in the position of the experimental animal is kept to a minimum, and the two image sets (usually in DICOM format) can be subsequently coregistered with specific software. In order to coregister a PET and CT image, it is necessary to have at least three reference points to guarantee a correct slice-by-slice alignment. These reference points must be external to the animal, radioactive for PET imaging, radiopaque for CT imaging, and positioned on the multimodality bed before initiation of the imaging session.

APPLICATIONS OF SMALL ANIMAL PET/MR IMAGING

As small animal CT is naturally connected to the small animal PET scanner for physical reasons and through the widespread use of clinical PET/CT scanners, MR imaging has been considered as a parallel method to CT. Only in the last few years have attempts been made to produce PET/MR imaging hybrid scanners. These scanners are difficult to integrate for several physical reasons, one of which includes the potential for damage to the PET imaging components due to the high magnetic field of the MR imaging scanner. Despite this problem, some prototypes are already available, and it is not impossible to predict the future development of these clinical and preclinical hybrid scanners.[16]

The relative delay in the use of MR imaging in preclinical molecular imaging applications in comparison with other imaging techniques such as optical imaging and PET is generally due to the relatively low sensitivity of MR imaging to detect small amounts of targeted probes. Whereas PET can detect nanomolar concentrations of administered radiotracer in vivo, MR imaging can generally only visualize millimolar concentrations of an administered probe. Considering that in vivo molecular interactions occur at nanomolar concentrations, the sensitivity of MR imaging is considered suboptimal for molecular imaging, even though the high-resolution anatomic images provided by MR imaging are useful for imaging small animals.

In recent years, the introduction of superparamagnetic contrast agents (superparamagnetic iron oxide, very small paramagnetic iron oxide, and ultrasmall superparamagnetic iron oxide) has increased the number of potential applications of MR imaging in the field of molecular imaging.

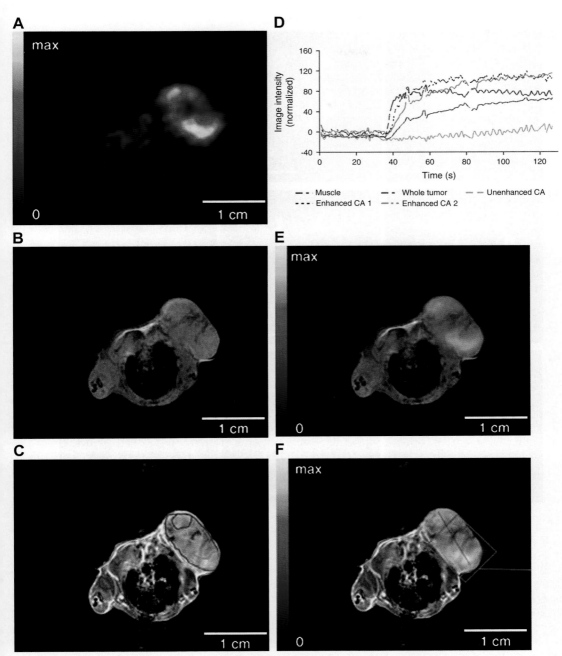

Fig. 1. PET/MR imaging in vivo tumor study. (A) FLT PET image of BALB/c mouse bearing CT26 colon carcinoma shows tumor areas with high radiotracer uptake corresponding to increased cell proliferation. (B, C) Pre- and postcontrast enhanced T1-weighted MR images, simultaneously acquired with PET, reveal macroscopic morphology. (D) Further analysis of contrast enhancement over time shows that the fast curve slopes and high amplitudes match areas of increased tumor proliferation on PET images. Areas in which the MR contrast agent enrichment rises slowly match areas of low FDG uptake on PET. (E, F) PET/MR images show that tumor areas of necrosis and inflammation have low enhancement on T1-weighted MR images and only faint FLT uptake on PET images. (Adapted from Judenhofer MS, Wehrl HF, Newport DF, et al. Simultaneous PET-MRI: a new approach for functional and morphologic imaging. Nat Med 2008;14:461; with permission.)

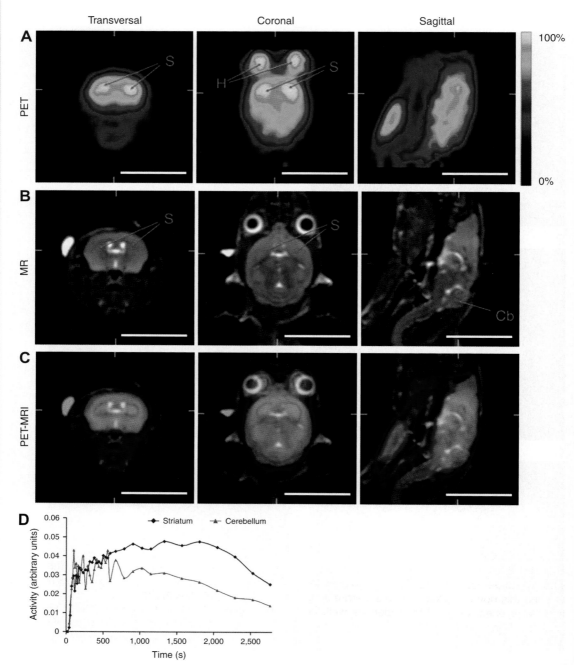

Fig. 2. PET/MR imaging in vivo brain study. (*A*) Dynamically acquired PET images from C57BL/6 mouse injected with [11C]-D-threo-methylphenidate show specific dopamine transporter binding in striatum (S) and nonspecific uptake in Harderian glands (H) (scale bars, 1 cm). (*B*) Simultaneously acquired three-dimensional turbo spin echo MR images reveal brain morphology (scale bars, 1 cm). (*C*) PET/MR images show enhanced radiotracer uptake matching morphology of striatum in MR imaging data (scale bars, 1 cm). (*D*) Time-activity curves, derived from PET data simultaneously acquired during MR imaging, allow further analysis such as kinetic modeling to determine dopamine transporter binding potential. Clear separation of striatum and cerebellum curves indicates more specific radiotracer binding in striatum than in cerebellum. Note that both curves include unbound radiotracer. (*Adapted from* Judenhofer MS, Wehrl HF, Newport DF, et al. Simultaneous PET-MRI: a new approach for functional and morphologic imaging. Nat Med 2008;14:462; with permission.)

These particles can be coupled to receptor targeted molecules or specific receptor ligands, creating a wide number of targeted probes for molecular imaging. Furthermore, the high number of iron atoms held within each particle dramatically increases MR imaging sensitivity for probe detection.[17,18]

Despite the introduction of these new targeted contrast agents, MR and PET imaging tend not to overlap. PET radiotracers are small physiologic molecules that can be used for the evaluation of metabolism as well as the analysis of tissue receptor expression. MR imaging targeted probes are much larger and are nonphysiologic molecules whose true potential is still undergoing evaluation. MR imaging also has the strengths of high spatial resolution and high soft tissue contrast resolution (in particular for bone marrow and solid organs) and provides the ability to make gross measurements of tissue composition through the use of magnetic resonance spectroscopy or of tissue or lesion perfusion through the use of dynamic image acquisition following the administration of intravenous contrast agents.

Based on these considerations, only a few reports in the literature are available regarding the combined use of both techniques for preclinical imaging. von Forstner and coworkers[19] analyzed an animal model of pancreatic carcinoma using three different PET probes and coregistered the PET images with MR images obtained on a separate scanner. MR imaging was essentially used to delineate tumor shape and to calculate tumor volume. Galie and coworkers used coregistered PET and MR imaging to analyze the relationship between PET FDG uptake and MR imaging tumor perfusion.[20] Lee and coworkers[21] developed a bifunctional iron oxide nanoparticle probe for PET and MR imaging scanners that, in a preliminary application, was able to detect tumor integrin $\alpha_v\beta_3$ expression. Despite this novel approach, two separate scanners were used for this application as well. Judenhofer and coworkers[22] have developed a three-dimensional animal PET scanner built into a 7-T MR imaging scanner. They demonstrated that both modalities preserve their functionality even when operated simultaneously (**Figs. 1** and **2**). Although PET/MR imaging in the preclinical setting is not yet well established, it will continue to undergo future development.

REFERENCES

1. Sossi V, Ruth TJ. Micropet imaging: in vivo biochemistry in small animals. J Neural Transm 2005;112(3): 319–30.

2. Aide N, Labiche A, Herlin P, et al. Usefulness of automatic quantification of immunochemical staining on whole tumor sections for correlation with oncological small animal PET studies: an example with cell proliferation, glucose transporter 1 and FDG. Mol Imaging Biol 2008;10(5):237–44.

3. Su H, Bodenstein C, Dumont RA, et al. Monitoring tumor glucose utilization by positron emission tomography for the prediction of treatment response to epidermal growth factor receptor kinase inhibitors. Clin Cancer Res 2006;12(19): 5659–67.

4. Nanni C, Di Leo K, Tonelli R, et al. FDG small animal PET permits early detection of malignant cells in a xenograft murine model. Eur J Nucl Med Mol Imaging 2007;34(5):755–62.

5. Apisarnthanarax S, Alauddin MM, Mourtada F, et al. Early detection of chemoradioresponse in esophageal carcinoma by 3'-deoxy-3'-3H-fluorothymidine using preclinical tumor models. Clin Cancer Res 2006;12(15):4590–7.

6. Dobrucki LW, Sinusas AJ. Molecular imaging: a new approach to nuclear cardiology. Q J Nucl Med Mol Imaging 2005;49(1):106–15.

7. Dobrucki LW, Sinusas AJ. Cardiovascular molecular imaging. Semin Nucl Med 2005;35(1):73–81.

8. Herrero P, Kim J, Sharp TL, et al. Assessment of myocardial blood flow using 15O-water and 1-11C-acetate in rats with small-animal PET. J Nucl Med 2006;47(3):477–85.

9. Cai W, Chen K, Mohamedali KA, et al. PET of vascular endothelial growth factor receptor expression. J Nucl Med 2006;47(12):2048–56.

10. Liu S. Radiolabeled multimeric cyclic RGD peptides as integrin alphavbeta3 targeted radiotracers for tumor imaging. Mol Pharmacol 2006; 3(5):472–87.

11. Cauchon N, Langlois R, Rousseau JA, et al. PET imaging of apoptosis with (64)Cu-labeled streptavidin following pretargeting of phosphatidylserine with biotinylated annexin-V. Eur J Nucl Med Mol Imaging 2007;34(2):247–58.

12. Yaghoubi SS, Couto MA, Chen CC, et al. Preclinical safety evaluation of 18F-FHBG: a PET reporter probe for imaging herpes simplex virus type 1 thymidine kinase (HSV1-tk) or mutant HSV1-sr39tk's expression. J Nucl Med 2006;47(4):706–15.

13. Fueger BJ, Czernin J, Hildebrandt I, et al. Impact of animal handling on the results of 18F-FDG PET studies in mice. J Nucl Med 2006;47(6):999–1006.

14. Jacobs AH, Li H, Winkeler A, et al. PET-based molecular imaging in neuroscience. Eur J Nucl Med Mol Imaging 2003;30(7):1051–65.

15. Ambrosini V, Nanni C, Pettinato C, et al. Assessment of a chemically induced model of lung squamous cell carcinoma in mice by 18F-FDG small-animal PET. Nucl Med Commun 2007;28(8):647–52.

16. Pichler BJ, Judenhofer MS, Pfannenberg C. Multi-modal imaging approaches: PET/CT and PET/MRI. Handb Exp Pharmacol 2008;(185 Pt 1):109–32.

17. Artemov D. Molecular magnetic resonance imaging with targeted contrast agents. J Cell Biochem 2003; 90(3):518–24.

18. Frank JA, Anderson SA, Kalsih H, et al. Methods for magnetically labeling stem and other cells for detection by in vivo magnetic resonance imaging. Cytotherapy 2004;6(6):621–5.

19. von Forstner C, Egberts JH, Ammerpohl O, et al. Gene expression patterns and tumor uptake of 18F-FDG, 18F-FLT, and 18F-FEC in PET/MRI of an orthotopic mouse xenotransplantation model of pancreatic cancer. J Nucl Med 2008;49(8): 1362–70.

20. Galie M, Farace P, Nanni C, et al. Epithelial and mesenchymal tumor compartments exhibit in vivo complementary patterns of vascular perfusion and glucose metabolism. Neoplasia 2007;9(11):900–8.

21. Lee HY, Li Z, Chen K, et al. PET/MRI dual-modality tumor imaging using arginine-glycine-aspartic (RGD)-conjugated radiolabeled iron oxide nanoparticles. J Nucl Med 2008;49(8):1371–9.

22. Judenhofer MS, Wehrl HF, Newport DF, et al. Simultaneous PET-MRI: a new approach for functional and morphological imaging. Nat Med 2008;14(4): 459–65.

Preclinical Multimodality Imaging in Vivo

David B. Stout, PhD[a], Habib Zaidi, PhD, PD[b],*

KEYWORDS
- Small-animals • Multimodality imaging
- Molecular imaging • Image fusion • Biomedical research

WHY MULTIMODALITY IMAGING?

The field of diagnostic imaging encompasses a wealth of modalities that are fundamental for assessing and managing patients requiring medical care. Conventional radiologic imaging modalities, such as plain film radiography, and modern techniques, such as CT[1] and MR imaging,[2] can be used to evaluate a patient's anatomy with submillimeter spatial resolution to distinguish structural abnormalities and to evaluate the location and extent of disease. These techniques also offer reasonably fast scan times, precise statistical characteristics, and good tissue contrast, especially when contrast media are administered to a patient. MR imaging can be combined with functional MR imaging[3] or magnetic resonance spectroscopy[4] to measure regional biochemical content and to assess metabolic status or the presence of neoplasia and other disease conditions in specific tissue areas.

In contrast to the anatomic imaging techniques, functional imaging modalities, including conventional 2-D planar scintigraphy, single photon emission CT (SPECT),[5] and positron emission tomography (PET),[6] assess regional differences in the biochemical status of biologic tissues and organs. This is performed by administering a biologically active molecule or pharmaceutical that is radiolabeled and accumulated in response to its biochemical attributes. That is, these techniques rely on the tracer principle in which a minute amount of a radiotracer is administered to assess physiologic function or the biomolecular status of a tissue, tumor, or organ within a patient. Similar to other biologic imaging techniques, such as optical imaging (OI),[7] PET can be used to study the cellular and molecular processes associated with disease. The lower spatial resolution and high statistical noise inherent to the procedure compared with anatomic imaging persuaded clinicians to allude to this modality as "unclear medicine," although this is becoming less true with new advances in submillimeter SPECT imaging.

The common practice is that patients receiving medical diagnosis typically undergo anatomic and functional imaging from commonly available stand-alone medical imaging systems. The anatomic images usually are viewed side by side or fused using image registration software with the functional images when desired. Nevertheless, many practitioners witnessed fundamental potential for multimodality imaging in the sense that it offers essential features for diagnostic studies and patient management.[8,9] First, the anatomic and functional information are complementary and not redundant. As noted previously, anatomic imaging is performed with techniques, such as CT or MR imaging, that have excellent spatial resolution and signal-to-noise characteristics, but that may offer low specificity for differentiating disease from normal structures. In contrast, nuclear imaging generally targets a specific functional or metabolic signature in a way that can be

This work was supported by grant no. SNSF 3100A0-116547 from the Swiss National Foundation.

a Crump Institute for Molecular Imaging, Department of Molecular and Medical Pharmacology, The David Geffen School of Medicine at UCLA, 570 Westwood Plaza, CNSI Building, Room 2151, Los Angeles, CA 90095, USA
b Division of Nuclear Medicine, Geneva University Hospital, CH-1211 Geneva, Switzerland
* Corresponding author.
E-mail address: habib.zaidi@hcuge.ch (H. Zaidi).

PET Clin 3 (2009) 251–273
doi:10.1016/j.cpet.2009.03.001

highly specific but generally lacks spatial resolution and anatomic cues, which often are needed to localize or stage a disease or plan therapy.[10,11] Similarly, the availability of correlated functional and anatomic images improves the detection of disease by highlighting areas of increased radiotracer uptake on the anatomic images, whereas regions that look abnormal on the anatomic images can draw attention to a potential area of disease where radiopharmaceutical uptake may be low. The information from CT or MR imaging supplements that from nuclear imaging and vice versa; therefore, it generally is advantageous to view CT and nuclear images side by side during diagnostic interpretation. In other cases, it can be valuable to view fused dual-modality images in which the SPECT or PET data are presented as a color overlay on gray-scale CT or MR images. Multimodality imaging can be used to guide radiation treatment planning, for example, by providing anatomic and functional data that are important for defining the target volume and indicating normal regions that should avoid irradiation.[12] Similar roles are played when the dual-modality data are used to guide surgery, biopsy, or other interventional procedures.[13]

In addition, multimodality imaging provides complementary information that cannot be discerned easily from one type of image modality alone. This is best illustrated in oncologic applications where anatomic imaging often is needed to differentiate whether or not a radiopharmaceutical has localized in sites of disease (eg, in the primary tumor, lymphatic system, or metastatic site) or as part of a benign process (eg, in the gastrointestinal tract, urinary system, or in sites of inflammation).[14] An example of combining multiple imaging modalities to address a basic research question is shown in **Fig. 1**, where OI, PET, and CT are used together, each playing to its own strengths, to demonstrate the feasibility of using recombinant human adenoviral vectors to detect nodal metastases in a human prostate cancer model.[15]

CLINICAL HISTORY OF MULTIMODALITY IMAGING

Traditionally, multimodality imaging was achieved through the use of software-based image registration and fusion to correlate anatomic (CT and MR imaging) and functional (SPECT-PET) information in clinical and research settings.[16,17] Depending on the application and regions of the body involved, this has been performed using rigid or nonrigid registration approaches. Rigid-body registration basically involves simple geometric transformations, such as translation and rotation, to match the two image data sets. These techniques have been successfully applied to brain studies, where the skull provides a rigid structure that preserves the geometric relationship of regions within the brain, and have been routinely used worldwide since the 1990s in clinical and research settings.[18–20] The solution to the image registration problem becomes more complicated, however, when applied to other regions of the body (eg, thorax and abdomen) where the body can bend and flex. This is true particularly when the functional (SPECT-PET) and anatomic (CT–MR imaging) data are acquired in separate sessions on stand-alone systems, often in different locations and on different days. In this case, geometric relationships between different anatomic regions might be affected by the shape of the patient bed; the orientation of the body and limbs (up or down) during scanning, which is dictated by the modality; internal organ shift between the two procedures; and the respiratory state of patients. In these situations, the image registration process might result in good matching of only one particular region of a patient's anatomy, not necessarily the whole scanned region. Nonrigid registration (warping) has been introduced as a technique to improve registration accuracy over a larger region of a patient's body. Software-based image registration is challenging and time consuming in most cases, thus limiting its use to academic institutions with advanced technical support that can accommodate the requirements of these procedures (scanning on both modalities on the same day using carefully matched anatomic positioning and respiration protocols).[21,22]

Although the introduction of clinical, hardware-based, dual-modality imaging systems in the clinic is fairly new, the prospective advantages of combining anatomical and functional imaging has been recognized by radiological scientists and physicians since the inception of medical imaging.[23] Many of the pioneers of nuclear medicine acknowledged that the capabilities of a radionuclide imaging system could be augmented by adding an external radioisotope source to acquire transmission data for anatomic correlation of the emission image. The conceptual designs were never reduced to practice or implemented in an experimental or a clinical setting, however, until Hasegawa and colleagues (University of California, San Francisco) pioneered in the 1990s the development of dedicated SPECT-CT[24,25] and, later, Townsend and coworkers (University of Pittsburgh) pioneered in 1998 the development of combined PET-CT imaging systems, which have the capability to record emission and transmission x-ray CT data for correlated functional/structural

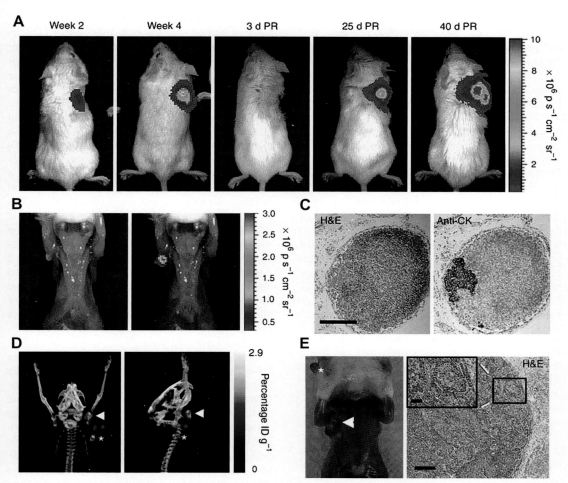

Fig. 1. (*A*) Representative images of mouse with LAPC-9–VEGF-C–GFP–RL tumor cells grafted on right shoulder to promote metastasis to brachial and axillary lymph nodes. Kinetics of tumor growth can be monitored by bioluminescence imaging of *Renilla* luciferase–expressing tumor cells. Color bar represents photons s^{-1} cm^{-2} sr^{-1} (p s^{-1}cm^{-2} sr^{-1}); PR, post resection. (*B*) Bioluminescence (*Renilla* luciferase activity) in exposed ipsilateral axillary lymph node of mouse with tumor 4 weeks after implantation: (*left*) photo; (*right*) overlay. (*C*) Histologic analysis of photon-emitting lymph node (*B*) shows subcapsular microscopic lesion as visualized by staining with hematoxylin-eosin (*left*) and with antibody to human cytokeratin (anti-CK) (*right*). (*D*) PET-CT imaging with F18-fluorothymidine at 30 days after resection of primary tumor shows extensive metastases (color bar represents percentage injected dose per gram, ID g^{-1}). (*E*) Photograph (*left*) of this mouse shows extensive metastases in ipsilateral primary axillary (*white arrowhead*) and accessory axillary (*red asterisk*) lymph nodes. Primary tumor regrowth (*white asterisk*) also is present. Hematoxylin-eosin staining (*right*) shows extensive infiltration by tumor cells, distending axillary lymph node. Higher magnification inset (*inset*) of boxed region shows that tumor cells make up most of population. Scale bars, 200 μm (*C, E [right]*), 50 μm (*E [right (inset)]*). p s^{-1} cm^{-2} sr^{-1}, photons per second per centimeter squared per steridian. (*Reprinted from* Burton JB, Johnson M, Sato M, et al. Adenovirus-mediated gene expression imaging to directly detect sentinel lymph node metastasis of prostate cancer. Nat Med 2008;14:882–8; with permission.)

imaging.[14,26] Thereafter, SPECT-CT and PET-CT dual-modality imaging systems were introduced by the major scanner manufacturers for routine clinical use in 2001. Since that time, the number of combined PET-CT units sold annually has increased steadily owing to their wide clinical acceptance, leading to manufacturers completely stop the production of stand-alone PET scanners, replacing them with combined PET-CT units since 2006.

Although virtually all commercial clinical dual-modality systems have been configured in the form of PET-CT or SPECT-CT, several investigators have proposed and constructed prototype preclinical systems that combine PET with MR imaging.[27–31] An overview of preclinical PET instrumentation is beyond the scope of this review. Readers are referred to the review by Levin and Zaidi.[32] Preclinical imaging entails difficult challenges for building systems with micrometer-level tolerances and sensitivity/resolution issues are not easily resolved. Much worthwhile research was performed to address the important challenges that must be overcome in implementing and operating combined PET–MR imaging or SPECT–MR imaging systems. One manufacturer developed a prototype PET–MR imaging system dedicated to high-resolution brain imaging,[33] and there are clear indications that several manufacturers are working toward the development of whole-body PET–MR imaging systems. In parallel, potential applications of this technology are being explored, as reported in the scientific literature.[33–35]

CHALLENGES IN PRECLINICAL SETTING
Animal Handling

Working with animals raises challenges not only in imaging system design and construction but also with related regulatory oversight and biosafety concerns. There are ongoing needs to train personnel in animal handling techniques, including surgical and injection skills needed to prepare and image animals. Space must be specifically configured for animal housing, with associated heating, light cycles, cage changing, and access control. In particular, biosafety control of carcinogenic or other hazardous materials may require considerable effort to address.

Several institutions have put the required training information online, including links to sites with information as to how training may be obtained.[36–38] Information about biosafety levels,[39–41] proper protection strategies, and garbing can be found online.[42,43] Advanced facilities have been designed with strong financial support by the National Institutes of Health[44] to establish a network of scientists active in collecting research data linked to small-animal models of human disease (eg, Mouse Models of Human Cancer Consortium[45]) to provide larger access to various mouse models to active investigators in the field.

Anesthesia and Heating

Most preclinical imaging systems require animals to remain motionless for several minutes to hours to obtain useful data; thus, some type of anesthesia is necessary. There is considerable interest in imaging without anesthesia, because conscious animals presumably have normal metabolic functions compared with those under anesthesia. Several groups have shown that this is feasible under some circumstances.[46–48] In particular, a group at Brookhaven National Laboratory (Upton, New York) has developed a rat conscious animal PET scanner (RatCAP), a complete 3-D tomograph designed to image the brain of an awake rat,[49] which incorporates the PET system into an integrated, compact arrangement of lutetium oxyorthosilicate/avalanche photodiode (LSO/APD) arrays with highly integrated electronics.[50] Nonetheless, most imaging work at present is conducted using anesthesia, and the type and injection route can play a significant role in the sedation and metabolic status of the animal.

Gas anesthesia is perhaps the most common method, offering safe, quick, and effective immobilization with quick recovery times. Isoflurane is commonly used; however, there also is increased interest in sevoflurane as it is becoming available as a generic brand at lower cost. There may be some advantage to using sevoflurane because it seems to have less effect on glucose levels compared with isoflurane.[51]

Injected anesthetics are common, although they need to be injected frequently or constantly infused to maintain a steady state of anesthesia. Commonly used injectibles include ketamine, midazolam, pentobarbital, and xylazine. These anesthetics are controlled substances and require a prescription. They must be kept under double lock and key and require careful tracking of their use. They are advantageous in that only a syringe and a vial of anesthetic are required for use. Any time animals are anesthetized, it is vital that proper heating be provided to maintain the core body temperature to prevent hypothermia. Heating is particularly important for peripheral tumors, where blood flow and, therefore, probe delivery are related to body temperature.[52]

Animal Access

Bringing detectors and collimators close to the animal offers certain advantages, including magnification, higher sensitivity, and possibly a smaller system size. Shielding for low-energy radiation, particularly with CT imaging, is necessary and requires an enclosed gantry. Unfortunately, this means that animals often are closely surrounded or sealed inside the system, leaving the animals hidden from view and access. This can be problematic for monitoring respiration and other motion problems and can make injection for probe and blood sampling difficult or impossible. Short-duration studies normally are not of concern, but longer-term studies lasting more than 30 minutes often require adjustments to anesthesia levels. It is important to monitor respiration, because with time the breathing can become labored, requiring reduction of anesthesia to prevent large movements due to agonistic breathing motions. Respiration can be monitored by camera, ventilator settings, and noninvasive probes that can measure inhalation indirectly.[53] Monitoring systems suitable for mouse work, where heart rates can go up to 1000 beats per minute, only recently have become widely available and suitable for molecular imaging research.

Injecting probes for immediate dynamic imaging poses another challenge for imaging within confined systems. For these studies, it is necessary to place animals in a scanner and begin acquisition before injecting an imaging probe. Because of the limited blood volume of mice, this species normally is limited to injection volumes of 250 μL or less and requires an insertion of a catheter in the animal, most commonly in the tail vein or in some cases the jugular vein or femoral artery. Catheters have what is often called a dead volume, which is the amount left inside the tubing and is related to the length and interior diameter. Although it is possible to flush out this volume into an animal, this often leads to a double-pulsed injection and may require too much volume due to the probe/saline valve dead volume. If a syringe is removed from the catheter to place a saline syringe for flush, there is risk for the radioactive probe coming back through the tubing due to backpressure in the line from the animal's blood pressure, which can lead to spills or inaccurate injection activity measurements.

Physiologic Monitoring

In some cases, monitoring physiologic parameters, such as heart rate, temperature, respiration, or blood pressure, may be necessary. Fortunately, several options are available to measure these in small rodents. Although visual measurement is possible in some imaging systems, a measurement system, preferably one that can generate computerized output files, often is preferable for tracking and storing the physiologic data.

Heart rate can be measured by needle probes inserted into the skin; by leads placed on the skin surface, pressure cuffs; or by infrared probes. Respiration can be measured using optical probes, cameras, or pressure cuffs. Temperature usually is assessed using a rectal thermocouple, but this is somewhat invasive and can lead to perforated bowel if not inserted carefully. One option for temperature is to carefully control the environment. Because anesthetized mice have

little heat capacity, they quickly equilibrate with ambient temperature at the ambient temperature. Often, monitoring systems suitable for one imaging modality are not ideal for other modalities, so that probes within the field of view must be appropriately selected to minimize artifacts and changes to the image data.

One area where respiration and heart rate measurements are essential is for gated acquisitions. Trigger signals for each breath or heart beat are sent to the imaging system, which trigger the acquisition or enable the image data to be divided up into various parts of the respiratory or heart rate cycles. These trigger signals can start or stop the image acquisition or can be put into the data stream for postprocessing.

Study Duration and Hydration

Modalities, such as PET and SPECT, allow static imaging and dynamic imaging over time. Static imaging, analogous to a snapshot at a given time, is useful for looking at the end-stage accumulation of probe after specific uptake and nonspecific clearance. Most common, perhaps, is F18-fluorodeoxyglucose (FDG) imaging approximately 1 hour after injection. This method allows many animals to be imaged in a short time period. For example a 10-minute imaging time allows 4 to 5 animals to be imaged per hour, making efficient use of the radioactive probe.

Dynamic imaging requires placing animals within a scanner and collecting data beginning from time of injection, typically for 60 to 90 minutes. Longer imaging times means fewer animals imaged per day and per radiochemistry synthesis. There also is the complication of injecting within the imaging system, where access to the animal likely is limited.

Despite the additional demands, dynamic imaging allows data to be obtained over time that can be used to estimate biodistribution, radiation dosimetry, and metabolic rate constants, which are true measures of biologic function rather than only endpoints. Whether or not using graphic methods (Patlak or Logan plots) or compartmental modeling, the blood and tissue time activity data are needed to estimate the rate constants.

In some instances, the endpoint may be the same in static and dynamic studies, but the process of getting there may differ and reveal insights to biologic processes. For example, intraperitoneal FDG injections compared with tail vein injections have different temporal and spatial probe distributions, but most organs have the same activity 1 hour after injection.[52] Another example is the tumor uptake of F18-fluorothymidine (FLT) and FDG after radiation therapy, where both were the same at 1 hour although the uptake paths were different between control and irradiated tumors.[54]

Maintenance of near normal physiologic conditions is important when conducting dynamic studies, because changes in temperature, anesthetic state, hydration, breathing, and heart rate can have an impact on the biologic process under investigation. Hypothermia and hyperthermia are serious concerns, especially in small animals that have little heat capacity. Depth of anesthesia plays a role in heart rate and, perhaps most importantly, in breathing. Rodents require less gas anesthesia with time and, if not checked, agonistic breathing can result, causing large breathing motions that degrade the resulting images. For long studies, more than 90 minutes, in small rodents, dehydration can result, especially with the dry, moisture-free gases used with gas anesthesia. For these studies, subcutaneous injections of saline or slow saline infusions often are helpful.

Submillimeter Level Accuracy

Preclinical imaging often challenges the spatial resolution of imaging systems by attempting to look at small objects, for example, brain anatomy in rats or mice. In these cases, spatial resolution often is not sufficient, leading to problems with spillover activity and partial volume effects. The challenge for makers of these imaging devices lies in obtaining submillimeter resolution while maintaining reasonable signal-to-noise characteristics and measurement sensitivity. In addition to resolution, the imaging systems ideally need to reproducibly place the animal into a known position for coregistration with other modalities and to match previous experiments with the same animal. Achieving submillimeter reproducible positioning is a mechanical challenge and is not a trivial endeavor.

Lack of Image Format Standard Across Modalities

In clinical environments, the need for standardized image formats to enable medical personnel to evaluate multiple image information sources led to the development of Digital Imaging and Communications in Medicine (DICOM), a semi-standardized format for radiologic and other types of medical information. Unfortunately, there is not yet a standardized format for preclinical information, in part because of the wide range of image data sources (ultrasound, PET, CT, MR imaging, and OI). Each imaging modality often has its own unique image information; thus, a unified image

format remains elusive. For example, optical data might require tracking light wavelengths, camera settings, stage height, and binning factors, whereas PET data require information about injected probe activity and type, dynamic framing sequences, voxel sizes, reconstruction parameters, and so forth. An image header format that attempted to include all divergent sources of information would quickly become far too large, and future information types will become necessary as new methods and modalities evolve.

Immunocompromised Animals, Biohazardous and Infectious Agents

One of the areas on which molecular imaging has had a huge impact is cancer imaging. Oncology research has greatly benefitted from the ability to image the same animals noninvasively over the course of a disease, treatment, or intervention. Understanding of rodent genomes and ability to create genetically modified strains has led to thousands of knockin and knockout deletions and insertions of specific genes or combinations of genes. Perhaps most fundamental are the nude and severe combined immunodeficiency mouse strains, which are missing the thymus and T cells or the thymus, T and B cells, and DNA repair mechanisms through a mutation in chromosome 16. These mice are extremely useful because they cannot reject implanted tumors, making it possible to study human xenografts over time and with various treatments. With suppression of the immune system comes the need to protect these animals from pathogens in the environment; thus, barrier facilities and imaging chambers are essential for maintaining the health of these animals.

Often investigators are interested in creating or treating animals using biohazardous or infectious agents. These might be viral vectors for gene insertion, chemotherapeutic agents, or perhaps bacteria or engineered cells. Certainly the activation and early response of the immune system is an interesting area of study, but this work is difficult to conduct given the necessity of protecting the researchers and other animals housed nearby. Use of these agents requires controlled environmental conditions, biosafety containment, and locating imaging systems within controlled areas or using sealed imaging chambers to isolate the hazardous agent.

COREGISTRATION OF SEPARATE DATA VERSUS SAME GANTRY ACQUISITION

As discussed previously, several techniques have been developed to coregister clinical multimodality medical imaging data (see articles by Maintz and Viergevera[55] and Pluim and colleagues[56] for review). Widely available image registration techniques developed specifically to address the needs of clinical imaging have yet to be translatable for small-animal imaging applications. Some investigators attempted to adapt popular image registration techniques using various combinations of functional and anatomic imaging data.[57,58] These studies reported various degrees of success when applying these algorithms in various scenarios.[59-66] Some of these techniques use external fiducial markers that are visible in the two-image datasets to be registered, which are attached to the animal body. Those techniques have been widely used for dual-modality image registration (eg, CT or MRI or, alternatively, SPECT or PET), although this is more challenging to accomplish for multimodality imaging where various modalities are involved. As PET and SPECT imaging probes become more targeted and nonspecific activity is eliminated, there may not be sufficient information contained in metabolic images to coregister with anatomic data. Inexpensive and easy-to-manufacture animal-specific molds also can be used for image registration of preclinical studies (accuracy within ±1–2 mm for sequential PET images).[67] Other possible solutions for sequential imaging with combined PET-CT imaging include imaging chambers that can be rigidly and reproducibly mounted on single-modality preclinical scanners with submillimeter accuracy (**Figs. 2** and **3**).[68] More refined immobilization devices also were suggested, with registration accuracy of approximately 0.2 to 0.3 mm.[69] Other strategies for the design of dual-modality systems, including a rail-with-sliding-bed approach and various rail-based, docking, and click-over approaches for anatomic-molecular imaging fusion, also are being explored.[70]

More sophisticated techniques rely on unsupervised algorithms that do not involve user interaction. The simplest form of automated image registration techniques uses a rigid body transformation where an affine transformation model, which permits only global translations, rotations, scaling along each of the three axes, and shearing deformations, is determined and applied to the floating image.[71] In this case, the solution to the image registration task yields 12 parameters that are embedded in a transformation matrix. The drawback of such techniques is that they tend to ignore organ deformation owing to issues discussed previously (differences between shapes of the gantry bed, internal organ shift, respiratory motion, and so forth). To address these limitations, nonrigid registration algorithms that permit compensation for perceived organ deformation for different modalities, or that even spatially coregister images of different animals, have been developed.[22,57,58] Several companies have recently begun offering chamber-based solutions, including m2m Imaging Corp. (Cleveland, Ohio), ASI (Eugene, Oregon), and Bioscan (Washington, DC). Notwithstanding the significant advancements in the field, robust multimodality image registration for small-animal imaging remains challenging and likely will continue to be an active research field for years to come.

The availability of multimodality imaging systems facilitates the process of acquiring functional and anatomic data from animals in a consistent configuration and during a single study in a way that is faster and more cost efficient than attempting to register the images by software after they are acquired on separate imaging systems. In this regard, recently introduced dual-modality techniques consisting of two hard-wired systems (eg, SPECT or PET and CT or MR imaging) offer a critical advantage over separate anatomic and radiotracer imaging systems in correlating anatomic and functional images without moving animals. Only table translation is required for sequential systems (eg, PET-CT) whereas most recent technologies (PET-MR imaging) allow simultaneous scanning given that the PET insert

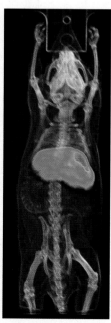

Fig. 2. Example of projection image showing all 3-D data for combined PET-CT scan using FDG in a tumor-bearing mouse. Using this view, all parts of data are visible as one image.

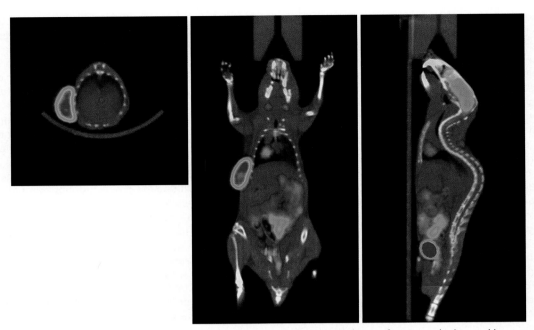

Fig. 3. Examples of transverse (*left*), coronal (*middle*), and sagittal (*right*) views of FDG uptake imaged in a mouse using PET and CT. These views enable detailed examination of all image data on slice-by-slice basis.

is introduced within the MR imaging scanner[30] (described later).

Multimodality imaging systems are designed to account consistently for differences in reconstruction diameter, offsets in isocenter, image reconstruction coordinates, and image format (eg, 512 × 512 versus 128 × 128) between the CT–MR and SPECT-PET image geometries to perform image coregistration and image fusion. Depending on the design of the system, image registration software may be needed to account for table sag or for misalignment when the animal moves between the CT-MR and SPECT-PET image scans. Generally, the coordinate systems implicit in the SPECT-PET and CT–MR image geometries are calibrated with respect to each other using fiducial markers that are scanned with both CT-MR and SPECT-PET imaging. The image registration must be confirmed to avoid misregistration errors in the multimodality images or in the SPECT-PET image reconstructed using CT- and, likely in the future, MR imaging–derived attenuation maps.

SIMULTANEOUS ACQUISITION VERSUS SEPARATE TEMPORAL DATA

Certain advantages exist with the acquisition of simultaneous data. As discussed previously, there would be no need to coregister separate datasets or worry about different experimental conditions. Metabolism (PET or SPECT),

functional activity (MR imaging), and anatomic (CT or MR) information could be acquired with temporal and spatial matching. The drawbacks of this approach have, until recently, been problematic, requiring giving up the optimal imaging capabilities of one or more modalities. For example, Goertzen and colleagues designed a simultaneous PET-CT system,[72] although the partial ring design reduced the PET sensitivity to make space for the CT source and detector.

Current designs of PET–MR systems using an insert approach exhibit no change in MR imaging signals while maintaining a good PET imaging capability.[27–30,73–75] The PET currently is somewhat limited for axial extent compared with stand-alone PET systems; however, this is likely to improve in the future. Another approach was to cut the MR imaging magnet in half and insert a PET ring;[76] however, this proved difficult and expensive to produce and required a specialized magnet. Use of a PET insert enables using existing MR imaging systems for research and no specialized production or limitations on the MR imaging system.

Currently, the majority of multimodality research acquires sequential images by moving a bed from one location to another within a common gantry or by moving a bed or chamber from one system to another. Many preclinical imaging systems are sold with multimodality capability. For example, the Inveon (Siemens, Knoxville, Tennessee) and GE Healthcare/Gamma Medica-Ideas Flex Triumph

(Northridge, California) and Bioscan NanoSPECT/CT systems have a common CT and SPECT or PET gantry that allows sequential acquisition without moving the bed. In a docked or multimodality gantry configuration, PET imaging is acquired by moving the bed to another location. The sequential approach almost always is required when using PET imaging, because this modality requires a ring of detectors. Other methods, such as CT and SPECT, often image by rotating the detectors, so more than one modality is possible at the same time or at least mounted to the same gantry.

Sequential imaging in a preclinical setting has existed for many decades. Prior to high-resolution systems currently available, research typically used larger primates, canines, pigs, and other large species. These animals were imaged in clinical systems, often with rudimentary attempts to position the animals in the same position for both imaging systems, often PET and CT or MR imaging. In the late 1990s and early 2000s, combination PET-CT clinical systems quickly took over the market. It took nearly 7 years for those same combinations to become prevalent in preclinical systems, in part because of the complexity of the systems and the often micrometer-level tolerances for construction and positioning.

One solution to sequential imaging was developed at the University of California, Los Angeles (UCLA), for using PET and CT together through the use of imaging chambers.[68,77] This approach integrated heating, anesthesia, and positioning within a chamber having a common mounting plate for PET and CT beds. This hardware, when positioned in the same location every time for imaging, enabled a fixed translational offset to coregister the data, eliminating the often difficult task of software registration. Further refinements with software enable automated processing to create the fused images without user interaction, thus simplifying the creation of data and lessening the burden of the imaging scientist.

The drawbacks to sequential imaging include the need to move animals between positions in a gantry or between imaging systems. This requires changing connections for heating and anesthesia and perhaps physiologic monitoring systems. There always is a risk in moving animals in that they no longer are in the same orientation as in the previous imaging work. There also are anesthesia and temporal changes that may alter the orientation or physiology of the animal and make coregistration problematic. A single gantry system would have slower throughput, as animals are imaged first in one, then another, modality. Separate systems enable higher throughput, but this may increase the chance of movement and doubles the work for investigators because more animals are imaged at the same time.

DATA COLLECTION STRATEGIES (DYNAMIC VERSUS STATIC INFORMATION)

Routine PET scanning protocols used in clinics usually involve data acquisition in a static mode where collected events are stored in a scanner-specific predefined projection or sinogram format. An image reconstruction algorithm is then applied to the data set to yield a static or sum image over the whole acquisition duration of the study. The advantage of this protocol is simplicity of use and acceptable image quality produced as a result of the good statistics that can be acquired over the whole study duration. The major drawback is the absence of information of tracer kinetics that prevents the extraction of physiologically relevant parameters, thus limiting the analysis to straightforward semiquantitative parameters, such as the standardized uptake value in oncologic imaging.

One important aspect of nuclear medicine imaging, including PET, is the inherent capability to perform dynamic imaging, taking advantage of the high sensitivity offered by high-end multiring PET systems. This is a remarkable capability, allowing measurements of change in the biodistribution of radiotracers within the tissues or organs of interest over time. This in turn provides valuable information about the underlying physiologic or metabolic processes being investigated, allowing extraction of relevant parameters using kinetic modeling techniques.[78]

Dynamic PET data acquisition can be performed using one of two common approaches. In the first and standard approach, the desired framing sequence is prespecified before data acquisition and the detected events are binned online in the sinogram corresponding to each frame. In this case, static images also can be obtained by summing the data acquired in image or in sinogram space. In the second approach, available on modern clinical and almost all preclinical PET scanners, the detected events are stored in a so-called list-mode format,[79,80] where the parameters characterizing each coincidence event (time of detection, spatial coordinates of interaction points, and energy if required) are written on disk. Therefore, the list-mode acquisition capability permits the extra flexibility to users by allowing the specification of the framing sequence post acquisition to optimize the framing sequence based on the probe kinetics. Another advantage of list-mode data acquisition is the possibility of applying direct list-mode reconstruction, which proved to have many added benefits compared with conventional reconstruction from binned projection data.[81] Alternatively, the standard approach for dynamic PET image reconstruction consists of independently reconstructing images corresponding to each dynamic frame. In either case, the result consists of a set of dynamic images containing information about tracer kinetics in the regions of interest.

OVERVIEW OF CURRENT SYSTEMS
Photograph Plus Data—Optical

A pseudomultimodality approach is used by several OI systems that use charge-coupled device (CCD) digital cameras to collect light information. Because these systems are suitable for low and high light flux uses, photographic images can be superimposed on top of the in vivo optical signals to provide a measure of spatial information. Despite using the same detector, the information obtained from the two methods comes from different sources. Photographs help with visual orientation of the subjects, whereas in vivo optical signals are related to the fluorophore or bioluminescent signal coming from within the animals.

Several manufacturers offer optical-photographic systems, including Caliper Life Sciences, Hopkinton, MA (formerly Xenogen), Carestream, Rochester, NY (formerly Kodak), and Cambridge Research and Instrumentation (Woburn, MA). The IVIS 3-D system (Caliper) takes the photographic information one step further and creates a spatial map in 3-D using transillumination to estimate the source of the light coming from the animals. IVIS fluorescent systems decode spectral information using a series of back to back image acquisitions using different filter wheels to separate auto fluorescence from specific signal. This method enables acquisition of divergent information using the same imaging system to gain additional information from a subject. The Maestro system (Cambridge Research and Instrumentation) uses a tunable liquid crystal to obtain multispectral wavelength information, enabling decoding of multiple fluorophores with one scan, which are then overlaid on photographic images for spatial orientation. Timing information can be used to decode the optical signal, such as the eXplore Optix system from Advanced Research Technologies (Montréal, Quebec).

PET-CT and SPECT-CT

Similar to commercial clinical dual-modality systems, which have been configured in the form of SPECT-CT or PET-CT scanners, several investigators proposed and in many cases have

implemented and tested prototype preclinical dual-modality systems that combine SPECT with CT and PET with CT.[82–84] The popularity of using animal models as models of human disease stimulated the growth of preclinical CT systems, which incorporate a low power x-ray tube and a phosphor-coupled CCD camera or similar 2-D x-ray imaging detector to achieve spatial resolutions as high as 25 μm or better.[85–88]

Taking advantage of the availability of high-resolution preclinical x-ray imaging systems, several investigators have developed and are continuing to develop dual-modality imaging systems specifically designed for imaging small animals. Cherry and coworkers have developed a combined preclinical PET-CT imaging system.[72] The PET detectors use an LSO scintillator coupled to a fiberoptic taper to a position-sensitive photomultiplier tube. These are placed on opposite sides of an animal with the annihilation photons from the positron emission detected in coincidence. The system includes a preclinical CT system having a microfocus x-ray tube and an amorphous selenium detector coupled to a flat panel thin film resistors readout array.[89] A second system was built later by the same group, who designed a novel preclinical CT scanner using photodiode detectors that have a flexible C-arm gantry design with adjustable detector positioning that was integrated with the microPET II scanner [2400].[90] A flexible design of a commercial system (Gamma Medica-Ideas) also can be configured as PET-CT (discussed later).

As an alternative to this design, the Sherbrooke group led by Lecomte is working toward a combined PET-CT system based on the LabPET scanner,[91] developed by the same group (now commercialized by Gamma Medica-Ideas), where PET and CT data are acquired using the same detector channels and electronics, thus allowing true simultaneous PET-CT scanning with the possibility to count and discriminate individual x-ray photons in CT mode.[92,93] This can be achieved by sampling the analog signal using high-speed analog-to-digital converters and digital processing in field-programmable gate arrays. The parallel architecture and fast digital processing electronics allow high count rates for PET and CT modes whereas the modularity of the system design allows extending the number of channels by 10^4 or more.

SPECT-CT systems designed specifically for small animal imaging are being developed by several investigators.[84,94–103] One of the first small animal SPECT-CT systems was developed by a consortium that included the Thomas Jefferson National Accelerator Facility (Jefferson

Laboratory), University of Virginia, and researchers at the College of William and Mary.[96–98] These systems use a compact scintillation camera that operates with multiple Hamamatsu R3292 position-sensitive photomultiplier tubes (PSPMTs) coupled to a pixelated array of cesium iodide crystals using pinhole and parallel-hole collimators. The x-ray data are acquired using a small fluoroscopic x-ray system (Lixi, Downers Grove, Illinois).[96]

Gamma Medica-Ideas has developed and introduced a small animal SPECT-CT system[95,100] with two compact scintillation cameras[104–106] and a high-resolution CT subsystem[100] for dual-modality imaging of rodents and other small animals. The SPECT camera can be operated with pinhole collimators that provide submillimeter spatial resolution in the reconstructed images or with parallel-hole collimators when higher detection sensitivity or whole body imaging is desired. The system includes a high-resolution preclinical CT subsystem[100] configured with a complementary metal-oxide semiconductor (CMOS) x-ray detector coupled to a gadolinium oxysulfide scintillator and a low-power x-ray tube. The preclinical CT system provides anatomic imaging with a spatial resolution of approximately 50 μm; the resulting x-ray data can be used for attenuation correction and for anatomic localization of the radionuclide data. In addition, the SPECT data can be acquired with respiratory and ECG gating for cardiovascular imaging applications where wall-motion abnormalities, ejection fraction calculations, or other assessments of ventricular function are necessary.

Another project, launched by Barrett from the Center for Gamma-Ray Imaging, University of Arizona, aimed to develop a high-resolution SPECT-CT system for small animal imaging.[99] High-resolution SPECT is performed with a modular semiconductor detector that consists of a $2.5 \times 2.5 \times 0.2$–$cm^3$ slab of cadmium zinc telluride (CZT) operated with a continuous gold electrode to apply bias on one side, and a 64×64 array of pixelated gold electrodes on the opposite side connected to an application-specific integrated circuit (ASIC) for readout of the individual pixel signals. The detector has a 380-mm pixel pitch and 330-mm–wide pixels coupled to a 7-mm–thick parallel-hole collimator for radionuclide imaging. The x-ray and radionuclide imaging subsystems are mounted with their image axes perpendicular to one another with the animal rotated vertically within the common field of view. The x-ray and radionuclide projection data are acquired sequentially and corrected for distortions and nonuniformities introduced by each of the detectors, then reconstructed with statistical iterative algorithms (OSEM).

The Inveon system, sold by Siemens, can be manufactured in the form of PET-CT, SPECT-CT, or all three (discussed later) in a single gantry system or docked PET with CT and/or SPECT. The Inveon PET system[107] uses block modules comprising 12×12 arrays of $1.5 \times 1.5 \times 10$ mm^3 LSO crystals, arranged in a 16.1-cm diameter ring, with a 12-cm diameter bore and 10-cm trans-axial and 12.7-cm axial field of view.

Positron Emission Tomography–MR Imaging and SPECT–MR Imaging

The history of combined PET–MR imaging dates to the mid-1990s, when image coregistration between separately acquired data was used to create postacquisition combined data sets.[108] At approximately the same time, an improvement in PET spatial resolution was characterized when positron annihilation takes place in a strong magnetic field.[109,110] The group from the University of Minnesota pioneered the design of the first combined system.[111] A collaborative effort between UCLA and Guy's and St Thomas' National Health Service Foundation Trust, London, followed, leading to the design of an MR imaging–compatible preclinical PET system modified to optically couple the detector crystals coupled to an external array of PSPMTs through 3-m–long fiber optics.[27,112] In this way, the combined system could acquire simultaneously PET and MR imaging data without measurable mutual interaction effects. More recently, other groups have used similar design approaches[28,29,113,114] or adopted more complex magnet designs, including a split magnet[76] or field-cycled MR imaging.[115]

A more attractive approach consists in using PET inserts that can be operated within existing MR magnets by designing suitable MR imaging–compatible PET systems using solid-state detectors that are insensitive to magnetic fields.[30,50,73–75] This includes APDs[116] and silicon photomultiplier tubes,[117,118] the latter of which look more promising for this application as they allow a significant reduction in the electronics required inside the MR imaging.[119] Several academic sites are equipped with PET inserts built using this technology that can be operated within a high-field MR imaging magnet.

Alternatively, the motivations for developing combined SPECT–MR imaging systems were addressed recently.[120] The availability of semiconductor-based SPECT detectors, such as CZT coupled with high-density low noise ASIC electronics to read out the semiconductor detectors, which are insensitive to magnetic fields, are enabling the design of integrated SPECT–MR imaging systems. The preclinical SPECT–MR imaging prototype constructed by Gamma Medica-Ideas consists of a polygonal ring of CZT detector with a field-of-view of 2.54 × 12.7 cm² fitted with a parallel-hole collimator. The materials used for fabrication (shielding, support, positioning, and cooling) were carefully selected to reduce their possible impact on magnetic field homogeneity. The design of the detector and front-end electronics were optimized for spectroscopic and timing performance, minimization of power dissipation, and low electromagnetic interference.[121]

Positron Emission Tomography–Optical Imaging

OI provides a sensitive method for examining gene expression due to the low background light levels. Unlike radioactivity imaging, where the radioactive signal is always "on," bioluminescent imaging creates light only where the inserted enzyme, substrate, oxygen, and ATP are present. This ability to see very small signals enables visualization of early expression and signal changes when compared with PET imaging. PET, however, is quantitative and can provide measurements of metabolic function with only minimal scatter and attenuation in rodents. The potential combination of these two modalities has been demonstrated by Chatziioannou (combined optical imaging and PET [OPET])[122,123] and Cherry, who used different instrumentation approaches. OPET uses the same detectors to image optical and radiation signals, whereas Cherry's system uses a conical mirror placed within a small animal PET scanner and a nearby separate optical detection camera.[124] A more recent design by the German Cancer Research Center (Heidelberg, Germany) uses a radial cylindric lattice of microlens arrays (115-mm diameter), which is mounted in front of PET detector blocks.[125] A network of optical fibers is allocated on a multihole plate such that the focal points of the individual microlenses correspond locally to single fiber–ending points.

Autoradiography Combined with other Modalities

The definitive method to determine the location of imaging probes remains autoradiography (AR), a modality capable of very high-resolution imaging, with localization possible at or below 10 μm. Given light scatter with OI and resolution limitations in SPECT, MR imaging, and PET systems, AR provides the best way of determining where the imaging probe is located within an animal. Unfortunately, this method requires freezing and slicing of the animals and thus is restricted to ex vivo single measurement points. Pairing AR with other nuclear medicine–based methods (PET or SPECT) and photographic images often is used to validate the findings in the nuclear based methods.

The AR images can provide additional information to determine the true location of PET probes in vivo. For example, recent work showing gut uptake of a newly labeled PET imaging probe was shown via AR to be located in the gastrointestinal lining, rather than in the gastrointestinal lumen (**Fig. 4**).[126] This was important information, because the lining required a bloodstream probe delivery rather than a gallbladder bile excretion route, which provided valuable insight concerning the metabolic fate of the imaging probe.

Optical Imaging–CT

The combination of OI with x-ray projection imaging pairs in vivo imaging information with anatomic information. This combination proves useful for imaging radiation exposure using gels, particularly in radiation therapy situations.[127] Carestream (formerly Kodak) markets an optical x-ray integrated system that uses the same detector system for x-ray photons and optical photons. Although both image sets are planar projections, the x-ray image provides some information about the location of lung, soft tissue, and bone that may be correlated to the optical signal source.[128] A more recent technique uses a time series of images acquired after injection of an inert dye where differences in the dye's in vivo biodistribution dynamics allow precise delineation and identification of major organs.[129]

MULTIPROBE IMAGING (MULTIMODALITY WITH DIFFERENT PROBES)
PET-SPECT

The demand for multiprobe molecular imaging of small animals using single-photon and positron-emitting radiotracers has stimulated the development of dedicated small-bore high-resolution systems for rodent imaging, allowing concurrent acquisition of SPECT and PET data. One system developed to match these needs is the yttrium aluminum perovskite (YAP)-(S)PET scanner.[130] The system consists of four rotating heads spaced 15 cm apart, each with an active area of 4 × 4 cm², containing a 20 × 20 array of 2 × 2 × 30 mm³ optically isolated YAP crystals coupled to PSPMTs, forming a 4-cm transaxial and axial field of view. Multiprobe scanning can be performed through energy discrimination, allowing acquisition of SPECT and PET data in different energy windows.

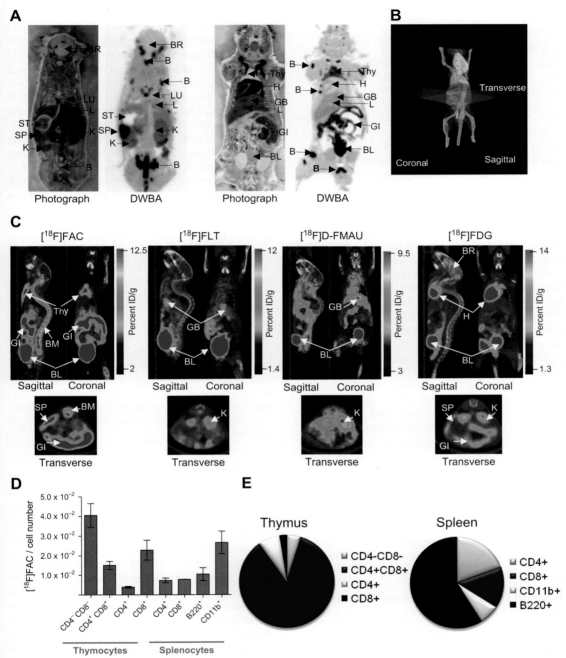

Fig. 4. (*A*) 18F-fluoroarabinofuranosyl cytosine (^{18}F-FAC) digital whole-body autoradiography shown along with corresponding tissue sections. B, bone; BL, bladder; BM, bone marrow; BR, brain; GB, gall bladder; GI, gastrointestinal tract; H, heart; K, kidney; L, liver; LU, lung; SP, spleen; ST, stomach; Thy, thymus. (*B, C*) C57/BL6 mice were scanned by microPET-CT using ^{18}F-FAC, F18-fluorothymidine (^{18}F-FLT), ^{18}F-D-FMAU, and ^{18}F-FDG. Mice were imaged 60 minutes after intravenous injection of probes. Orientation of sagittal, coronal, and transverse sections is depicted in 3-D microCT image in (*B*). Images are 1-mm thick. Percentage ID/g, percentage injected dose per gram of tissue. (*D*) ^{18}F-FAC retention/cell number in thymocytes and splenocytes. Error bars represent means ±SEM, and results are representative of two independent experiments. (*E*) Proportion of ^{18}F-FAC retention per cell lineage per lymphoid organ. (*Reprinted from* Radu CG, Shu CJ, Nair-Gill E, et al. Molecular imaging of lymphoid organs and immune activation by positron emission tomography with a new [18F]-labeled 2′-deoxycytidine analog. Nat Med 2008;14:783–8; with permission.)

SPECT with SPECT (Energy Discrimination)

Dual-tracer imaging using SPECT, where multiple energy windows are used for simultaneous imaging of radiotracers using radionuclides emitting γ-rays at different energies, is one of the unique advantages inherent to SPECT technology. Examples of this include (1) [99m]Tc (140 keV) sestamibi stress and [201]Tl (75 keV/167 keV) rest myocardial perfusion imaging and (2) simultaneous use of a [99m]Tc (140 keV)–labeled perfusion agent and an [123]I (159 keV)–labeled neurotransmitter agent (eg, in neurodegenerative diseases). The use of simultaneous acquisition reduces the overall acquisition time and, therefore, the duration of anesthesia to the animal. Another significant advantage is that the resulting images from the different radiotracers are perfectly registered in space and time.

A complication with dual-tracer imaging is the presence of crosstalk between the multiple energy windows. In the case of, for instance, imaging with [99m]Tc (140 keV) and [201]Tl (75 keV/167 keV), the lower-energy ^{201}Tl energy window is contaminated by ^{99m}Tc photons scattered in patients or collimator (referred to as down-scatter) and lead x-rays generated by scattered and unscattered ^{99m}Tc photons in the collimator. In addition, the ^{99m}Tc data are contaminated by scattered (approximately 135 keV) and unscattered (167 keV) ^{201}Tl photons. To address these difficulties, current research has focused on optimization of multiple energy-window acquisition parameters[131,132] and modeling of crosstalk effects (ie, down-scatter and collimator x-ray generation) in the reconstruction task.[133–135] Combinations of these methods and detailed clinical evaluation are still required to make dual-tracer SPECT imaging an acceptable protocol for small laboratory animal research.

Positron Emission Tomography–Positron Emission Tomography

Multiprobe imaging has been used for several decades[136] to look at multiple information sources using the same imaging modality. A prime example is in cardiac imaging with the use of radiolabeled ammonia (NH_3) for blood flow and FDG for energy use using PET imaging.[137] The short half-life of NH_3 (10 minutes) enables a scan to be followed up with a second (stress versus rest) or alternative (FDG) imaging probe. In the case of NH_3-FDG, this shows where cardiac blood is flowing versus viable tissue, which is of great value to cardiac surgeons who would like to know before surgery whether or not a bypass procedure would have any benefit to patients. More often, the same subject or patient undergoes imaging a day or two apart. With adequate control over reproducible positioning, this method can provide imaging information from any combination of probes. Recently, Wu and colleagues[138] have shown that signals from serially injected probes using the same F18 isotope can be temporally decoded in mice, enabling sequential imaging without moving the subject between the two probe injections. This reduces changes in position and potentially in biologic status. Similar efforts are under examination in clinical settings.[139]

The dual-tracer approach is not straightforward for use in PET imaging because the detected events emanating from all radiotracers used have the same energy (511 keV). Despite the difficulties, few groups are investigating the feasibility of scanning multiple PET radiotracers using dynamic imaging techniques, where the signals from each tracer are separated based on differences in tracer half-life, kinetics, and distribution.[140–142] The single tracer components then can be assessed through multivariate analysis tools, such as principal component analysis. This field is an area of active research and to be successful, the approach deserves further research and development efforts and additional evaluation for potential clinical use.[143,144]

Optical Fluorescence–Wavelength-specific Probes

Similar to SPECT probe discrimination by energy, multiple fluorophores can be imaged in vivo using wavelength separation. Several companies have systems with this feature, including the Maestro, IVIS Spectrum, and others. The fluorophores can be excited using different filters or excitation lasers. Separation of the resulting signals can be by a series of specific band pass filters or, in the case of the Maestro, by a tunable liquid crystal display that sweeps through the spectral range. The goal is to separate nonspecific autofluorescence background (hemoglobin, fur, chow, and collagen) from the specific fluorophore signals. Each fluorophore has its own heterogeneous background signal, which can make specific signal detection difficult. Because light has to go into and out of an animal and activates any endogenous fluorescent molecules, fluorescent imaging is inherently less sensitive due to background than bioluminescent imaging. Nonetheless, fluorescent imaging enables following the expression or signal movement of multiple sources at the same time. In the biologic realm, where multiple factors are involved with any biologic process under investigation, the more information that can be obtained at the same time about various states, the better the system can be accurately characterized. A distinct advantage of fluorescence imaging is that the temporal movement of fluorophores can be followed, because there is no substrate injected that is delivered and consumed over time.[7,145]

TRIMODALITY OPTIONS
Positron Emission Tomography–SPECT–CT

In response to the need of integrated multimodality platforms for multiprobe imaging, it was conjectured that the availability of a trimodality imaging system, allowing combining three modalities and recording quasisimultaneously complementary information gathered from SPECT, PET, and CT, might offer many advantages in some situations. Currently available commercial trimodality systems include the Inveon (Siemens) and the FLEX Triumph platform (developed by Gamma Medica-Ideas).[146] The Inveon is the current generation system of Siemens microPET product line.[107] The Siemens preclinical SPECT-CT system has been out for several years and the Inveon now can be bought within the same gantry as the SPECT-CT. The FLEX system uses the SPECT and CT sys-tems (described previously) and can be configured with the X-PET[147] or the LabPET[148] as a PET subsystem. It also has been argued that the APD-based detector module proposed by Saoudi and Lecomte[149] is particularly attractive for the design of compact multimodality (PET-SPECT-CT) imaging systems.

MR Imaging–Functional MR Imaging–Positron Emission Tomography

Recent developments with insert-based PET scanners that can be placed within MR imaging magnets[30,31] enable the combination of PET imaging with MR imaging and functional MR imaging. Anatomic MR images provide excellent soft tissue contrast that can be used to correct PET images for attenuation.[150–152] Using functional MR imaging, it is possible to measure blood flow and brain activation, typically using nonradioactive gadolinium contrast agents. Spectroscopic magnetic resonance measurements can distinguish probes and their metabolites, potentially eliminating the need for blood sampling to establish a metabolism profile. Metabolite analysis, especially in mice, remains a challenge in small animals due to their limited blood pool and need for taking samples at multiple time points.

Combined with radioactive PET probes, MR imaging and functional MR imaging can be used at the same time to observe a metabolic process (PET) separate from blood flow and anatomic measurements.

The primary advantage of combining these systems together is the ability to acquire simultaneous information from an animal in vivo. This eliminates the need to coregister divergent and often different image data, removes the need to move the animal between imaging systems, and ensures that the biologic state is the same for all measurements. The combination of nanomolar tracer metabolism measurements using PET with exquisite anatomic information from MR imaging makes a powerful combination for in vivo research, particularly when paired with functional MR imaging for metabolite analysis. PET and MR imaging have cost and safety concerns, which may limit the widespread use of this combination, although this approach remains the best option for neuroscience research.

SPECT–CT–Optical Imaging

A trimodality (SPECT-CT-OI) small animal imaging system is being developed at the German Cancer Research Center.[125,153] The SPECT component consists of a compact detector of a 2×2 array of PSPMTs, which are connected to a 66×66 array of optode-coupled $1.3 \times 1.3 \times 6–mm^3$ sodium iodide crystals. The optical subsystem consists of a high-resolution CCD camera containing a progressive scan interline CCD chip. Various laser sources, selected by wavelength and light power requirements, can be mounted on the gantry. The x-ray CT component uses an x-ray tube having a 35-μm focal spot size and a cone angle of 24° whereas the x-ray detector consists of a $49.2 \times 98.6–mm^2$ gadolinium oxysulfide scintillator screen placed in direct contact with a CMOS photodiode array with 48-μm sensor pixel size. The modular design allows mounting of the subsystems on a common gantry, enabling a wide range of applications to be performed.

CHALLENGES FACED
Maintaining Image Quality, Low Dose, and Quantitation

There are several challenges facing the use of preclinical multimodality imaging, which may represent inherent limitations in these techniques. These include appropriate selection of an imaging modality or combination of multiprobe imaging modalities and the design of optimal task–specific acquisition and processing protocols. In this respect, small-animal imaging poses many challenges when it comes to maintaining image quality and improving quantitative accuracy compared with clinical studies. Image quality in preclinical studies should be carefully optimized taking into account the physical performance characteristics of the imaging system used and the purposes of the experiment.

Multimodality molecular imaging has a long tradition of incorporating quantitative analysis in research protocols. Until recently, the analysis was based on functional or metabolic images as the sole input although the importance of the complementary information available from other anatomic modalities or from earlier scans has long been recognized. In addition, the visual quality and quantitative accuracy of small-animal imaging can be improved using anatomic imaging techniques to guide the reconstruction procedure[154] and to correct the radionuclide data for physical errors contributed by photon attenuation,[155] scatter radiation,[156] and partial volume effects[157] due to the limited spatial resolution of the nuclear imaging system. CT-based attenuation correction usually requires x-ray CT scanning of a cylindric phantom containing cylindric holes filled with a mixed solution of potassim phosphate and water with varying concentrations to simulate biologic tissues with different densities (**Fig. 5**). The calibration curve obtained then can be used for conversion of CT images of the animal to an attenuation map that can be used for attenuation correction purposes (**Fig. 6**). Alternatively, absolute quantification using PET generally requires accurate measurement of activity concentrations in arterial blood, which provides the input function to the kinetic model used. Although many dedicated blood sampling devices have been designed specifically for this purpose (eg,[158,159]),

it remains a challenging task in small-animal imaging.

The radiation dose delivered to animals is a critical issue in preclinical imaging and can be high depending on the experiments and should be carefully monitored as it might change tumor characteristics; induce significant biologic effects, thus changing the animal model being studied; or even cause lethality.[160,161] The same applies to other imaging modalities, such as CT,[162] particularly when performed on multimodality imaging systems where the resulting absorbed dose is the sum of the individual contributions of each modality. Although much worthwhile effort has been devoted toward the assessment of radiation dose delivered to human subjects, few research studies addressed this issue for small animals.[160,162–164] High-resolution CT implies high radiation dose to the animal. If only a low-resolution scan is acquired, then the majority of the radiation dose comes from the PET tracer. Thus, increasing the sensitivity of preclinical PET systems might allow injecting lower activities and thus reducing the absorbed dose in the animal.

Creating and Timing Protocols to Obtain Simultaneous Data

One of the challenges to simultaneous and independent imaging procedures is recognizing when imaging data are informative and interesting. In static imaging situations, where there are no fast temporal changes of signal, it is simple to acquire data such that precise timing of the acquisition rarely is essential. With dynamic imaging, signals may change rapidly, such as with the first pass of a probe or contrast agent through the tissue bloodstream. There may be difficulties in starting

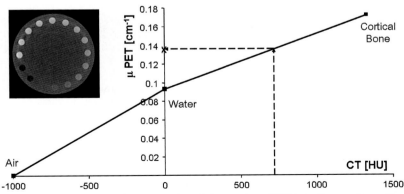

Fig. 5. Typical bilinear calibration curve for conversion of CT numbers (HU) into linear attenuation coefficients at 511 keV for preclinical PET-CT scanner. The in-house designed polyethylene cylindric phantom containing 16 cylindric holes is shown in upper left corner. Samples contained mixed solutions of K2HPO4 and water with concentrations varying between 80 mg/μL and 1000 mg/μL to simulate cortical bone with different densities.

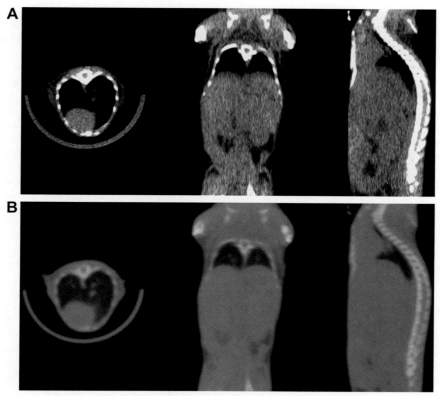

Fig. 6. Representative slices of original CT image in Hounsfield units (*A*) and generated attenuation map (*B*). Procedure involved the following steps: down-sampling from 512 × 512 to 256 × 256, followed by energy mapping by transforming CT numbers into linear attenuation coefficients at 511 keV using bilinear calibration curve shown in **Fig. 5**, and finally gaussian smoothing to match spatial resolution of preclinical PET scanner.

acquisitions at exact times, delays due to configuration of files, activation of injection systems, or simply having to start two separate computers at the same time. There also is a challenge to create images that have specific information from a certain period of time. An example might be an image showing optimal contrast or probe localization in one region of space that has a fast temporal change. This sort of optimization of the image might require considerable reprocessing of the data (or even specific timing of the acquisition) to get the best possible image. Often offline processing is desirable so that this optimization process does not tie up the imaging systems. Wherever possible, automation of the acquisition and processing can greatly facilitate optimal image timing and generation.

FUTURE TRENDS

The future of preclinical multimodality imaging lies in the creation of systems that make imaging simple, easy, and reproducible. The target information is not actually pretty images but rather the information content related to how much probe went to which specific location. Preclinical imaging systems will expand to incorporate systems for positioning; physiologic support, such as heating and anesthesia; enclosures for immunodeficient or infected animals; and operation and use by minimally trained personnel. The process of creating fused coregistered images from multiple sources will become increasingly automated and requires less user interaction. The images themselves will become increasingly less emphasized as the content becomes the focus, shifting from pictures to relevant data about timing and uptake information (parametric). It is possible that one day images will disappear, replaced by an automated process that maps uptake data onto standardized mouse or rat atlases. The future will likely see a shift toward the end user, typically a biologist, as the primary user with little or no support required to operate and analyze the imaging-based data.

One issue remains clear, which is that the more information that can be obtained, sequentially or simultaneously, the better a biologic system can be understood. Often the imaging modalities are complementary, providing different pieces of information about the same animal; thus, the multimodality approach is likely to become the standard way that imaging-based research is conducted in the future.

REFERENCES

1. Kalender WA. X-ray computed tomography. Phys Med Biol 2006;51:R29–43.
2. Holdsworth SJ, Bammer R. Magnetic resonance imaging techniques: fMRI, DWI, and PWI. Semin Neurol 2008;28:395–406.
3. Matthews PM, Honey GD, Bullmore ET. Applications of fMRI in translational medicine and clinical practice. Nat Rev Neurosci 2006;7:732–44.
4. Prost RW. Magnetic resonance spectroscopy. Med Phys 2008;35:4530–44.
5. Madsen MT. Recent advances in SPECT imaging. J Nucl Med 2007;48:661–73.
6. Muehllehner G, Karp JS. Positron emission tomography. Phys Med Biol 2006;51:R117–37.
7. Ntziachristos V. Fluorescence molecular imaging. Annu Rev Biomed Eng 2006;8:1–33.
8. Phelps ME. PET: the merging of biology and imaging into molecular imaging. J Nucl Med 2000;41:661–81.
9. Bar-Shalom R, Yefemov N, Guralnik L, et al. Clinical performance of PET/CT in evaluation of cancer: additional value for diagnostic imaging and patient management. J Nucl Med 2003;44:1200–9.
10. Vogel WV, Oyen WJ, Barentsz JO, et al. PET/CT: panacea, redundancy, or something in between? J Nucl Med 2004;45(Suppl 1):15S–24S.
11. Macapinlac HA. Clinical applications of positron emission tomography/computed tomography treatment planning. Semin Nucl Med 2008;38:137–40.
12. Zaidi H, Vees H, Wissmeyer M. Molecular PET/CT imaging-guided radiation therapy treatment planning. Acad Radiol 2009, in press.
13. Schoder H, Ong SC. Fundamentals of molecular imaging: rationale and applications with relevance for radiation oncology. Semin Nucl Med 2008;38:119–28.
14. Townsend DW. Multimodality imaging of structure and function. Phys Med Biol 2008;53:R1–39.
15. Burton JB, Johnson M, Sato M, et al. Adenovirus-mediated gene expression imaging to directly detect sentinel lymph node metastasis of prostate cancer. Nat Med 2008;14:882–8.
16. Hutton BF, Braun M. Software for image registration: algorithms, accuracy, efficacy. Semin Nucl Med 2003;33:180–92.
17. Maes F, Vandermeulen D, Suetens P. Medical image registration using mutual information. Proceedings of the IEEE 2003;91:1699–722.
18. Pelizzari CA, Chen GT, Spelbring DR, et al. Accurate three-dimensional registration of CT, PET, and/or MR images of the brain. J Comput Assist Tomogr 1989;13:20–6.
19. Pietrzyk U, Herholz K, Fink G, et al. An interactive technique for three-dimensional image registration: validation for PET, SPECT, MRI and CT brain studies. J Nucl Med 1994;35:2011–8.
20. Woods RP, Grafton ST, Holmes CJ, et al. Automated image registration: I. General methods and intrasubject, intramodality validation. J Comput Assist Tomogr 1998;22:139–52.
21. Krishnasetty V, Fischman AJ, Halpern EL, et al. Comparison of alignment of computer-registered data sets: combined PET/CT versus independent PET and CT of the thorax. Radiology 2005;237:635–9.
22. Slomka PJ. Software approach to merging molecular with anatomic information. J Nucl Med 2004;1(45 Suppl):36S–45S.
23. Hasegawa B, Zaidi H. Dual-modality imaging: more than the sum of its components. In: Zaidi H, editor. Quantitative analysis in nuclear medicine imaging. New York: Springer; 2006. p. 35–81.
24. Hasegawa BH, Gingold EL, Reilly SM, et al. Description of a simultaneous emission-transmission CT system. Proc Soc Photo Opt Instrum Eng 1990;1231:50–60.
25. Hasegawa BH, Iwata K, Wong KH, et al. Dual-modality imaging of function and physiology. Acad Radiol 2002;9:1305–21.
26. Beyer T, Townsend D, Brun T, et al. A combined PET/CT scanner for clinical oncology. J Nucl Med 2000;41:1369–79.
27. Shao Y, Cherry SR, Farahani K, et al. Simultaneous PET and MR imaging. Phys Med Biol 1997;42:1965–70.
28. Mackewn JE, Strul D, Hallett WA, et al. Design and development of an MR-compatible PET scanner for imaging small animals. IEEE Trans Nucl Sci 2005;52:1376–80.
29. Raylman RR, Majewski S, Velan SS, et al. Simultaneous acquisition of magnetic resonance spectroscopy (MRS) data and positron emission tomography (PET) images with a prototype MR-compatible, small animal PET imager. J Magn Reson 2007;186:305–10.
30. Judenhofer MS, Wehrl HF, Newport DF, et al. Simultaneous PET-MRI: a new approach for functional and morphological imaging. Nat Med 2008;14:459–65.
31. Pichler BJ, Wehrl HF, Kolb A, et al. Positron emission tomography/magnetic resonance imaging: the next generation of multimodality imaging? Semin Nucl Med 2008;38:199–208.
32. Levin CS, Zaidi H. Current trends in preclinical PET system design. PET Clinics 2007;2:125–60.

33. Schlemmer HP, Pichler BJ, Schmand M, et al. Simultaneous MR/PET imaging of the human brain: feasibility study. Radiology 2008;248:1028–35.

34. Gaa J, Rummeny EJ, Seemann MD. Whole-body imaging with PET/MRI. Eur J Med Res 2004;30:309–12.

35. Seemann MD. Whole-body PET/MRI: the future in oncological imaging. Technol Cancer Res Treat 2005;4:577–82.

36. Small Animal Imaging Workshop at Stanford. Available at: http://radiologycme.stanford.edu/2008smallanimal/. Accessed November 30th, 2008.

37. Small Animal Imaging Workshop at Tuebingen. Available at: http://89.110.144.29:8080/4th-small-animal-imaging-workshop-2009. Accessed November 30th, 2008.

38. In vivo small animal imaging at UCDavis. In vivo small animal imaging. Available at: http://imaging.bme.ucdavis.edu/events.html. Accessed November 30th, 2008.

39. Richmond JY, Hill RH, Weyant RS, et al. What's hot in animal biosafety? ILAR J 2003;44:20–7.

40. Pritt S, Hankenson FC, Wagner T, et al. The basics of animal biosafety and biocontainment training. Lab Anim (NY) 2007;36:31–8.

41. Richmond JY. The 1, 2, 3's of biosafety levels. Available at: http://www.cdc.gov/OD/ohs/symp5/jyrtext.htm. Accessed November 30th, 2008.

42. Johns Hopkins Animal Care and Use. Animal care and use training. Available at: http://www.jhu.edu/animalcare/training3.html. Accessed November 30th, 2008.

43. Howard Hughes Medical Institute. Lab safety training materials. Available at: http://www.hhmi.org/about/research/training.html. Accessed November 30th, 2008.

44. Peters LL, Robledo RF, Bult CJ, et al. The mouse as a model for human biology: a resource guide for complex trait analysis. Nat Rev Genet 2007;8:58–69.

45. Mouse Models of Human Cancer Consortium. Available at: http://mouse.ncifcrf.gov/. Accessed November 30th, 2008.

46. Wang YX, Betton G, Floettmann E, et al. Imaging kidney in conscious rats with high-frequency ultrasound and detection of two cases of unilateral congenital hydronephrosis. Ultrasound Med Biol 2007;33:483–6.

47. Ferris CF, Febo M, Luo F, et al. Functional magnetic resonance imaging in conscious animals: a new tool in behavioural neuroscience research. J Neuroendocrinol 2006;18:307–18.

48. Kyme AZ, Zhou VW, Meikle SR, et al. Real-time 3D motion tracking for small animal brain PET. Phys Med Biol 2008;53:2651–66.

49. Vaska P, Woody CL, Schlyer DJ, et al. RatCAP: miniaturized head-mounted PET for conscious rodent brain imaging. IEEE Trans Nucl Sci 2004;51:2718–22.

50. Woody C, Schlyer D, Vaska P, et al. Preliminary studies of a simultaneous PET/MRI scanner based on the RatCAP small animal tomograph. Nucl Instr Meth A 2007;571:102–5.

51. Flores JE, McFarland LM, Vanderbilt A, et al. The effects of anesthetic agent and carrier gas on blood glucose and tissue uptake in mice undergoing dynamic FDG-PET imaging: sevoflurane and isoflurane compared in air and in oxygen. Mol Imaging Biol 2008;10:192–200.

52. Fueger BJ, Czernin J, Hildebrandt I, et al. Impact of animal handling on the results of 18F-FDG PET studies in mice. J Nucl Med 2006;47:999–1006.

53. Star Life Sciences probe. White paper. 2008?

54. Pan MH, Huang SC, Liao YP, et al. FLT-PET imaging of radiation responses in murine tumors. Mol Imaging Biol 2008;10:325–34.

55. Maintz JB, Viergever MA. A survey of medical image registration. Med Image Anal 1998;2:1–36.

56. Pluim JP, Maintz JB, Viergever MA. Mutual-information-based registration of medical images: a survey. IEEE Trans Med Imaging 2003;22:986–1004.

57. Zanzonico PB. Broad-spectrum multi-modality image registration: from PET, CT, and MRI to autoradiography, microscopy, and beyond. Conf Proc IEEE Eng Med Biol Soc 2006;1:1584–8.

58. Zanzonico PB, Nehmeh SA. Introduction to clinical and laboratory (small-animal) image registration and fusion. Conf Proc IEEE Eng Med Biol Soc 2006;1:1580–3.

59. Cross DJ, Minoshima S, Nishimura S, et al. Three-dimensional stereotactic surface projection analysis of macaque brain PET: development and initial applications. J Nucl Med 2000;41:1879–87.

60. Shimada Y, Uemura K, Ardekani BA, et al. Application of PET-MRI registration techniques to cat brain imaging. J Neurosci Methods 2000;101:1–7.

61. Vaquero JJ, Desco M, Pascau J, et al. PET, CT, and MR image registration of the rat brain and skull. IEEE Trans Nucl Sci 2001;48:1440–5.

62. Humm JL, Ballon D, Hu YC, et al. A stereotactic method for the three-dimensional registration of multi-modality biologic images in animals: NMR, PET, histology, and autoradiography. Med Phys 2003;30:2303–14.

63. Jan M-L, Chuang K-S, Chen G-W, et al. A three-dimensional registration method for automated fusion of micro PET-CT-SPECT whole-body images. IEEE Trans Med Imaging 2005;24:886–93.

64. Fei B, Wang H, Muzic J, et al. Deformable and rigid registration of MRI and microPET images for photodynamic therapy of cancer in mice. Med Phys 2006;33:753–60.

65. Deroose CM, De A, Loening AM, et al. Multimodality imaging of tumor xenografts and metastases in

mice with combined small-animal PET, small-animal CT, and bioluminescence imaging. J Nucl Med 2007;48:295–303.

66. Pascau J, Gispert JD, Michaelides M, et al. Automated method for small-animal PET image registration with intrinsic validation. Mol Imaging Biol 2009;11(2):107–13.

67. Zanzonico P, Campa J, Polycarpe-Holman D, et al. Animal-specific positioning molds for registration of repeat imaging studies: comparative microPET imaging of F18-labeled fluoro-deoxyglucose and fluoro-misonidazole in rodent tumors. Nucl Med Biol 2006;33:65–70.

68. Chow PL, Stout DB, Komisopoulou E, et al. A method of image registration for small animal, multi-modality imaging. Phys Med Biol 2006;51:379–90.

69. Christian N, Lee JA, Bol A, et al. Immobilization device for in vivo and in vitro multimodality image registration of rodent tumors. Radiother Oncol 2008;87:147–51.

70. Beekman F, Hutton B. Multi-modality imaging on track. Eur J Nucl Med Mol Imaging 2007;34:1410–4.

71. Collins DL, Neelin P, Peters TM, et al. Automatic 3D intersubject registration of MR volumetric data in standardized Talairach space. J Comput Assist Tomogr 1994;18:192–205.

72. Goertzen AL, Meadors AK, Silverman RW, et al. Simultaneous molecular and anatomical imaging of the mouse in vivo. Phys Med Biol 2002;21:4315–28.

73. Catana C, Wu Y, Judenhofer MS, et al. Simultaneous acquisition of multislice PET and MR images: Initial results with a MR-compatible PET scanner. J Nucl Med 2006;47:1968–76.

74. Pichler BJ, Judenhofer MS, Catana C, et al. Performance test of an LSO-APD detector in a 7-T MRI scanner for simultaneous PET/MRI. J Nucl Med 2006;47:639–47.

75. Judenhofer MS, Catana C, Swann BK, et al. Simultaneous PET/MR images, acquired with a compact MRI compatible PET detector in a 7 Tesla magnet. Radiology 2007;244:807–14.

76. Lucas AJ, Hawkes RC, Ansorge RE, et al. Development of a combined microPET-MR system. Technol Cancer Res Treat 2006;5:337–41.

77. Suckow C, Kuntner C, Chow P, et al. Multimodality rodent imaging chambers for use under barrier conditions with gas anesthesia. Mol Imaging Biol 2008;10(2):114–20.

78. Bentourkia MH, Zaidi H. Tracer kinetic modeling in PET. PET Clinics 2007;2:267–77.

79. Snyder DL. Parameter estimation for dynamic studies in emission-tomography systems having list-mode data. IEEE Trans Nucl Sci 1984;31:925–31.

80. Rahmim A, Lenox M, Reader AJ, et al. Statistical list-mode image reconstruction for the high resolution research tomograph. Phys Med Biol 2004;49:4239–58.

81. Reader AJ, Zaidi H. Advances in PET image reconstruction. PET Clinics 2007;2:173–90.

82. Cherry SR. Multimodality in vivo imaging systems: twice the power or double the trouble? Annu Rev Biomed Eng 2006;8:35–62.

83. Del Guerra A, Belcari N. State-of-the-art of PET, SPECT and CT for small animal imaging. Nucl Instr Meth A 2007;583:119–24.

84. Franc BL, Acton PD, Mari C, et al. Small-animal SPECT and SPECT/CT: Important tools for preclinical investigation. J Nucl Med 2008;49:1651–63.

85. Paulus MJ, Gleason SS, Kennel SJ, et al. High resolution X-ray computed tomography: an emerging tool for small animal cancer research. Neoplasia 2000;2:62–70.

86. Ritman EL. Micro-computed tomography-current status and developments. Annu Rev Biomed Eng 2004;6:185–208.

87. Kiessling F, Greschus S, Lichy MP, et al. Volumetric computed tomography (VCT): a new technology for noninvasive, high-resolution monitoring of tumor angiogenesis. Nat Med 2004;10:1133–8.

88. Vaquero JJ, Redondo S, Lage E, et al. Assessment of a new high-performance small-animal X-ray tomograph. IEEE Trans Nucl Sci 2008;55:898–905.

89. Andre MP, Spivey BA, Martin PJ, et al. Integrated CMOS-selenium x-ray detector for digital mammography. Proc Soc Photo Opt Instrum Eng 1998;3336:204–9.

90. Liang H, Yang Y, Yang K, et al. A microPET/CT system for in vivo small animal imaging. Phys Med Biol 2007;52:3881–94.

91. Dumouchel T, Bergeron M, Cadorette J, et al. Initial performance assessment of the LabPET™ APD-based digital PET scanner [abstract]. J Nucl Med 2007;48:39P.

92. Fontaine R, Belanger F, Cadorette J, et al. Architecture of a dual-modality, high-resolution, fully digital positron emission tomography/computed tomography (PET/CT) scanner for small animal imaging. IEEE Trans Nucl Sci 2005;52:691–6.

93. Bérard P, Riendeau J, Pepin C, et al. Investigation of the LabPETTM detector and electronics for photon-counting CT imaging. Nucl Instr Meth A 2007;571:114–7.

94. Iwata K, Wu MC, Hasegawa BH. Design of combined x-ray CT and SPECT systems for small animals. IEEE Nuclear Science Symposium and Medical Imaging Conference Record 1999;3:1608–12.

95. Iwata K, Hwang AB, Wu MC, et al. Design and utility of a small animal CT/SPECT system. IEEE Nuclear Science Symposium and Medical Imaging Conference Record 2002;3:1849–52.

96. Williams MB, Zhang G, More MJ, et al. Integrated CT-SPECT system for small animal imaging. Proc Soc Photo Opt Instrum Eng 2000;4142:265–74.

97. Welsh RE, Brewer P, Bradley EL, et al. An economical dual-modality small animal imaging system with application to studies of diabetes. IEEE Nuclear Science Symposium and Medical Imaging Conference Record 2002;3:1845–8.

98. Weisenberger AG, Wojcik R, Bradley EL, et al. SPECT-CT system for small animal imaging. IEEE Trans Nucl Sci 2003;50:74–9.

99. Kastis GA, Furenlid LR, Wilson DW, et al. Compact CT/SPECT small-animal imaging system. IEEE Trans Nucl Sci 2004;51:63–7.

100. MacDonald LR, Iwata K, Patt BE, et al. Evaluation of x-ray detectors for dual-modality CT-SPECT animal imaging. Proc Soc Photo Opt Instrum Eng 2002;4786:91–102.

101. Song X, Frey EC, Tsui BMW. Development and evaluation of a microCT system for small animal imaging. IEEE Nuclear Science Symposium and Medical Imaging Conference Record 2002;3: 1600–4.

102. Hwang AB, Iwata K, Sakdinawat AE, et al. Gantry specifications for a dual modality imaging system for small animals. IEEE Nuclear Science Symposium and Medical Imaging Conference Record 2003;2:1303–7.

103. Hasegawa BH, Wu MC, Iwata K, et al. Applications of penetrating radiation for small animal imaging. Proc Soc Photo Opt Instrum Eng 2002; 4786:80–90.

104. MacDonald LR, Patt BE, Iwanczyk JS, et al. Pinhole SPECT of mice using the LumaGEM gamma camera. IEEE Trans Nucl Sci 2001;48:830–6.

105. MacDonald LR, Iwanczyk JS, Patt BE, et al. Development of new high resolution detectors for small animal SPECT imaging. IEEE Nuclear Science Symposium and Medical Imaging Conference Record 2002;3:21/75.

106. McElroy DP, MacDonald LR, Beekman FJ, et al. Performance evaluation of A-SPECT: a high resolution desktop pinhole SPECT system for imaging small animals. IEEE Trans Nucl Sci 2002;49:2139–47.

107. Visser EP, Disselhorst JA, Brom M, et al. Spatial resolution and sensitivity of the Inveon small-animal PET scanner. J Nucl Med 2009;50:139–47.

108. Lin K-P, Sung-Cheng H, Baxter LR, et al. A general technique for interstudy registration of multifunction and multimodality images. IEEE Trans Nucl Sci 1994;41:2850–5.

109. Rickey D, Gordon R, Huda W. On lifting the inherent limitations of positron emission tomography by using magnetic fields (MagPET). Automedica 1992;14:355–69.

110. Hammer BE, Christensen NL, Heil BG. Use of a magnetic field to increase the spatial resolution of positron emission tomography. Med Phys 1994; 21:1917–20.

111. Christensen NL, Hammer BE, Heil BG, et al. Positron emission tomography within a magnetic field using photomultiplier tubes and light-guides. Phys Med Biol 1995;40:691–7.

112. Slates R, Cherry SR, Boutefnouchet A, et al. Design of a small animal MR compatible PET scanner. IEEE Trans Nucl Sci 1999;46:565–70.

113. Yamamoto S, Takamatsu S, Murayama H, et al. A block detector for a multislice, depth-of-interaction MR-compatible PET. IEEE Trans Nucl Sci 2005;52: 33–7.

114. Raylman RR, Majewski S, Lemieux SK, et al. Simultaneous MRI and PET imaging of a rat brain. Phys Med Biol 2006;51:6371–9.

115. Handler WB, Gilbert KM, Peng H, et al. Simulation of scattering and attenuation of 511 keV photons in a combined PET/field-cycled MRI system. Phys Med Biol 2006;51:2479–91.

116. Renker D. Geiger-mode avalanche photodiodes, history, properties and problems. Nucl Instr Meth A 2006;567:48–56.

117. Dolgoshein B, Balagura V, Buzhan P, et al. Status report on silicon photomultiplier development and its applications. Nucl Instr Meth A 2006;563: 368–76.

118. McElroy DP, Saveliev V, Reznik A, et al. Evaluation of silicon photomultipliers: a promising new detector for MR compatible PET. Nucl Instr Meth A 2007;571:106–9.

119. Moehrs S, Del Guerra A, Herbert DJ, et al. A detector head design for small-animal PET with silicon photomultipliers (SiPM). Phys Med Biol 2006;51:1113–27.

120. Wagenaar DJ, Kapusta M, Li J, et al. Rationale for the combination of nuclear medicine with magnetic resonance for pre-clinical imaging. Technol Cancer Res Treat 2006;5:343–50.

121. Wagenaar D, Nalcioglu O, Muftuler L, et al. A multiring small animal CZT system for simultaneous SPECT/MRI imaging. J Nucl Med 2007;48:89P, –c-.

122. Prout DL, Silverman RW, Chatziioannou A. Detector concept for OPET-A combined PET and optical imaging system. IEEE Trans Nucl Sci 2004;51: 752–6.

123. Douraghy A, Rannou FR, Silverman RW, et al. FPGA electronics for OPET: a dual-modality optical and positron emission tomograph. IEEE Trans Nucl Sci 2008;55:2541–5.

124. Li C, Mitchell GS, Yang Y, et al. Simultaneous PET and multispectral three-dimensional fluorescence optical tomography imaging system for small animals. World Molecular Imaging Conference (WMIC), Nice, France, 10–13, Sept 2008.

125. Peter J, Semmler W. vECTlab-A fully integrated multi-modality Monte Carlo simulation framework

for the radiological imaging sciences. Nucl Instr Meth A 2007;580:955–9.

126. Radu CG, Shu CJ, Nair-Gill E, et al. Molecular imaging of lymphoid organs and immune activation by positron emission tomography with a new [18F]-labeled 2'-deoxycytidine analog. Nat Med 2008;14: 783–8.

127. Oldham M, Kim L, Hugo G. Optical-CT imaging of complex 3D dose distributions. J Phys 2005;5745: 138–46.

128. McLaughlin W, Douglas V. Kodak in vivo imaging system: precise co registration of molecular imaging with anatomical X-ray imaging in animals. Available at: http://www.carestreamhealth.com/WorkArea/showcontent.aspx?id=360874. Accessed November 30th, 2008.

129. Hillman EMC, Moore A. All-optical anatomical co-registration for molecular imaging of small animals using dynamic contrast. Nat Photonics 2007;1: 526–30.

130. Del Guerra A, Bartoli A, Belcari N, et al. Performance evaluation of the fully engineered YAP-(S)PET scanner for small animal imaging. IEEE Trans Nucl Sci 2006;53:1078–83.

131. Du Y, Frey E, Wang W, et al. Optimization of acquisition energy windows in simultaneous 99mTc/123I brain SPECT. IEEE Trans Nucl Sci 2003;50: 1556–61.

132. Wang W, Tsui B, Lalush D, et al. Optimization of acquisition parameters for simultaneous 201Tl and 99mTc dual-isotope myocardial imaging. IEEE Trans Nucl Sci 2005;52:1227–35.

133. de Jong HW, Beekman FJ, Viergever MA, et al. Simultaneous (99m)Tc/(201)Tl dual-isotope SPET with Monte Carlo-based down-scatter correction. Eur J Nucl Med Mol Imaging 2002;29:1063–71.

134. Song X, Frey E, Wang W, et al. Validation and evaluation of model based crosstalk compensation method in simultaneous 99mTc stress and 201Tl rest myocardial perfusion SPECT. IEEE Trans Nucl Sci 2004;51:72–9.

135. Ouyang J, El Fakhri G, Moore SC. Fast Monte Carlo based joint iterative reconstruction for simultaneous 99mTc/123I SPECT imaging. Med Phys 2007;34:3263–72.

136. Phelps M, Huang S, Hoffman E, et al. Cerebral extraction of N-13 ammonia: its dependence on cerebral blood flow and capillary permeability—surface area product. Stroke 1981;12:607–19.

137. Schelbert HR, Henze E, Phelps ME, et al. Assessment of regional myocardial ischemia by positron-emission computed tomography. Am Heart J 1982;103.

138. Wu H-M, Yu AS, Lin H-D, et al. The feasibility of performing longitudinal measurements in mice using small animal PET imaging and a microfluidic blood sampling device. IEEE Nucl Sci Symp Conf Rec NSS '07, Honolulu, Hawai, Oct. 26-Nov. 3 2007, 2007;6:4174–5.

139. Tian J, Yang X, Yu L, et al. A multicenter clinical trial on the diagnostic value of dual-tracer PET/CT in pulmonary lesions using 3'-Deoxy-3'-18F-Fluorothymidine and 18F-FDG. J Nucl Med 2008;49: 186–94.

140. Kadrmas DJ, Rust TC. Feasibility of rapid multi-tracer PET tumor imaging. IEEE Trans Nucl Sci 2005;52:1341–7.

141. Rust TC, DiBella EVR, McGann CJ, et al. Rapid dual-injection single-scan 13N-ammonia PET for quantification of rest and stress myocardial blood flows. Phys Med Biol 2006;51:5347–62.

142. Black NF, McJames S, Rust TC, et al. Evaluation of rapid dual-tracer (62)Cu-PTSM + (62)Cu-ATSM PET in dogs with spontaneously occurring tumors. Phys Med Biol 2008;53:217–32.

143. Verhaeghe J, D'Asseler Y, De Winter O, et al. Simultaneous dual tracer NH3/FDG cardiac PET imaging: a simulation study [abstract]. J Nucl Med 2005;46:56P.

144. El Fakhri G, Sitek A, Guérin B. Simultaneous dual tracer PET using generalized factor analysis of dynamic sequences. Proc. IEEE Nuclear Science Symposium and Medical Imaging Conference, San Diego, CA, 2006:2128–30.

145. Park JM, Gambhir SS. Multimodality radionuclide, fluorescence, and bioluminescence small-animal imaging. Proceedings of the IEEE 2005;93: 771–83.

146. Parnham KB, Chowdhury S, Li J, et al. Second-generation, tri-modality pre-clinical imaging system. IEEE Nucl Sci Symp Conf Rec 2006;3:1802–5.

147. Xie S, Ramirez R, Liu Y, et al. A pentagon photo-multiplier-quadrant-sharing BGO detector for a rodent research PET (RRPET). IEEE Trans Nucl Sci 2005;52:210–6.

148. Bergeron M, Cadorette J, Beaudoin JF, et al. Performance evaluation of the LabPET™; APD-based digital PET scanner. IEEE Nucl Sci Symp Conf Rec 2007;6:4185–91.

149. Saoudi A, Lecomte R. A novel APD-based detector module for multi-modality PET/SPECT/CT scanners. IEEE Trans Nucl Sci 1999;46:479–84.

150. Zaidi H, Montandon M-L, Slosman DO. Magnetic resonance imaging-guided attenuation and scatter corrections in three-dimensional brain positron emission tomography. Med Phys 2003; 30:937–48.

151. Zaidi H. Is MRI-guided attenuation correction a viable option for dual-modality PET/MR imaging? Radiology 2007;244:639–42.

152. Hofmann M, Steinke F, Scheel V, et al. MRI-based attenuation correction for PET/MRI: a novel approach combining pattern recognition and Atlas registration. J Nucl Med 2008;49:1875–83.

153. Peter J, Semmler W. A modular design triple-modality SPECT-CT-ODT small animal imager [abstract]. Eur J Nucl Med Mol Imaging 2007;34: S158.

154. Baete K, Nuyts J, Van Paesschen W, et al. Anatomical-based FDG-PET reconstruction for the detection of hypo-metabolic regions in epilepsy. IEEE Trans Med Imaging 2004;23:510–9.

155. Zaidi H, Montandon M-L, Alavi A. Advances in attenuation correction techniques in PET. PET Clinics 2007;2:191–217.

156. Zaidi H, Montandon M-L. Scatter compensation techniques in PET. PET Clinics 2007;2:219–34.

157. Rousset O, Rahmim A, Alavi A, et al. Partial volume correction strategies in PET. PET Clinics 2007;2: 235–49.

158. Convert L, Morin-Brassard G, Cadorette J, et al. A new tool for molecular imaging: the microvolumetric {beta} blood counter. J Nucl Med 2007;48: 1197–206.

159. Wu HM, Sui G, Lee CC, et al. In vivo quantitation of glucose metabolism in mice using small-animal PET and a microfluidic device. J Nucl Med 2007; 48:837–45.

160. Funk T, Sun M, Hasegawa BH. Radiation dose estimate in small animal SPECT and PET. Med Phys 2004;31:2680–6.

161. Taschereau R, Chatziioannou AF. Monte Carlo simulations of absorbed dose in a mouse phantom from 18-fluorine compounds. Med Phys 2007;34:1026–36.

162. Taschereau R, Chow PL, Chatziioannou AF. Monte Carlo simulations of dose from microCT imaging procedures in a realistic mouse phantom. Med Phys 2006;33:216–24.

163. Stabin MG, Peterson TE, Holburn GE, et al. Voxel-based mouse and rat models for internal dose calculations. J Nucl Med 2006;47:655–9.

164. Hindorf C, Ljungberg M, Strand SE. Evaluation of parameters influencing S values in mouse dosimetry. J Nucl Med 2004;45:1960–5.

The Clinical Role of Fusion Imaging Using PET, CT, and MR Imaging

Habib Zaidi, PhD, PD[a],*, Marie-Louise Montandon, PhD[a],
Abass Alavi, MD, PhD (Hon), DSc (Hon)[b]

KEYWORDS
- Multimodality imaging • Image fusion
- PET/CT • PET/MRI • Quantification

Medical imaging has evolved rapidly during the last 2 decades, and we are now observing radical changes in the way medicine is practiced as a logical consequence of this growth. Nowadays, clinical diagnosis is rarely done without imaging, which makes molecular imaging an essential component of the clinical decision-making tree. Contemporary molecular imaging technologies now represent the leading component of any health care institution and have a pivotal role in the daily clinical management of patients.[1]

X-ray projection imaging, ultrasonography, CT, and MR imaging differentiate disease from normal tissue by revealing structural differences or differences in regional perfusion of the administered contrast media. The interpretation of the images can be complicated when normal perfusion patterns are disrupted by prior surgery or radiotherapy, which can lead to tissue damage or necrosis where contrast patterns can mimic those associated with neoplasia. This effect presents a significant challenge when imaging techniques are used to define the anatomic extent of disease, such as for planning highly conformal radiation treatment or highly targeted therapeutic regimens.[2]

In comparison with anatomic imaging techniques, functional imaging methods including planar scintigraphy, single-photon emission computed tomography (SPECT), positron emission tomography (PET), and MR spectroscopy assess regional differences in the biochemical status of tissues. In nuclear medicine, including SPECT and PET, this assessment is done by administering a biologically active molecule or pharmaceutical to the patient which is radiolabeled and accumulated in response to its biochemical attributes. The realization that the information provided by anatomic (CT and MR) and molecular (SPECT and PET) imaging modalities is complementarity spurred the development of various strategies for multimodality image registration and fusion. Correlative or fusion functional-anatomic imaging is now well established and its clinical value widely recognized.

Several investigators proposed and in most cases developed techniques to improve the correlation between the anatomic and physiologic information obtained using these anatomic and functional imaging studies. These methods include software-based image registration in which two or more sets of images from two or more different studies are fused following their separate acquisition on stand-alone imaging systems. Commonly, image registration techniques produce a single "fused" or "combined" image in which the functional SPECT or PET image is displayed in color over a gray-scale CT or MR image of the same anatomic region. Alternatively, hardware-based, dual-modality imaging systems including SPECT/CT, PET/CT, and, in the future, PET/MR imaging, more successfully achieve this

This work was supported by grant SNSF 3100A0-116547 from the Swiss National Foundation.
[a] Division of Nuclear Medicine, Geneva University Hospital, CH-1211 Geneva, Switzerland
[b] Division of Nuclear Medicine, Hospital of the University of Pennsylvania, 3400 Spruce Street, Philadelphia, PA 19104, USA
* Corresponding author.
E-mail address: habib.zaidi@hcuge.ch (H. Zaidi).

PET Clin 3 (2009) 275–291
doi:10.1016/j.cpet.2009.03.002

goal, which underlies their wider clinical acceptance by the medical imaging community.

This article discusses recent advances in clinical multimodality imaging and the role of correlative fusion imaging in the clinical setting. Future opportunities and challenges facing the adoption of multimodality imaging are also addressed.

SOFTWARE-BASED IMAGE REGISTRATION AND FUSION

Software image fusion can be challenging to perform on a routine basis in the clinical setting because it requires exceptional digital communication in medicine (DICOM) connectivity, compatibility between the scanning protocols used by various imaging modalities, and outstanding collaboration between various clinical departments. These challenges may be overcome by the use of combined PET/CT systems described in the following section, although software-based coregistration offers greater flexibility and might in some cases offer some complementary advantages to hardware-based approaches.[3,4]

Achieving a high degree of accuracy for a spatial transformation between image sets can be complicated. Physical factors such as noise, limited spatial resolution, attenuation, scatter, and partial volume effect (PVE) and biologic factors such as persistent activity in the blood pool and nonspecific uptake may decrease the contrast and blur the images; therefore, it can be difficult to locate consistent landmarks. The coregistration problem in the brain is different from the situation in whole-body imaging. Furthermore, diagnostic CT images are usually taken using breath-holding techniques, whereas PET data are acquired during a relatively long time period with the resultant reconstructed image set being an average of all phases of respiration.[5] PET/CT investigations involving imaging of the thorax, abdomen, or pelvis, where organ motion exists, result in inconsistent image sets. This inconsistency can cause complications, for example, if the body boundaries of the CT data and the PET can be registered but the internal structures still differ significantly. Various PET/CT scanning protocols performed for a short period but with a similar breathing pattern have been designed to avoid the breath-holding problem.[6] The CT data acquired allow for both attenuation correction and registration of PET/CT data for accurate localization of metabolic abnormalities. Despite their difficulties, many semi- or fully automated registration methods have been developed and used with various degrees of success in research and clinical settings. An in-depth overview of software-based

registration techniques and algorithms is beyond the scope of this review. For a detailed survey of the algorithms developed so far, the reader is referred to recent comprehensive reviews.[7–10]

Two main strategies have emerged in the literature to perform so-called "rigid registration," such as brain PET-MR imaging registration of images of the same patient. The first strategy is based on the identification of similar structures in both images and subsequent minimization of a "distance measure" between them. The second strategy uses a voxel-per-voxel similarity measure of the full three-dimensional data set as a matching criterion (where *voxel* stands for a *volume element*, ie, a three-dimensional image point). The criterion that drives the registration algorithm is known as the "similarity measure." The most popular similarity measures find their origin in information theoretic approaches. These approaches include minimization of histogram dispersion,[11] maximization of mutual information,[12] or maximization of the correlation ratio.[13] The most widely used criterion is mutual information, an intensity-based similarity measure, and many variants to this approach (eg, normalized mutual information) have subsequently been proposed in the literature. Nonrigid registration approaches are usually required to correlate images of the thorax and abdomen. These approaches are usually combined with linear registration techniques to correct for changes in body configuration, differences in breathing patterns, or internal organ motion and associated displacements. Within the context of the assessment of response to treatment in which intrapatient registration of pre- and post-treatment whole-body PET images may be required to automate the analysis of lesion size and uptake,[14,15] nonrigid registration with position-dependent rigidity approaches have been suggested. These techniques assign a high degree of rigidity to some regions (eg, lesions, brain) that will remain unchanged following the registration process.[16]

HARDWARE-BASED MULTIMODALITY IMAGING
Combined PET/CT Instrumentation

The historical development of multimodality imaging is marked by various significant technical and scientific accomplishments driven by an unprecedented collaboration between multidisciplinary groups of investigators. Even though the introduction of commercial PET/CT units in a clinical setting is a recent feature, the prospective benefits of correlative multimodality imaging have been well established since the early years of medical imaging. Many pioneering radiologic scientists and physicians recognized that the capabilities of a radionuclide imaging system could be improved by adding an external source to allow acquisition of transmission data for anatomic correlation of the emission image.[2] Interestingly, the derived theoretical concepts that were occasionally patented[17,18] never materialized in practice until the late Dr. Bruce Hasegawa and colleagues at the University of California, San Francisco[19,20] pioneered in the 1990s the development of dedicated SPECT/CT. Dr. Hasegawa is the person to credit for the conception and design of the first combined SPECT/CT unit, which now stands as a wonderful tribute to his memory.[21] Later, Dr. Townsend and coworkers at the University of Pittsburgh[22,23] pioneered in 1998 the development of combined PET/CT imaging systems, which have the capability to record both PET emission and x-ray transmission data for correlated functional/structural imaging. More compact and cost-effective designs of dual-modality systems have been explored more recently. One such approach uses a rail-with-sliding-bed design in which a sliding CT bed is placed on a track in the floor and linked to a flexible SPECT camera.[24]

A variety of rail-based, docking, and click-over concepts for correlating functional and anatomic images are also being considered with the goal of offering a more economic approach to multimodality imaging for institutions with limited resources.[25]

Among the many advantages offered by PET/CT is a reduction in the overall scanning time, allowing one to increase patient throughput by approximately 30%[26] owing to the use of fast CT-based attenuation correction when compared with lengthy procedures involving the use of external transmission rod sources. **Fig. 1** illustrates the timeline for various stand-alone PET and combined PET/CT scanning protocols following tracer injection and the typical 1-hour waiting time for ^{18}F-fluorodeoxyglucose (FDG). The patient is prepared for imaging by administering the radiopharmaceutical, typically 370 to 555 MBq (10 to 15 mCi) of ^{18}F-FDG in adults. A pre-injection transmission scan is usually performed on stand-alone PET scanners before tracer injection to reduce spillover of emission data into the transmission energy window, although post-injection transmission scanning

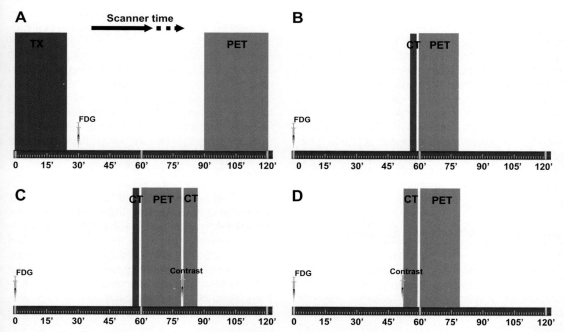

Fig. 1. Timeline for various stand-alone PET and PET/CT scanning protocols following tracer injection and typical 1 hour waiting time for ^{18}F-FDG. (A) The pre-injection transmission scan required on conventional stand-alone PET scanners (approximately 3 minutes per bed position on full-ring systems) is usually acquired before tracer injection. On contemporary combined PET/CT scanners equipped with fast detectors, the acquisition time is practically half the time required on conventional detectors. A low-dose CT for attenuation correction (B) or a study combined with a diagnostic quality contrast-enhanced CT (C) is usually performed depending on the clinical indication. The latter can also be used for attenuation correction but might result in artifacts in some cases by overcorrecting for attenuation in regions containing contrast medium (D). PET/CT allows one to reduce the overall scanning time, thus increasing patient throughput.

protocols have been successfully used in the clinic with the use of contemporary PET scanners.[27] When using combined PET/CT units, the patient is asked to remove all metal objects that could introduce artifacts in the CT scan and is then positioned on the table of the dual-modality imaging system. The patient undergoes an "overview" or "scout" scan during which x-ray projection data are obtained from the patient to identify the axial extent of the CT and PET study. The patient then undergoes a low-dose spiral CT acquisition followed by the PET study starting approximately 1 hour after FDG administration. The CT and PET data are reconstructed and registered, with the CT data used for attenuation correction of the reconstructed PET images. Depending on institutions and agreements between clinical departments and clinical requirements,[28–30] the images might be interpreted in tandem by a radiologist and nuclear medicine physician who can view the CT scan, the PET images, and the fused PET/CT data, followed by preparation of the associated clinical report. Some clinical indications commonly require administration with contrast media to acquire a relatively high-dose diagnostic quality CT scan.[31] The latter scan can be performed either before or following the PET study. In the former case, the contrast-enhanced CT is also used to correct the PET data for photon attenuation, and the low-dose CT scan is no longer needed. Care should be taken to avoid hot-spot artifacts in the attenuation-corrected PET images that might be caused by overcorrection of radiodense oral and intravenous contrast agents. As a rule of thumb, examination of the uncorrected images is recommended to distinguish technical artifacts from physiologic/pathologic hypermetabolism. Alternatively, post-processing correction methods have been proposed in the literature.[32,33]

Combined PET/MR Imaging Instrumentation

The interest in PET scanning within strong magnetic fields was first motivated by the need to reduce the distance positrons travel before annihilation (positron range) through magnetic confinement of the emitted positrons.[34–36] Indeed, Monte Carlo simulation studies predicted improvements in spatial resolution for high-energy positron emitters ranging between 18.5% (2.73 mm instead of 3.35 mm) for ^{68}Ga and 26.8% (2.68 mm instead of 3.66 mm) for ^{82}Rb for a magnetic field strength of 7 T.[36] These improvements are in agreement with the results obtained using another Monte Carlo code in which a 27% improvement in spatial resolution for a PET

scanner incorporating a 10 T magnetic field was reported.[37]

The history of combined PET/MR imaging dates back to the mid-1990s even before the advent of PET/CT.[35,37,38] Early attempts to design MR-compatible PET units relied on slight modification of PET detector blocks of a preclinical PET scanner to keep the photomultiplier tubes (PMTs) at a reasonable distance from the strong magnetic field of a clinical MR imaging unit.[39–43] The detectors were coupled to long optical fibers (4–5 m), leading the weak scintillation light outside the fringe magnetic field to position-sensitive PMTs. Despite the limitations of this design, similar approaches were adopted by other investigators.[44–47] Other related design concepts based on conventional PMT-based PET detectors rely on more complex magnet designs, including a split magnet[48] or field-cycled MR imaging.[49]

Other investigators have developed PET/MR imaging systems configured with suitable solid-state detectors that can be operated within a magnetic field for PET imaging. These systems include avalanche photodiodes (APDs)[50] and Geiger-mode avalanche photodiodes (G-APDs).[51,52] APD-based readout has already been implemented on a commercial preclinical PET system, the LabPET scanner,[53] 10 years after the development of the first prototype based on this technology.[54] Various MR-compatible preclinical PET prototypes have been designed using both APD-based[55–60] and G-APD based[61,62] technologies. Other promising technologies that might be used for the design of future generation PET/MR imaging systems include amorphous selenium avalanche photodetectors, which have an excellent quantum efficiency, a large avalanche gain, and a rapid response time.[63,64]

Most of these systems have been tested within a high field (up to 9.7 T) and have produced PET and MR images that appear to be free of distortion, consolidating the hypothesis that there is no significant interference between the two systems, and that each modality is virtually invisible to the other.

The promising results obtained on preclinical systems have encouraged one of the major industrial players (Siemens Medical Solutions, Knoxville, TN) to develop the first clinical PET/MR imaging prototype (BrainPET), dedicated for simultaneous brain imaging, in collaboration with the University of Tuebingen in Germany.[65] **Fig. 2** illustrates the conceptual design and a photograph of the integrated MR/PET scanner, showing isocentric layering of the MR head coil, PET detector ring, and MR magnet tunnel together with concurrently acquired clinical MR, PET, and fused MR/PET images. The system is being assessed in a clinical setting by

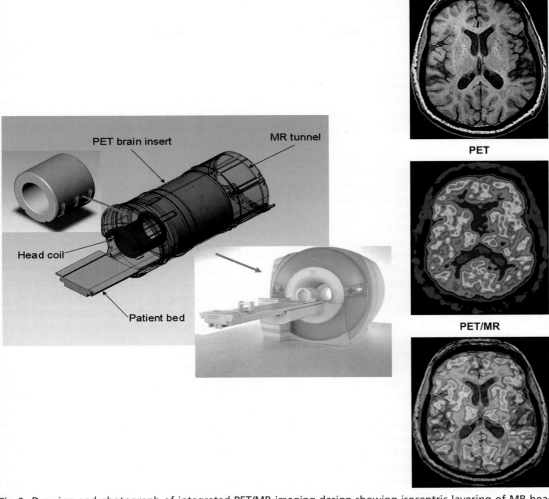

Fig. 2. Drawing and photograph of integrated PET/MR imaging design showing isocentric layering of MR head coil, PET detector ring, and MR magnet tunnel (*left*). Simultaneously acquired MR images, PET, and fused combined PET/MR images of 66-year-old man after intravenous injection of 370 MBq of FDG are shown. Tracer distribution was recorded for 20 minutes at steady state after 120 minutes. (*Adapted from* Schlemmer HP, Pichler BJ, Schmand M, et al. Simultaneous MR/PET imaging of the human brain: feasibility study. Radiology 2008; 248:1030; with permission.)

exploiting the full potential of anatomic MR imaging in terms of high soft-tissue contrast sensitivity in addition to the many other possibilities offered by this modality, including blood oxygenation level dependant (BOLD) imaging, functional MR imaging, diffusion-weighted imaging, perfusion-weighted imaging, and diffusion tensor imaging.[66] The prospective applications of a hypothetical whole-body PET/MR imaging system are being explored in the literature.[67–70] Such a system would allow one to exploit, in addition to the previously discussed applications, the power of MR spectroscopy to measure the regional biochemical content and to assess the metabolic status or the presence of neoplasia and other diseases in specific tissue areas.[71]

CLINICAL ROLE OF CORRELATIVE FUSION IMAGING

The clinical role of correlative imaging encompasses a wide variety of applications. It is now performed routinely with commercially available radiopharmaceuticals to answer important clinical questions in oncology,[72] cardiology,[73] neurology, and psychiatry.[74,75] As discussed previously, much of the early image registration effort was restricted to intrasubject brain applications, where the confinement of compact brain tissues within the skull renders a rigid-body model a satisfactory approximation.[76,77] Correlative fusion imaging techniques were introduced in the clinic, mostly for neuroimaging applications, well before the advent of hardware-based, dual-modality imaging. Multimodality imaging had a pivotal role in the assessment of central nervous system disorders such as seizures, Alzheimer's and Parkinson's disease, head injury, and inoperable brain tumors.[78–80]

Brain SPECT imaging using ^{99m}Tc-labeled perfusion ligands shows a sharp increase during an epileptic seizure (ictal scan) at the position of the epileptogenic focus, whereas most epileptic foci show a diminished perfusion on the interictal scan. By means of ictal/interictal subtraction studies, with subsequent coregistration onto MR imaging (Subtraction *I*ctal SPECT *Co*registered to *MR* imaging [SISCOM]), a predictive value up to 97% for the correct localization of an epileptic focus has been reported,[81] which is higher than any other competing modality. **Fig. 3** shows an example of a ^{99m}Tc-labelled ethylene cysteine dimer (ECD) perfusion SPECT and FDG-PET studies of the same patient coregistered to an anatomic T1-weighted MR imaging study for the evaluation of epilepsy. The two ^{99m}Tc-ECD scans were performed during seizure (ictal) and when the patient was seizure free (interictal) the following day. Both SPECT studies and a three-dimensional, T1-weighted MR imaging study were coregistered using the normalized mutual information criterion, which is similar to mutual information but usually more robust and efficient in finding the correct fitting transform.[82] The differences between the ictal and interictal SPECT studies were overlaid on transaxial slices of the MR imaging study to permit accurate localization of the focus of the epilepsy. A coregistered FDG-PET study superimposed on the MR imaging study is also shown. This type of image registration and fusion technique has been a standard component of many clinical practices for the last 2 decades and is used routinely in the authors' institution. Corresponding techniques for other regions of the body have not achieved the same widespread clinical use.

Another example from the neuro-oncology field shows a patient with a glioblastoma (WHO IV) in the left temporal and frontal areas (**Fig. 4**). A similar registration approach as for **Fig. 3** was used for coregistration of an ^{18}F-fluoro-ethyl-tyrosine (^{18}F-FET) brain PET scan and gadolinium-enhanced, T2-weighted MR imaging. This study showed that PET frequently detected tumors that were not visible on MR imaging. Moreover, substantial differences in terms of gross tumor volume delineation were reported when compared with MR imaging–guided treatment planning.[83]

A plethora of novel tracers are used routinely for assessing tumor metabolism and other biologic and physiologic parameters associated with many diseases.[84,85] These tracers have clearly demonstrated the enormous potential of PET/CT as an emerging modality in the field of molecular imaging. Multiple studies have demonstrated unequivocally the role of PET/CT, especially for oncologic applications.[72,86] Nevertheless, the limited role of PET/CT in some clinical indications, including central nervous system disorders, orthopedic infections, and inflammatory disorders, and in the evaluation and follow-up of metastatic disease has been advocated as a serious concern against the decision of vendors to stop manufacturing less expensive stand-alone PET systems for clinical use, which are more affordable for economically depressed nations.[87,88]

Molecular imaging in its broad definition represents methodologies and probes that allow visualization of events at the cellular and molecular levels.[89] The intended targets for this purpose include cells surface receptors, transporters, intracellular enzymes, or messenger RNA. The source of the signal detected by these techniques could originate directly from the molecule or its surrogates. In both clinical and research studies involving control subjects or volunteers, an accurate estimate of the tracer biodistribution and its pharmacokinetics is frequently a goal to understand the biochemical behavior of the probe and its suitability for the task at hand. This assessment also allows radiation dosimetry estimates to be performed to assess potential radiation risks associated with novel tracers before their administration to patients. **Fig. 5** shows typical biodistributions of ^{18}F-choline and ^{11}C-acetate probes in a subject. The CT scan can be used for attenuation correction of the PET data and for anatomic localization of tracer uptake and organ/tissue volumetric estimation, which is also required for dosimetry calculations. FDG-PET has limited impact in many malignancies presenting with low FDG avidity (eg, prostate cancer, hepatic metastases, and associated lymph nodes), where more specific tracers should be used. **Fig. 6** shows a clinical PET/CT study illustrating the limitations of ^{18}F-FDG for the detection of hepatic metastases and lymph node involvement which are clearly visible on the ^{18}F-FDopa study. In addition, the high sensitivity and specificity of FDG-PET for lymph node involvement and the capacity to better discriminate between

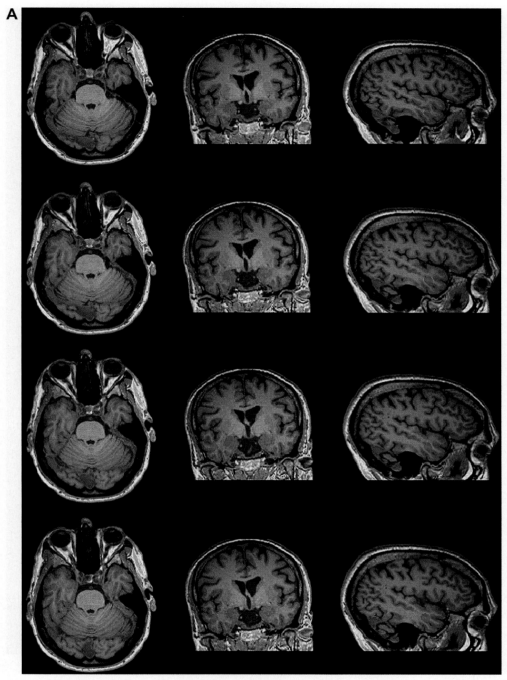

Fig. 3. Representative slices of a patient showing an example of SPECT/PET and MR imaging registration and fusion for the evaluation of epilepsy. Two ^{99m}Tc-ECD scans performed during seizure (ictal) and when the patient was seizure free (interictal) the following day are shown. Both SPECT studies and a three-dimensional, T1-weighted MR imaging study were coregistered using the normalized mutual information criterion. (*A*) The differences between the ictal and interictal SPECT studies are overlaid on transaxial slices of the MR imaging study to permit accurate localization of the focus of the epilepsy. (*B*) A coregistered FDG-PET study superimposed on the MR imaging study is also shown.

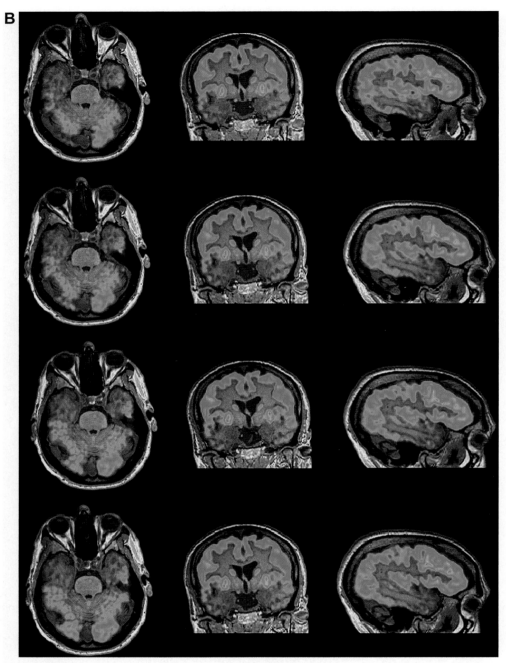

Fig. 3. (*continued*)

tumor extent and atelectasis may substantially alter the delineation of target volumes in radiotherapy.[86,90–94] **Fig. 7** shows an example where PET allowed excluding associated atelectasis that was impossible to differentiate using CT alone.[94]

ADVANCES IN ANATOMICALLY GUIDED QUANTIFICATION OF PET DATA

The primary motivation for multimodality imaging has been image fusion of functional and anatomic data to facilitate anatomic localization of functional

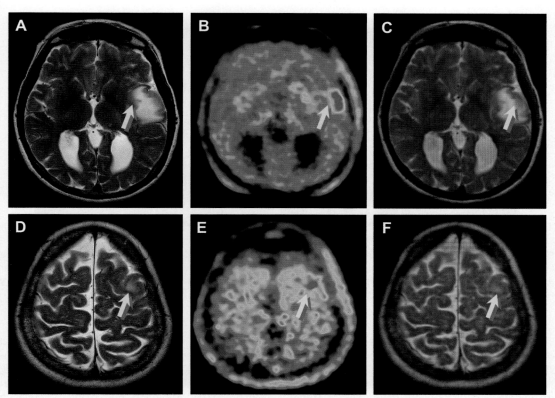

Fig. 4. Example of a patient with a glioblastoma (WHO IV) (*arrows*) in the left temporal and frontal areas. The images shown on the top row (temporal area) correspond to gadolinium-enhanced, T2-weighted MR imaging (*A*), coregistered ^{18}F-FET (*B*), and fused PET/MR imaging (*C*) of the first study. The same images are shown in the bottom row for the frontal area (*D*, *E*, and *F*). The ^{18}F-FET PET study revealed an additional lesion missed on MR imaging. In addition, the T2-weighted MR image and the ^{18}F-FET PET show substantially different gross tumor volume extension for radiotherapy treatment planning.

abnormalities and to assist region-of-interest (ROI) definition for quantitative analysis. The anatomic information also can be useful for many other tasks, including attenuation compensation, transmission-based scatter modeling, motion detection, and correction, introducing a priori anatomic information into reconstruction of the PET emission data and partial volume correction.[95]

Anatomically Guided PET Attenuation and Scatter Compensation

The use of CT-based[96,97] and, more recently, MR imaging–guided[98,99] attenuation compensation has received a great deal of attention in the scientific literature. As discussed earlier, the former has many advantages when compared with conventional transmission-based scanning, which is now considered obsolete following the advent of hybrid systems.[100] Nevertheless, CT-based attenuation correction has many drawbacks that need

to be addressed through research, including polychromaticity of x-ray photons and the beam-hardening effect, misregistration between CT and PET images resulting from respiratory motion, truncation artifacts, the presence of oral and intravenous contrast medium, metallic implants, x-ray scatter in CT images, and other CT artifacts from any source.[97] MR imaging–guided attenuation correction is in its infancy and remains challenging for whole-body imaging.[98,99] This very active research topic will certainly impact the future of hybrid PET/MR imaging technology.

Traditionally, approximate scatter compensation techniques in PET have been applied in which the scatter component is estimated from measurements using additional energy windows placed adjacent to the photopeak window used to acquire the primary PET emission data. The expanding diagnostic and therapeutic applications of quantitative PET imaging have motivated the development of scatter correction techniques, which

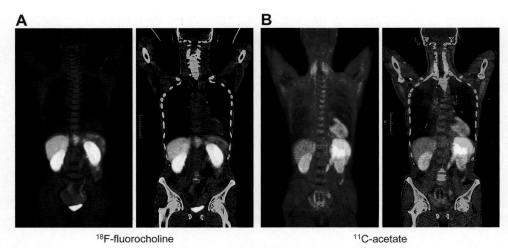

¹⁸F-fluorocholine   ¹¹C-acetate

Fig. 5. Role of PET/CT in novel tracer biodistribution studies showing typical biodistributions for ¹⁸F-fluorocholine (*A*) and ¹¹C-acetate (*B*) in the same subject. The CT scan is used for attenuation correction of the PET data and for anatomic localization of tracer uptake and organ/tissue volumetric estimation which is required for dosimetry calculations.

incorporate patient-specific attenuation maps derived from either transmission scans or CT imaging and the physics of interaction and detection of emitted photons to estimate the scatter magnitude and distribution accurately.[101] Transmission-based scatter correction methods use an attenuation map to define the inhomogeneous properties of the scattering object and derive a distribution of scattered events using line integrals calculated as part of the attenuation correction method. Algorithms belonging to this class of model-based methods have been successfully applied in a clinical setting.[102–105] Although computationally intensive, more refined algorithms that use a patient-specific attenuation map, an estimate of the emission image, and Monte Carlo–based radiation transport calculations to estimate the magnitude and spatial distribution of Compton scattered events that would be detected have also been considered.[106–108]

Anatomically Guided PET Image Reconstruction

An undesirable property of the statistical iterative reconstruction techniques including the popular maximum likelihood–expectation maximization (ML-EM) algorithm is that large numbers of iterations increase the noise content of the reconstructed PET images.[109] The noise characteristics can be controlled by incorporating a prior distribution to describe the statistical properties of the unknown image and thus produce a posteriori probability distributions from the image conditioned upon the data. Bayesian reconstruction methods form a powerful extension of the ML-EM algorithm. Maximization of the a posteriori (MAP) probability over the set of possible images results in the MAP estimate.[110] This approach has many advantages because the various components of the prior, such as the pseudo-Poisson nature of statistics, nonnegativity of the solution, local voxel correlations (local smoothness), or known existence of anatomic boundaries, may be added one by one into the estimation process, assessed individually, and used to guarantee a fast working implementation of preliminary versions of the algorithms. A Bayesian model also can incorporate prior anatomic information derived from a registered CT[111] or MR[112,113] image in the reconstruction of PET data with the aim of avoiding resolution loss due to the regularization, exploiting the superior resolution of the anatomic images.

This class of algorithms incorporates a coupling term in the reconstruction procedure that favors the formation of edges in the PET data that are associated with the location of noteworthy anatomic edges from the anatomic images. A Gibbs prior distribution is usually used to encourage the piece-wise smoothness of reconstructed PET images. A Gibbs prior of piece-wise smoothness can also be incorporated in the bayesian model. Some groups have published preliminary promising results with segmentation-free anatomic priors based on measures similar to mutual information, but further investigation is required. In this way, the development of dual-modality imaging systems producing accurately

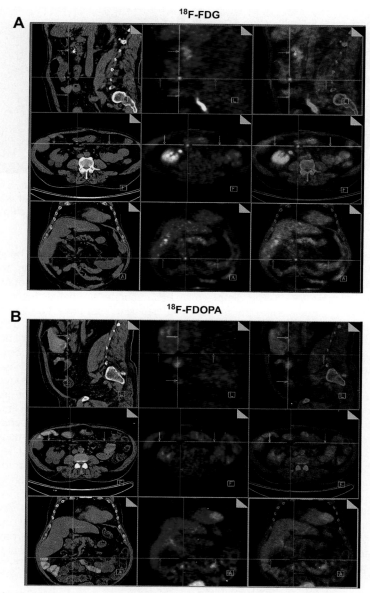

Fig. 6. Illustration of a clinical PET/CT study showing the limitations of ^{18}F-FDG for the detection of hepatic metastases and lymph node involvement, which are clearly visible on the ^{18}F-FDopa study.

registered anatomic and functional image data[23,114] is motivating the further investigation of the potential of bayesian MAP reconstruction techniques.

Anatomically Guided Partial Volume Correction in PET

The quantitative accuracy of PET is hampered by the low spatial resolution capability of currently available clinical scanners. The well-accepted criterion is that one can accurately quantify the activity concentration for sources having dimensions equal to or larger than twice the system's spatial resolution measured in terms of its full-width-at-half-maximum (FWHM). Sources of smaller size only partly occupy this characteristic volume, and, as such, the counts are spread over a larger volume than the physical size of the object owing to the limited spatial resolution of the imaging system. The total number of counts is conserved in the corresponding PET images. In this case, the resulting PET images reflect the total amount of the activity within the object but

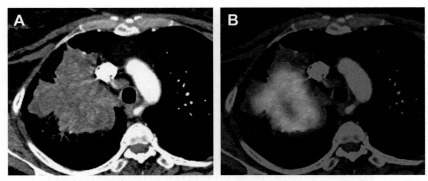

Fig. 7. Transaxial CT (*left*) and FDG-PET (*right*) images of a clinical PET/CT study of a patient with non-small cell lung cancer of the right upper lobe. PET/CT allowed excluding associated atelectasis that was impossible using a diagnostic quality CT alone, modifying the gross tumor volume delineated for radiotherapy treatment planning.

not the actual activity concentration. This phenomenon is referred to as the PVE and can be corrected using one of the various strategies developed for this purpose.[115,116] The simplest technique uses recovery coefficients determined in a calibration measurement for objects of simple geometric shape.[117] This technique works relatively well for objects that can be approximated by simple geometric shapes (eg, tumors of spherical shape).[118] More sophisticated anatomy-based, post-reconstruction approaches have also been developed to correct for this effect knowing the size and shape of corresponding structures as assessed by structural imaging (MR imaging or CT).[119,120]

Fig. 8 shows the principle of the MR imaging–guided partial volume correction approach in functional brain PET imaging. The procedure used follows the approach described by Matsuda and colleagues,[121] which involves realigning the PET and MR image volumes followed by segmenting the MR image into white and gray matter using the statistical parametric mapping (SPM5)

segmentation toolbox.[122] The next step of this correction method consists in convolving the segmented white and gray matter images by the PET scanner's spatial resolution modeled by a gaussian response function. The gray matter PET image is then obtained by subtraction of the convolved PET white matter image from the original PET image. The PVE corrected gray matter PET image is then obtained by dividing the gray matter PET image by the convolved gray matter MR image. A binary mask for gray matter is finally applied. The accuracy of MR imaging–guided PVE correction in PET largely depends on the accuracy achieved by the PET–MR imaging coregistration procedure and MR imaging segmentation algorithm. The impact of image misregistration and segmentation errors has been assessed by some investigators.[119,123–127]

More recent techniques using multi-resolution synergetic approaches that combine functional and anatomic information from various sources appear promising and should be investigated further in a clinical setting.[128] The corrections for

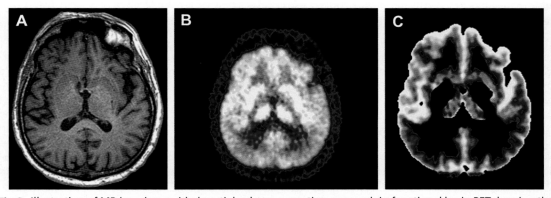

Fig. 8. Illustration of MR imaging–guided partial volume correction approach in functional brain PET showing the original T1-weighted MR image (*A*) and PET image before (*B*) and after (*C*) voxel-by-voxel PVE correction.

the PVE can also be applied during the reconstruction process by incorporating a mathematical model for PVE along with other physical perturbations (photon attenuation, scattered radiation, and other physical effects) directly into the reconstruction algorithm.[129]

SUMMARY AND FUTURE PROSPECTS

This article has attempted to summarize important themes of ongoing advancements by providing an overview of current state-of-the art developments in software- and hardware-based multimodality imaging combining PET with other structural imaging modalities (PET/CT and PET/MR imaging). Clearly, multimodality imaging has changed drastically over the last 2 decades. The pace of change has accelerated rapidly in the last decade driven by the introduction and widespread acceptance of combined PET/CT units in the clinic and the likely deployment of compact PET/MR imaging systems in the near future. Navigating beyond the sixth dimension is now becoming possible with recent progress in multidimensional and multiparametric multimodality imaging combining the latest advances in sophisticated software to make use of existing advanced hardware.[130] A controversy arose recently regarding the future role of SPECT in the era of PET.[131–134] Time will determine whether these predictions are wrong or will come true. Given that the role of any molecular imaging technology is established with respect to the benefits conveyed to patients, dual-modality imaging systems using PET as the key component are here to stay and will definitely maintain an exclusive standing in clinical diagnosis, the assessment of response to treatment, and the delivery of personalized treatments and targeted therapies.

ACKNOWLEDGEMENTS

The authors would like to thank Dr. C. Steiner for providing some of the clinical illustrations used in this manuscript.

REFERENCES

1. Webb S. Combating cancer in the third millennium: the contribution of medical physics. Phys Med 2008;24:42–8.
2. Hasegawa B, Zaidi H. Dual-modality imaging: more than the sum of its components. In: Zaidi H, editor. Quantitative analysis in nuclear medicine imaging. New York: Springer; 2006. p. 35–81.
3. Pietrzyk U. Does PET/CT render software fusion obsolete? Nuklearmedizin 2005;44:S13–7.
4. Weigert M, Pietrzyk U, Muller S, et al. Whole-body PET/CT imaging: combining software- and hardware-based co-registration. Z Med Phys 2008; 18:59–66.
5. Nehmeh SA, Erdi YE. Respiratory motion in positron emission tomography/computed tomography: a review. Semin Nucl Med 2008;38:167–76.
6. Slomka PJ, Dey D, Przetak C, et al. Automated 3-dimensional registration of stand-alone (18)F-FDG whole-body PET with CT. J Nucl Med 2003; 44:1156–67.
7. Hill DL, Batchelor PG, Holden M, et al. Medical image registration. Phys Med Biol 2001;46:R1–45.
8. Hutton BF, Braun M. Software for image registration: algorithms, accuracy, efficacy. Semin Nucl Med 2003;33:180–92.
9. Maes F, Vandermeulen D, Suetens P. Medical image registration using mutual information. Proceedings of the IEEE 2003;91:1699–722.
10. Slomka PJ. Software approach to merging molecular with anatomic information. J Nucl Med 2004; 45(Suppl 1):36S–45S.
11. Hill DLG, Studholme C, Hawkes DJ. Voxel similarity measures for automated image registration. In: Robb R, editor, Visualization in biomedical computing, vol 2359. Bellingham (DC): SPIE Press; 1994. p. 205–16.
12. Maes F, Collignon A, Vandermeulen D, et al. Multimodality image registration by maximization of mutual information. IEEE Trans Med Imaging 1997;16:187–98.
13. Lau YH, Braun M, Hutton BF. Non-rigid image registration using a median-filtered coarse-to-fine displacement field and a symmetric correlation ratio. Phys Med Biol 2001;46:1297–319.
14. Juweid ME, Cheson BD. Positron-emission tomography and assessment of cancer therapy. N Engl J Med 2006;354:496–507.
15. Weber WA, Figlin R. Monitoring cancer treatment with PET/CT: does it make a difference? J Nucl Med 2007;48:36S–44.
16. De Moor K, Nuyts J, Plessers L, et al. Non-rigid registration with position dependent rigidity for whole body PET follow-up studies. Proceedings of the Nuclear Science Symposium and Medical Imaging Conference. San Diego, CA; 2006. p. 3502–6.
17. Mirshanov DM. Transmission-emission computer tomograph. USSR Patent No. 621.386:616–073 20.01.87-SU-181935, 1987.
18. Kaplan CH. Transmission/emission registered image (TERI) computed tomography scanners. International Patent No. PCT/US90/03722, 1989.
19. Hasegawa BH, Gingold EL, Reilly SM, et al. Description of a simultaneous emission-transmission CT system. Proc Soc Photo Instrum Eng 1990;1231:50–60.
20. Hasegawa BH, Iwata K, Wong KH, et al. Dual-modality imaging of function and physiology. Acad Radiol 2002;9:1305–21.

21. Jones EF, Gould RG, VanBrocklin HF. Bruce H. Hasegawa, PhD, 1951–2008. J Nucl Med 2008;49:37N–8N.

22. Beyer T, Townsend D, Brun T, et al. A combined PET/CT scanner for clinical oncology. J Nucl Med 2000;41:1369–79.

23. Townsend DW. Multimodality imaging of structure and function. Phys Med Biol 2008;53:R1–39.

24. Bailey D, Roach P, Bailey E, et al. Development of a cost-effective modular SPECT/CT scanner. Eur J Nucl Med Mol Imaging 2007;34:1415–26.

25. Beekman F, Hutton B. Multi-modality imaging on track. Eur J Nucl Med Mol Imaging 2007;34:1410–4.

26. Steinert HC, von Schulthess GK. Initial clinical experience using a new integrated in-line PET/CT system. Br J Radiol 2002;73:S36–8.

27. Luk WR, Digby WD, Jones WF, et al. An analysis of correction methods for emission contamination in PET postinjection transmission measurement. IEEE Trans Nucl Sci 1995;42:2303–8.

28. Coleman RE, Delbeke D, Guiberteau MJ, et al. Concurrent PET/CT with an integrated imaging system: intersociety dialogue from the joint working group of the American College of Radiology, the Society of Nuclear Medicine, and the Society of Computed Body Tomography and Magnetic Resonance. J Nucl Med 2005;46:1225–39.

29. Bischof Delaloye A, Carrio I, Cuocolo A, et al. White paper of the European Association of Nuclear Medicine (EANM) and the European Society of Radiology (ESR) on multimodality imaging. Eur J Nucl Med Mol Imaging 2007;34:1147–51.

30. Stegger L, Schäfers M, Weckesser M, et al. EANM-ESR white paper on multimodality imaging. Eur J Nucl Med Mol Imaging 2008;35:677–80.

31. Antoch G, Freudenberg LS, Beyer T, et al. To enhance or not to enhance? 18F-FDG and CT contrast agents in dual-modality 18F-FDG PET/CT. J Nucl Med 2004;45(Suppl 1):56S–65S.

32. Mawlawi O, Erasmus JJ, Munden RF, et al. Quantifying the effect of IV contrast media on integrated PET/CT: clinical evaluation. AJR Am J Roentgenol 2006;186:308–19.

33. Ahmadian A, Ay MR, Bidgoli JH, et al. Correction of oral contrast artifacts in CT-based attenuation correction of PET images using an automated segmentation algorithm. Eur J Nucl Med Mol Imaging 2008;35:1812–23.

34. Rickey D, Gordon R, Huda W. On lifting the inherent limitations of positron emission tomography by using magnetic fields (MagPET). Automedica 1992;14:355–69.

35. Hammer BE, Christensen NL, Heil BG. Use of a magnetic field to increase the spatial resolution of positron emission tomography. Med Phys 1994;21:1917–20.

36. Wirrwar A, Vosberg H, Herzog H, et al. Muller-Gartner H-W 4.5 Tesla magnetic field reduces range of high-energy positrons: potential implications for positron emission tomography. IEEE Trans Nucl Sci 1997;44:184–9.

37. Raylman RR, Hammer BE, Christensen NL. Combined MRI-PET scanner: a Monte-Carlo evaluation of the improvements in PET resolution due to the effects of a static homogeneous magnetic field. IEEE Trans Nucl Sci 1996;43:2406–12.

38. Christensen NL, Hammer BE, Heil BG, et al. Positron emission tomography within a magnetic field using photomultiplier tubes and light guides. Phys Med Biol 1995;40:691–7.

39. Shao Y, Cherry SR, Farahani K, et al. Simultaneous PET and MR imaging. Phys Med Biol 1997;42:1965–70.

40. Shao Y, Cherry SR, Farahani K, et al. Development of a PET detector system compatible with MRI/NMR systems. IEEE Trans Nucl Sci 1997;44:1167–71.

41. Slates R, Cherry SR, Boutefnouchet A, et al. Design of a small animal MR compatible PET scanner. IEEE Trans Nucl Sci 1999;46:565–70.

42. Slates R, Farahani K, Shao Y, et al. A study of artifacts in simultaneous PET and MR imaging using a prototype MR compatible PET scanner. Phys Med Biol 1999;44:2015–27.

43. Marsden PK, Strul D, Keevil SF, et al. Simultaneous PET and NMR. Br J Radiol 2002;75:S53–9.

44. Mackewn JE, Strul D, Hallett WA, et al. Design and development of an MR-compatible PET scanner for imaging small animals. IEEE Trans Nucl Sci 2005;52:1376–80.

45. Yamamoto S, Takamatsu S, Murayama H, et al. A block detector for a multislice, depth-of-interaction MR-compatible PET. IEEE Trans Nucl Sci 2005;52:33–7.

46. Raylman RR, Majewski S, Lemieux SK, et al. Simultaneous MRI and PET imaging of a rat brain. Phys Med Biol 2006;51:6371–9.

47. Raylman RR, Majewski S, Velan SS, et al. Simultaneous acquisition of magnetic resonance spectroscopy (MRS) data and positron emission tomography (PET) images with a prototype MR-compatible, small animal PET imager. J Magn Reson 2007;186:305–10.

48. Lucas AJ, Hawkes RC, Ansorge RE, et al. Development of a combined micro-PET-MR system. Technol Cancer Res Treat 2006;5:337–41.

49. Handler WB, Gilbert KM, Peng H, et al. Simulation of scattering and attenuation of 511 keV photons in a combined PET/field-cycled MRI system. Phys Med Biol 2006;51:2479–91.

50. Renker D. Properties of avalanche photodiodes for applications in high energy physics, astrophysics and medical imaging. Nucl Instr Meth A 2002;486:164–9.

51. Renker D. Geiger-mode avalanche photodiodes, history, properties and problems. Nucl Instr Meth A 2006;567:48–56.

52. Llosa G, Battiston R, Belcari N, et al. Novel silicon photomultipliers for PET applications. IEEE Trans Nucl Sci 2008;55:877–81.

53. Pepin CM, St-Pierre C, Forgues J-C, et al. Physical characterization of the LabPET, LGSO, and LYSO scintillators. Nuclear Science Symposium Conference Record 2007;3:2292–5.

54. Lecomte R, Cadorette J, Rodrigue S, et al. Initial results from the Sherbrooke avalanche photodiode positron tomograph. IEEE Trans Nucl Sci 1996;43:1952–7.

55. Pichler BJ, Judenhofer MS, Catana C, et al. Performance test of an LSO-APD detector in a 7-T MRI scanner for simultaneous PET/MRI. J Nucl Med 2006;47:639–47.

56. Catana C, Wu Y, Judenhofer MS, et al. Simultaneous acquisition of multislice PET and MR images: initial results with a MR-compatible PET scanner. J Nucl Med 2006;47:1968–76.

57. Catana C, Procissi D, Wu Y, et al. Simultaneous in vivo positron emission tomography and magnetic resonance imaging. Proc Natl Acad Sci U S A 2008;105:3705–10.

58. Woody C, Schlyer D, Vaska P, et al. Preliminary studies of a simultaneous PET/MRI scanner based on the RatCAP small animal tomograph. Nucl Instr Meth A 2007;571:102–5.

59. Judenhofer MS, Catana C, Swann BK, et al. Simultaneous PET/MR images, acquired with a compact MRI compatible PET detector in a 7 Tesla magnet. Radiology 2007;244:807–14.

60. Judenhofer MS, Wehrl HF, Newport DF, et al. Simultaneous PET-MRI: a new approach for functional and morphological imaging. Nat Med 2008;14:459–65.

61. Moehrs S, Del Guerra A, Herbert DJ, et al. A detector head design for small-animal PET with silicon photomultipliers (SiPM). Phys Med Biol 2006;51:1113–27.

62. Hong SJ, Song IC, Ito M, et al. An investigation into the use of Geiger-mode solid-state photomultipliers for simultaneous PET and MRI acquisition. IEEE Trans Nucl Sci 2008;55:882–8.

63. Reznik A, Lui BJ, Rowlands JA. An amorphous selenium based positron emission mammography camera with avalanche gain. Technol Cancer Res Treat 2005;4:61–7.

64. Reznik A, Baranovskii SD, Rubel O, et al. Avalanche multiplication in amorphous selenium and its utilization in imaging. Journal of Non-Crystalline Solids 2008;354:2691–6.

65. Schlemmer HP, Pichler BJ, Schmand M, et al. Simultaneous MR/PET imaging of the human brain: feasibility study. Radiology 2008;248:1028–35.

66. Holdsworth SJ, Bammer R. Magnetic resonance imaging techniques: fMRI, DWI, and PWI. Semin Neurol 2008;28:395–406.

67. Gaa J, Rummeny EJ, Seemann MD. Whole-body imaging with PET/MRI. Eur J Med Res 2004;30:309–12.

68. Seemann MD. Whole-body PET/MRI: the future in oncological imaging. Technol Cancer Res Treat 2005;4:577–82.

69. Schlemmer HP, Pichler BJ, Krieg R, et al. An integrated MR/PET system: prospective applications. Abdom Imaging, in press.

70. Hicks RJ, Lau EW. PET/MRI: a different spin from under the rim. Eur J Nucl Med Mol Imaging 2009;36:10–4.

71. Payne GS, Leach MO. Applications of magnetic resonance spectroscopy in radiotherapy treatment planning. Br J Radiol 2006;79:S16–26 (Spec No 1).

72. Czernin J, Allen-Auerbach M, Schelbert HR. Improvements in cancer staging with PET/CT: literature-based evidence as of September 2006. J Nucl Med 2007;48:78S–88S.

73. Di Carli MF, Dorbala S, Meserve J, et al. Clinical myocardial perfusion PET/CT. J Nucl Med 2007;48:783–93.

74. Costa DC, Pilowsky LS, Ell PJ. Nuclear medicine in neurology and psychiatry. Lancet 1999;354:1107–11.

75. Tatsch K, Ell PJ. PET and SPECT in common neuropsychiatric disease. Clin Med 2006;6:259–62.

76. Pelizzari CA, Chen GT, Spelbring DR, et al. Accurate three-dimensional registration of CT, PET, and/or MR images of the brain. J Comput Assist Tomogr 1989;13:20–6.

77. Woods RP, Mazziotta JC, Cherry SR. MRI-PET registration with automated algorithm. J Comput Assist Tomogr 1993;17:536–46.

78. Gilman S. Imaging the brain. N Engl J Med 1998;338:812–20.

79. Viergever MA, Maintz JB, Niessen WJ, et al. Registration, segmentation, and visualization of multimodal brain images. Comput Med Imaging Graph 2001;25:147–51.

80. Muzik O, Chugani DC, Zou G, et al. Multimodality data integration in epilepsy. Int J Biomed Imaging 2007;2007:13963.

81. O'Brien TJ, Miles K, Ware R, et al. The cost-effective use of 18F-FDG PET in the presurgical evaluation of medically refractory focal epilepsy. J Nucl Med 2008;49:931–7.

82. Studholme C, Hill DLG, Hawkes DJ. An overlap invariant entropy measure of 3D medical image alignment. Pattern Recognit 1999;32:71–86.

83. Vees H, Senthamizhchelvan S, Miralbell R, et al. Assessment of various strategies for 18F-FET PET-guided delineation of target volumes in high-grade glioma patients. Eur J Nucl Med Mol Imaging 2009;36:182–93.

84. Antoni G, Langstrom B. Radiopharmaceuticals: molecular imaging using positron emission tomography. Handb Exp Pharmacol 2008;185:177–201.

85. Kumar R, Dhanpathi H, Basu S, et al. Oncologic PET tracers beyond [(18)F]FDG and the novel quantitative approaches in PET imaging. Q J Nucl Med Mol Imaging 2008;52:50–65.

86. Lardinois D, Weder W, Hany TF, et al. Staging of non-small-cell lung cancer with integrated positron-emission tomography and computed tomography. N Engl J Med 2003;348:2500–7.

87. Zaidi H. The quest for the ideal anato-molecular imaging fusion tool. Biomed Imaging Interv J 2006;2:e47.

88. Alavi A, Mavi A, Basu S, et al. Is PET-CT the only option? Eur J Nucl Med Mol Imaging 2007;34:819–21.

89. Weissleder R, Mahmood U. Molecular imaging. Radiology 2001;219:316–33.

90. De Ruysscher D, Wanders S, Minken A, et al. Effects of radiotherapy planning with a dedicated combined PET-CT-simulator of patients with non-small cell lung cancer on dose limiting normal tissues and radiation dose-escalation: a planning study. Radiother Oncol 2005;77:5–10.

91. Nestle U, Walter K, Schmidt S, et al. 18F-deoxyglucose positron emission tomography (FDG-PET) for the planning of radiotherapy in lung cancer: high impact in patients with atelectasis. Int J Radiat Oncol Biol Phys 1999;44:593–7.

92. Messa C, Ceresoli GL, Rizzo G, et al. Feasibility of [18F]FDG-PET and coregistered CT on clinical target volume definition of advanced non-small cell lung cancer. Q J Nucl Med Mol Imaging 2005;49:259–66.

93. Luketich JD, Friedman DM, Meltzer CC, et al. The role of positron emission tomography in evaluating mediastinal lymph node metastases in non-small-cell lung cancer. Clin Lung Cancer 2001;2:229–33.

94. Zaidi H, Vees H, Wissmeyer M. Molecular PET/CT imaging-guided radiation therapy treatment planning. Acad Radiol 2009, in press.

95. Basu S, Zaidi H, Houseni M, et al. Novel quantitative techniques for assessing regional and global function and structure based on modern imaging modalities: implications for normal variation, aging and diseased states. Semin Nucl Med 2007;37:223–39.

96. Kinahan PE, Hasegawa BH, Beyer T. X-ray–based attenuation correction for positron emission tomography/computed tomography scanners. Semin Nucl Med 2003;33:166–79.

97. Zaidi H, Montandon M-L, Alavi A. Advances in attenuation correction techniques in PET. PET Clinics 2007;2:191–217.

98. Zaidi H. Is MRI-guided attenuation correction a viable option for dual-modality PET/MR imaging? Radiology 2007;244:639–42.

99. Hofmann M, Pichler B, Scholkopf B, et al. Towards quantitative PET/MRI: a review of MR-based attenuation correction techniques. Eur J Nucl Med Mol Imaging 2009;36:93–104.

100. Zaidi H. Is radionuclide transmission scanning obsolete for dual-modality PET/CT systems? Eur J Nucl Med Mol Imaging 2007;34:815–8.

101. Zaidi H, Montandon M-L. Scatter compensation techniques in PET. PET Clinics 2007;2:219–34.

102. Watson CC. New, faster, image-based scatter correction for 3D PET. IEEE Trans Nucl Sci 2000;47:1587–94.

103. Watson CC, Casey ME, Michel C, et al. Advances in scatter correction for 3D PET/CT. Nuclear Science Symposium Conference Record, 19-22 October 2004, Rome, Italy 5:3008–12.

104. Wollenweber SD. Parameterization of a model-based 3-D PET scatter correction. IEEE Trans Nucl Sci 2002;49:722–7.

105. Accorsi R, Adam L-E, Werner ME, et al. Optimization of a fully 3D single scatter simulation algorithm for 3D PET. Phys Med Biol 2004;49:2577–98.

106. Levin CS, Dahlbom M, Hoffman EJ. A Monte Carlo correction for the effect of Compton scattering in 3-D PET brain imaging. IEEE Trans Nucl Sci 1995;42:1181–8.

107. Zaidi H. Comparative evaluation of scatter correction techniques in 3D positron emission tomography. Eur J Nucl Med 2000;27:1813–26.

108. Holdsworth CH, Levin CS, Janecek M, et al. Performance analysis of an improved 3-D PET Monte Carlo simulation and scatter correction. IEEE Trans Nucl Sci 2002;49:83–9.

109. Reader AJ, Zaidi H. Advances in PET image reconstruction. PET Clinics 2007;2:173–90.

110. Green PJ. Bayesian reconstructions from emission tomography data using a modified EM algorithm. IEEE Trans Med Imaging 1990;9:84–93.

111. Comtat C, Kinahan PE, Fessler JA, et al. Clinically feasible reconstruction of 3D whole-body PET/CT data using blurred anatomical labels. Phys Med Biol 2002;47:1–20.

112. Gindi G, Lee M, Rangarajan A, et al. Bayesian reconstruction of functional images using anatomical information as priors. IEEE Trans Med Imaging 1993;12:670–80.

113. Baete K, Nuyts J, Van Paesschen W, et al. Anatomical-based FDG-PET reconstruction for the detection of hypo-metabolic regions in epilepsy. IEEE Trans Med Imaging 2004;23:510–9.

114. Pichler BJ, Wehrl HF, Kolb A, et al. Positron emission tomography/magnetic resonance imaging: the next generation of multimodality imaging? Semin Nucl Med 2008;38:199–208.

115. Rousset O, Rahmim A, Alavi A, et al. Partial volume correction strategies in PET. PET Clinics 2007;2:235–49.

116. Soret M, Bacharach SL, Buvat I. Partial-volume effect in PET tumor imaging. J Nucl Med 2007;48:932–45.

117. Kessler RM, Ellis JR, Eden M. Analysis of emission tomographic scan data: limitations imposed by resolution and background. J Comput Assist Tomogr 1984;8:514–22.

118. Geworski L, Knoop BO, de Cabrejas ML, et al. Recovery correction for quantitation in emission tomography: a feasibility study. Eur J Nucl Med 2000;27:161–9.

119. Quarantelli M, Berkouk K, Prinster A, et al. Integrated software for the analysis of brain PET/SPECT studies with partial-volume-effect correction. J Nucl Med 2004;45:192–201.

120. Da Silva AJ, Tang HR, Wong KH, et al. Absolute quantification of regional myocardial uptake of 99mTc-sestamibi with SPECT: experimental validation in a porcine model. J Nucl Med 2001;42:772–9.

121. Matsuda H, Ohnishi T, Asada T, et al. Correction for partial-volume effects on brain perfusion SPECT in healthy men. J Nucl Med 2003;44:1243–52.

122. Ashburner J, Friston KJ. Unified segmentation. Neuroimage 2005;26:839–51.

123. Rousset OG, Collins DL, Rahmim A, et al. Design and implementation of an automated partial volume correction in PET: application to dopamine receptor quantification in the normal human striatum. J Nucl Med 2008;49:1097–106.

124. Meltzer CC, Kinahan PE, Greer PJ, et al. Comparative evaluation of MR-based partial-volume correction schemes for PET. J Nucl Med 1999;40:2053–65.

125. Frouin V, Comtat C, Reilhac A, et al. Correction of partial volume effect for PET striatal imaging: fast implementation and study of robustness. J Nucl Med 2002;43:1715–26.

126. Zaidi H, Ruest T, Schoenahl F, et al. Comparative evaluation of statistical brain MR image segmentation algorithms and their impact on partial volume effect correction in PET. Neuroimage 2006;32:1591–607.

127. Rousset O, Zaidi H. Correction of partial volume effects in emission tomography. In: Zaidi H, editor. Quantitative analysis of nuclear medicine images. New York: Springer; 2006. p. 236–71.

128. Shidahara M, Tsoumpas C, Hammers A, et al. Functional and structural synergy for resolution recovery and partial volume correction in brain PET. Neuroimage 2009;44:340–8.

129. Baete K, Nuyts J, Laere KV, et al. Evaluation of anatomy based reconstruction for partial volume correction in brain FDG-PET. Neuroimage 2004;23:305–17.

130. Zaidi H. Navigating beyond the 6th dimension: a challenge in the era of multi-parametric molecular imaging. Eur J Nucl Med Mol Imaging, in press.

131. Rahmim A, Zaidi H. PET versus SPECT: strengths, limitations and challenges. Nucl Med Commun 2008;29:193–207.

132. Alavi A, Basu S. Planar and SPECT imaging in the era of PET and PET–CT: can it survive the test of time? Eur J Nucl Med Mol Imaging 2008;35:1554–9.

133. Mariani G, Bruselli L, Duatti A. Is PET always an advantage versus planar and SPECT imaging? Eur J Nucl Med Mol Imaging 2008;35:1560–5.

134. Seret A. Will high-resolution/high-sensitivity SPECT ensure that PET is not the only survivor in nuclear medicine during the next decade? Eur J Nucl Med Mol Imaging 2009;36:533–5.

PET and MR Imaging of Brain Tumors

Michael F. Goldberg, MD, MPH*, Sanjeev Chawla, PhD,
Abass Alavi, MD, PhD (Hon), DSc (Hon), Drew A. Torigian, MD, MA,
Elias R. Melhem, MD, PhD

KEYWORDS

- Brain tumor • Neoplasm
- Positron emission tomography
- Single photon emission computed tomography
- Computed tomography
- Magnetic resonance imaging • PET/CT • PET/MR Imaging

Intracranial brain neoplasms can be classified as primary or secondary. The basic classification of primary brain neoplasms by the World Health Organization (WHO) relies on their cellular origin.[1] The incidence of primary brain neoplasms varies between subtypes, with the most common primary brain neoplasms in adults being gliomas and meningiomas.

Gliomas are classified into astrocytomas, oligodendrogliomas, mixed oligoastrocytomas, ependymal tumors, and tumors of the choroid plexus, based on histologic features. Malignancy or grade is generally assessed according to the WHO criteria, taking into account the presence of nuclear changes, mitotic activity, endothelial proliferation, and necrosis.[2,3] The most fatal and common primary brain neoplasm is the glioblastoma multiforme (GBM), which corresponds to WHO grade IV. Despite aggressive multimodal treatment regimens of conventional therapies (surgery, radiation, and chemotherapy), the disease invariably leads to death over months or years. A complex series of molecular events occur during tumor growth, resulting in dysregulation of the cell cycle, alterations in apoptosis and cell differentiation, neovascularization, and tumor-cell migration and invasion into the normal brain parenchyma. Genetic alterations also play an important role in the development of glioma, including a loss, mutation, or hypermethylation of a tumor suppressor gene, such as PTEN or p53, or other genes involved in the regulation of the cell cycle. During progression from low-grade to high-grade, stepwise accumulation of genetic alterations occurs. Growth of certain tumors seems to be related to the presence of viruses and familial diseases that accelerate the progression of molecular alterations, or to exposure to environmental chemicals, pesticides, herbicides, and fertilizers.[4,5] A better understanding of tumorigenesis is crucial for the development of specific molecular therapies that specifically target the neoplasm and reduce patient morbidity and mortality.

Positron emission tomography (PET) measures a wide range of physiologic processes critical for understanding the pathophysiology of brain neoplasms with high sensitivity. Different radiotracers have been used with PET to help in the diagnosis and management of patients with brain neoplasms.[6,7] These tracers may be classified into three groups: the markers of energetic metabolic pathways, the markers of protein and nucleic acid synthetic pathways, and the radioligands for receptor imaging.[8–10] Depending on the radiotracer, various molecular processes can be visualized and quantified by PET, most of them relating to an increased cell proliferation within gliomas.

Radiolabeled 2-[18F]-fluoro-2-deoxy-D-glucose (FDG), methyl-[11C]-L-methionine (MET), and

Department of Radiology, Hospital of the University of Pennsylvania, 3400 Spruce Street, Philadelphia, PA 19104, USA
* Corresponding author.
E-mail address: Michael.Goldberg@uphs.upenn.edu (M.F. Goldberg).

PET Clin 3 (2009) 293–315
doi:10.1016/j.cpet.2009.02.001
1556-8598/09/$ – see front matter

3-deoxy-3-[18F]-fluoro-L-thymidine (FLT) are taken up by proliferating gliomas depending on tumor grade as a reflection of increased activity of membrane transporters for glucose, amino acids, and nucleosides, respectively. More recently, methyl-[11C]-choline (CHO) was introduced as another novel agent to evaluate different aspects of tumor physiology, as will be discussed below.[11,12] PET can also assess the expression of endogenous or exogenous gene coding for enzymes or receptors by measuring the accumulation or binding of the respective enzyme substrates or receptor-binding compounds.[13,14]

Continuous developments in PET provide new insights into the diagnosis, classification, and pathophysiology of brain neoplasms. As such, PET has played an increasingly important role in the staging of brain neoplasms, image-guided therapy planning, and treatment monitoring. Multimodality imaging has brought about a new perspective into the field of neuro-oncology, as PET complements the more conventional anatomic imaging modalities of computed tomography (CT) and MR imaging. In selected situations, PET is used in conjunction with CT[15] and MR imaging[16,17] to better define the extent of neoplasm.

Recent research has concentrated on the fusion of PET and MR imaging technologies into one single machine. The goal of this development is to integrate the PET detectors into the MR imaging scanner, which would allow simultaneous data acquisition, resulting in combined functional and morphologic images with excellent soft-tissue contrast, spatial and temporal resolution, and improved coregistration of the fused images. Because advanced MR imaging techniques, such as perfusion-weighted imaging, diffusion-weighted imaging, blood oxygenation level-dependent imaging, and proton magnetic resonance spectroscopy provide physiologic and metabolic information, fusion of PET with MR imaging may provide more insight into the pathophysiology of brain neoplasms in vivo.[18,19] This article addresses the most commonly used agents in PET imaging of brain tumors.

FDG

Although there is great potential for other newer radiotracers, the vast majority of clinical PET is still based on FDG, an analog of glucose. Because of its relatively simple synthesis, long half-life (approximately 2 hours), and well-understood mechanism of action, FDG is commonly used in neuro-oncology.

Malignant cells generally have elevated glucose metabolism compared with nonmalignant cells, and therefore exhibit increased glycolytic activity.[20] The increase in glucose transport rate is not simply related to the accelerated tumor growth rate, but also to malignant transformation[21] and increased membrane-glucose transport capability.[22] There is a significant increase in the number of functional glucose transporters at the transformed cell's surface, and nearly all mitogens and cellular oncogenes activate glucose transport.[23] Six mammalian glucose transporters have been identified and over-expression of both GLUT-1 and GLUT-3 has been demonstrated in brain tumors, with a higher ratio of GLUT-3 seen in more aggressive neoplastic lesions.[24]

FDG is metabolized similarly to glucose, as FDG enters a cell via glucose transporter proteins, competes with glucose for hexokinase, and is phosphorylated. In contrast to glucose-6-phosphate, however, FDG-6-phosphate is metabolically trapped within tumor cells in proportion to the glucose metabolic rate, and thus PET can detect its accumulation. The FDG uptake into malignant cells is a consequence of a tumor cell's increased expression of glucose transport and glycolytic activity. The primary exception to the metabolic trapping is in the liver, where the large concentration of phosphatase enzymes results in de-phosphorylation of the FDG-6-phosphate and subsequent clearance of FDG from the liver.

CLINICAL APPLICATIONS OF FDG-PET IN NEURO-ONCOLOGY

FDG-PET has been used for differentiating neoplastic from nonneoplastic tissue, as well as for the diagnosis, grading, and prognosis of gliomas. FDG-PET can also be used to classify brain neoplasms, evaluate treatment response, and assist in treatment planning. The basic steps of FDG-PET imaging include the following: (i) greater than or equal to 4 hours of patient fasting, (ii) intravenous administration of the radiotracer (with dose based on body weight, with a typical usual dose of 10 mCi) after the patient relaxes for 5 minutes in a dimly lit room, (iii) patient rest for about 60 minutes after the injection, and (iv) subsequent acquisition of imaging data.

Detection

Distinguishing nonneoplastic from neoplastic lesions can be challenging based on anatomic imaging. FDG-PET has been shown to be of limited value in distinguishing between neoplastic and nonneoplastic ring-enhancing intracranial lesions, as observed on MR imaging. High FDG uptake may occur in cases of neoplasm, brain abscess, and in acute inflammatory demyelination.[25] Multiple reports have shown that lesions with a high concentration of inflammatory cells, such as neutrophils and activated macrophages, also show increased uptake of FDG that can be mistaken for malignant neoplasm.[26] In general, inflammatory cells often exhibit lower levels of FDG uptake compared with malignant cells. However, despite low levels of FDG uptake by inflammatory cells in the resting state, glucose metabolic activity of these cells can increase dramatically, making the distinction from tumor difficult.

Kubota and colleagues[27] first showed that newly formed granulation tissue around a neoplasm contained high concentrations of macrophages and showed a higher uptake of FDG than the viable neoplastic cells. This phenomenon may be explained by the fact that, in addition to neoplastic cells, inflammatory cells also have increased expression of glucose transporters, particularly after cellular stimulation by multiple cytokines.[28–30] Cytokines and growth factors have been shown to acutely increase the affinity of glucose transporters in inflammatory cells to deoxyglucose, and this up-regulation involves both tyrosine kinases and protein kinase C activity.[31]

Delineation of Tumor

Both high-grade gliomas and gray-matter structures take up FDG avidly. Thus, when tumors are in or near gray matter, it may be difficult to distinguish between the two.[32] The limited delineation between tumor and normal gray matter by FDG-PET may be improved by scanning at delayed intervals (3–7 hours) after tracer injection.[33] It has been demonstrated that the rate constant of FDG-6-phosphate degradation was not significantly different between tumor and normal brain tissue at early imaging times, but was lower in tumor than normal brain tissue at extended time intervals between FDG administration and PET data acquisition. This suggests that greater FDG-6-phosphate degradation at delayed time points may be responsible for higher excretion of FDG from normal tissue relative to neoplasm.

In a group of 10 patients with astrocytomas (WHO grades II and III), Herholz and colleagues[34] found that cell density, but not nuclear polymorphism, correlated significantly with FDG uptake. Standardized uptake values (SUV) in the brain do not correlate well with regional metabolic rates of glucose use, and are less effective in characterizing primary brain neoplasms than neoplasm-to-white matter or neoplasm-to-cortex ratios.[35]

FDG uptake is not specific for cancer, as FDG accumulation has been observed in inflammatory

cells and granulation issue.[27] Furthermore, there are some reports that have failed to show a relationship between FDG uptake and Ki-67 index, a histologic index for cell proliferation.[36,37]

Grading

In general, low-grade gliomas and high-grade gliomas have metabolic activity similar to white matter and gray matter, respectively. A glioma-to-white matter ratio of greater than 1.5 and a glioma-to-gray matter ratio of greater than 0.6 have been found to be indicative of high-grade gliomas with high sensitivity (94%) and limited specificity (77%) (**Fig. 1**).[38] Kaschten and colleagues[39] proposed a cutoff value of 0.8 and 1.1 for tumor-to-mean cortical uptake to differentiate grade II from grade III and grade III from grade IV gliomas, respectively. Several other reports[39,40] have also shown significant correlation between glioma grade and FDG uptake, with the exception of a few studies.[41]

Mechanisms leading to glucose hypermetabolism in high-grade gliomas are not fully understood. Possible explanations may derive from increased energetic demands related to proliferative processes,[34] increased expression of glucose transporters in response to oncogene expression, or the deregulation of the hexokinase enzymatic activity.[42,43]

Oligodendroglial tumors harboring combined 1p and 19q chromosomal deletions are characterized by a favorable prognosis and response to treatment. In a recent article, authors investigated the potential of FDG uptake to predict 1p/19q loss preoperatively. Positive FDG uptake was identified in six of eight grade II gliomas with 1p/19q loss, but in none of the eight grade II gliomas without 1p/19q loss.[44]

Prognosis

In high-grade gliomas, some studies have claimed that FDG-PET has predictive value of survival independent from the histologic classification.[45–47] Barker and colleagues[48] studied the prognostic value of FDG-PET in 55 patients with malignant glioma. In univariate analysis, the FDG-PET score was a significant predictor of survival time after FDG-PET scanning ($P = .005$). Median survival was 10 months for patients with FDG-PET uptake scores of 2 or 3, and 20 months for those with low uptake scores of 0 or 1. Padma and colleagues[49] also observed similar findings, and the median survival of patients with high-uptake scores in their study was 11 months, as compared with 28 months in patients with low-uptake scores.

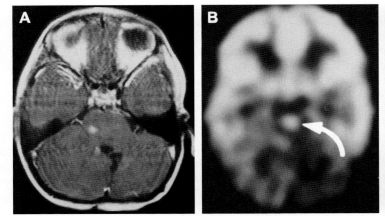
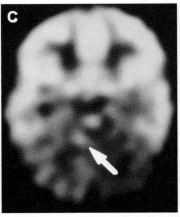

Fig. 1. Axial postcontrast T1-weighted image (*A*) demonstrates contrast-enhancing lesion at junction of pons and midbrain. Corresponding axial FDG-PET images (*B* and *C*) show avid uptake of FDG characteristic of malignant high-grade tumor (*arrows*).

Survival differed significantly between patients with low versus high uptake of FDG (*P* = .001).

Other groups have reported significant correlation between FDG-PET score and survival in patients with malignant gliomas imaged at various times in the course of their disease. Alavi and colleagues[46] reported median survivals of 7 and 33 months in patients with hypermetabolic and hypometabolic lesions, respectively (*P* = .0007). Patronas and colleagues[50] reported median survival of 5 and 19 months in patients with hypermetabolic and hypometabolic lesions, respectively (*P*<.001). Not all studies have confirmed the high predictive ability of FDG-PET with regard to grade of pathology or survival. Tyler and colleagues[51] found variable FDG uptake rates without correlation to neoplastic grade and size, and low FDG uptake in several patients with high-grade gliomas. Janus and colleagues[32] found that decreased uptake of FDG suggested prolonged survival in their study of 30 patients with primary brain neoplasms, but that increased uptake of FDG did not predict survival. Rozenthal and colleagues[52] found that neither the baseline glucose-uptake ratio nor the visual tumor grade accurately predicted length of survival.

Lower sensitivity and specificity of FDG-PET in the prediction of pathology grade and survival may be because of multiple factors. One possible reason may be volume averaging from necrotic portions of a heterogeneous neoplasm and surrounding edema. Alternatively, some neoplasms may be so hypovascular that their metabolic rates are limited by the undersupply of glucose. Moreover, cystic and calcified regions are also hypovascular. Relatively benign neoplasms with a high FDG uptake include pilocytic astrocytoma and ganglioglioma. Pilocytic astrocytomas have a good prognosis despite exhibiting high FDG uptake because of the presence of metabolically active fenestrated endothelial cells.

Classification of Brain Neoplasms

FDG-PET has been useful in differentiating common enhancing malignant brain neoplasms, such as lymphomas, from high-grade gliomas, lymphomas from brain metastases, and high-grade gliomas from brain metastases.[53] However, FDG-PET is limited in differentiating oligodendrogliomas from astrocytomas of the same grade.[54] On the other hand, using FDG-PET, it is also possible to differentiate grade I from grade II or III meningiomas.[55]

Meningiomas represent 10% to 15% of primary intracranial neoplasms. They are usually benign, curable neoplasms but can occasionally recur and demonstrate aggressive behavior.[56] Di Chiro and colleagues[45] found that the glucose metabolic rate of meningiomas correlates with tumor growth and aggressive behavior. In their study, an atypical meningioma had the highest metabolic rate greater than that of cerebral cortex.

Hemangiopericytomas are richly vascularized mesenchymal tumors that are derived from pericytes. Kracht and colleagues[57] observed low glucose use in a case of hemangiopericytoma in spite of high cellularity and proliferation rate.

Effectiveness of Therapy

Differentiation of after-therapy radiation necrosis from residual or recurrent brain neoplasm remains a challenging diagnostic problem. Because of the relatively high background activity, especially in the cortical regions, FDG-PET is not suited to evaluate residual/recurrent neoplasm after therapy.[58,59] However, the effects of radiation and chemotherapy can be visualized by FDG-PET only after several weeks,[60] with a possible transient increase of FDG-uptake in the initial phase, most likely because of infiltration of macrophages.[61,62] At further follow-up, however, recurrent neoplasm and progression from low-grade to high-grade glioma can be visualized by the new appearance of hypermetabolism.[63,64]

It has been reported that FDG-PET had a sensitivity of 81% to 86% and a specificity of 40% to 94% for distinguishing between radiation necrosis and residual or recurrent neoplasm (**Figs 2** and **3**).[65] Attempts to use the ratio of tumor uptake to contralateral normal white matter or gray matter have yielded poor results.[66] This finding was a subject of controversy, however, because one research group achieved good results using receiver-operating characteristic curve analysis.[67] The difficulty with using the ratio approach to

diagnose residual or recurrent neoplasm was because of the fact that an area of treated brain has a wide range of background metabolic activity and usually is of lower metabolic activity than the normal untreated brain. Residual and recurrent neoplasms can have similarly varied degrees of metabolic activity that also can frequently be lower than that of the normal brain. It should be emphasized that in patients receiving corticosteroids, evaluation with FDG-PET might be hampered by a reduced cortex-to-white matter ratio.[68]

Coregistration of FDG-PET images with MR imaging greatly improves the performance of FDG-PET, and as such it is critical to have the MR image available while the FDG-PET images are interpreted.[69] Because residual and recurrent neoplasm may show FDG uptake equal to or lower than uptake in the normal cortex, reference to the MR image delineates the area of interest. In the area of interest on MR imaging, any FDG uptake higher than the expected background level in the adjacent brain may be considered recurrent neoplasm, even though the uptake may be equal

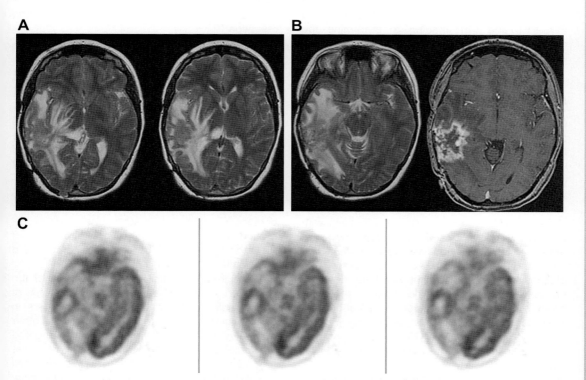

Fig. 2. A 22-year-old woman diagnosed with grade III anaplastic astrocytoma underwent radiation therapy and surgery. Axial T2-weighted images (*A*) show ill-defined hyperintense mass with extensive fingerlike edema in the right parieto-occipital lobe. There is heterogeneous contrast enhancement within the mass on the corresponding axial postcontrast T2-weighted image (*B, left panel*) and axial FDG-PET image (*B, right panel*). (*C*) show ring-shaped areas of increased FDG uptake corresponding to enhancing areas. Significant cerebral dysfunction caused by edema adjacent to tumor is also visible as decreased FDG uptake.

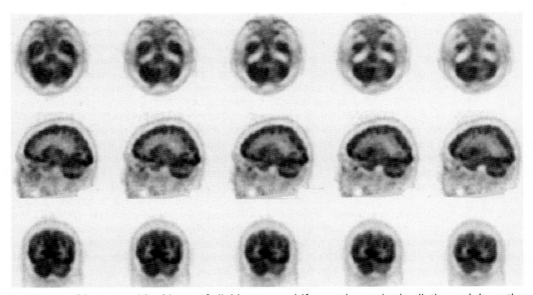

Fig. 3. A 45-year-old woman with a history of glioblastoma multiforme who received radiation and chemotherapy following surgery. MR imaging (not shown) showed enhancing lesion within the brain. However, multiplanar FDG-PET images demonstrate no evidence of residual neoplastic tissue, consistent with radiation injury.

to or less than that in normal cortex.[70] A recent report has also advocated the use of coregistered FDG-PET and MR imaging to determine the residual or recurrent neoplasm viability by the enhancing regions of the tumor.[71]

Imaging for Planning Stereotactic Biopsy

Gliomas are histologically heterogeneous, with components that include varying degrees of cellularand nuclear pleomorphism, mitotic activity, vascular proliferation, and necrosis.[2,3] Thus, low-grade and high-grade regions may be present within the same tumor. These regional variations cannot be distinguished on conventional anatomic imaging, such as MR imaging or CT, even with intravenous contrast administration.[72] Therefore, target selection may lead to a significant sampling error and understaging. Accurate grading and diagnosis are especially important for directing the therapeutic approach and providing the prognosis in patients with nonresectable neoplasms. Stereotactic biopsy aims for tumor sites with the highest tumor grade. FDG-PET-guided stereotactic brain biopsy has proven to be useful for improved delineation of anaplastic regions,[73–75] and better identification of neoplastic residues,[45] thereby increasing the diagnostic yield of brain biopsy. However, integration of MR imaging with PET provides complementary information that helps in the assessment of neoplastic extent and surgical planning better than either technique

alone. This combined information has been exploited in accomplishing maximum neoplastic resection.[17,76]

Pitfalls of FDG-PET

FDG-PET imaging of brain neoplasms provides information on neoplastic grade and patient prognosis. Compared with other organ systems, the brain presents unique challenges because of the high background-glucose metabolism of normal gray matter structures. Coregistration of MR (or CT) and FDG-PET images is essential for accurate evaluation of brain neoplasms. Other tracers, such as MET and CHO, avidly accumulate in brain neoplasms and have the advantage of low-background cortical activity. Other major limitations of PET are its relatively poor spatial resolution and low specificity.

Although FDG, which takes advantage of the increased glucose transport and glycolysis of cancer cells, is the most widely used agent in PET imaging of brain neoplasms, there are other potential metabolic pathways that can be targeted for imaging. The metabolic imaging of other processes, such as protein metabolism, cell membrane turnover, DNA synthesis, and hypoxia, has been shown to provide alternative valuable information for the evaluation of brain tumors. To this end, other radiotracers have been used, including amino acids, cell membrane components, and nucleosides.

RADIOLABELED AMINO ACIDS

Radiolabeled amino acids are particularly helpful in the brain, a location in which FDG-PET has two key limitations: (1) Because of the brain's relatively increased baseline physiologic glucose metabolism, there is a high background level of FDG uptake that limits contrast resolution and, therefore, sensitivity for detecting pathologic FDG uptake; and (2) Because of increased FDG metabolism in inflammatory cells, FDG-PET is limited in distinguishing neoplastic from inflammatory processes.

Proteins play a critical role in nearly every biologic process within the body. Amino acids, the building blocks of proteins, are either produced via metabolic processes or obtained via dietary ingestion. Fundamental to their ability to be a target of metabolic imaging, they can serve as components in metabolic cycles, many of which are up-regulated in cells with increased proliferative activity, such as in the setting of cancer. Amino acids enter cells either through passive diffusion or, more commonly, active diffusion via the L-amino acid transporter.

What makes amino acids attractive for the most common form of radiolabeling is that the substitution of [11C] for a nonradioactive [12C] carbon atom does not alter the amino acid's chemical characteristics. Certain amino acids have gained more popularity than others as metabolic imaging agents because of differences in relative ease and cost of production, biodistribution, and formation of radiolabeled metabolites. The most studied radiolabeled amino acid for PET evaluation of brain tumors is MET. However, because of the short half-life of [11C] (20 minutes), [18F]-labeled aromatic amino acid analogs have been developed for tumor imaging including O-2-[18F]-fluoroethyl-L-tyrosine (FET) and L-3,4-dihydroxy-6-[18F]-fluoro-phenylalanine (FDOPA). Other radiolabeled amino acids include L-1-[11C]-tyrosine (TYR), and L-3-[18F]-fluoro-α-methyltyrosine (FMT). L-3-[123I]-iodo-α-methyltyrosine (IMT) is a promising radiolabeled amino acid for use in single photon emission computed tomography (SPECT) imaging.[77]

MET

MET is a radiolabeled amino acid that has been studied as a potential PET agent for the evaluation of brain neoplasms. The molecular basis of MET-PET's role in tumor imaging is controversial. Based on the physiology of amino acid metabolism and protein synthesis, one theory is that increased uptake of MET is a reflection of a cancer cell's increased protein synthesis.[78] More recent studies, however, have shown that the increased activity of a brain tumor on a MET-PET study may be an indicator of activation of carrier-mediated cell transport at the blood-brain barrier, rather than solely protein synthesis.[77–80]

MET is the most frequently used radiolabeled amino acid in PET evaluation of brain neoplasms.[77] This is largely because of its relative ease of production that lacks complicated purification steps. MET uptake correlates with cell proliferation, in vitro Ki-67 expression, proliferating cell nuclear antigen, and microvessel density, making it a potential biomarker for active tumor proliferation.[81]

MET-PET has been studied to determine its value in a variety of roles in the evaluation of neoplasms, including detection, delineation of tumor, grading, prognosis, and effectiveness of therapy.

Detection

MET accumulates in gliomas, as demonstrated by multiple prior studies, and MET-PET has repeatedly demonstrated that it is a very sensitive tool for detection of brain neoplasms.[39,82–86] The sensitivities for malignant neoplasms have ranged from 61% to 97%, with higher rates for higher grade neoplasms.[85] As will be discussed in greater depth below, increased uptake of MET was also seen in neoplasms in which there was little or absent contrast enhancement on MR imaging and low uptake on FDG-PET, findings typical of low-grade gliomas.[87]

Delineation

Multiple studies have shown that MET-PET shows earlier and more accurate delineation of neoplastic extent than anatomic imaging, such as with CT or MR imaging alone.[16,75,88–90]

In a study of 10 patients with pathologically proven GBM, Miwa and colleagues[16] performed both contrast-enhanced MR imaging and MET-PET before treatment to better assess the relationship between abnormalities seen on both modalities. Coregistration of the anatomic and metabolic images was performed with a commercial software package using a previously published method.[91] This study found that in 100% of cases, the area of abnormal MET uptake (MET area) was larger than the gadolinium-enhancing area (Gd area). In 90% of cases, the MET area was located within a 3-cm radius of the Gd area. This distance was positively correlated with tumor size. In 100% cases, the area of T2 prolongation surrounding the tumor was larger than the MET area, suggesting that peritumoral edema extends beyond the margins of the neoplasm (**Fig. 4**). This study also showed that MET-PET was more sensitive for the earlier detection of tumor recurrence than MR imaging. In total, this study concluded that with a better understanding of the discrepancies between MET-PET and MR imaging, the combined use of these modalities could be helpful for surgical and radiation planning.

The discrepancy between MR imaging and MET-PET is likely because of the inherent differences in the modalities and the processes they are imaging. For example, to assess the extent of neoplasm, T1-weighted MR imaging detects the morphologic abnormalities in brain structures secondary to mass effect from a neoplasm, a relatively insensitive technique, especially in the case of low-grade or infiltrative neoplasms. The addition of intravenous contrast material does not significantly increase accuracy in assessing the extent of neoplasm, as contrast enhancement is dependent upon breakdown of the blood-brain barrier, a finding usually only seen in the most aggressive

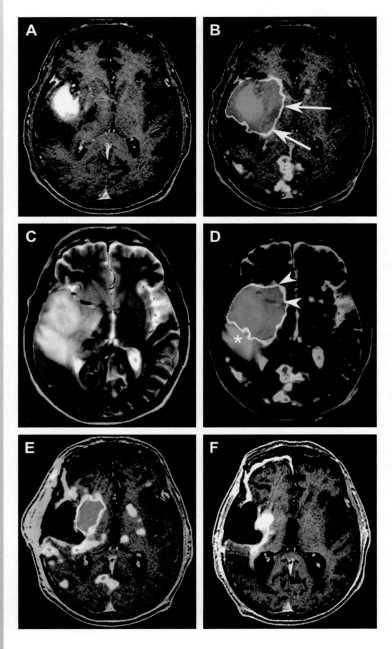

Fig. 4. Axial postcontrast T1-weighted MR image (*A* and *F*), postcontrast T1-weighted MR images coregistered with MET-PET images (*B* and *E*), T2-weighted MR image (*C*), and T2-weighted MR image coregistered with MET-PET image (*D*). Red indicates MET area (*B*, *D*, and *E*). MET area was larger than Gd area, completely encompassing it (*B*). Arrows indicate points at which MET area extended beyond Gd area (*B*). Part of MET area existed outside T2 high signal-intensity area (*arrowheads*), but T2 high signal-intensity area existed without increased MET accumulation (***) (*D*). Gd area was completely resected but residual MET area can be seen in right basal ganglia on postcontrast T1-weighted MR image coregistered with MET-PET image after surgery (*E*). Postcontrast T1-weighted MR image 8 months after first examination (*F*) showing development of new Gd area in right basal ganglia at which MET area had extended outside Gd area on first examination. (*Reproduced from* Miwa K, Shinoda J, Yano H, et al. Discrepancy between lesion distributions on methionine PET and MR images in patients with glioblastoma multiforme: insight from a PET and MR fusion image study. J Neurol Neurosurg Psychiatry 2004;75(10):1459; with permission.)

components of a neoplasm. T2-weighted MR imaging can show increased signal intensity surrounding a neoplasm, which can help in defining the extent of a neoplasm, although this suffers from low specificity because edema has an identical appearance. Conversely, MET-PET relies on the greater metabolic needs of the tumor, rather than on the associated morphologic or blood-brain barrier abnormalities, to create a more accurate depiction of neoplastic extent.

Grading

In addition to detection, MET-PET has also been shown to be a valuable tool for the grading of brain neoplasms.[40,82,83,85,87,92,93] MET-PET's ability to serve in this role is likely because of the correlation between MET uptake and markers of neoplastic aggressiveness, including cell proliferation in vitro, the expression of Ki-67, and proliferating cell nuclear antigen, as well as to microvessel density.[81]

The use of neoplastic grading by MET-PET has been of particular interest for low-grade tumors, which are not only difficult to detect on contrast-enhanced MR imaging and FDG-PET, but also difficult to differentiate from nonneoplastic lesions. In the largest study of this topic, Herholz and colleagues[87] evaluated 196 consecutive patients suspected of having low-grade gliomas. The study found that MET-PET could differentiate between high-grade gliomas, low-grade gliomas, and chronic or subacute nonneoplastic lesions (**Fig. 5**). This ability was independent from contrast-enhancement on CT or MR imaging, as expected, given that MET uptake, unlike contrast enhancement, does not rely on breakdown of the blood-brain barrier.

Prognosis

MET-PET has also been used as a tool for prognosis in patients with cerebral gliomas.[37,39,94,95] Currently, the standard prognostic factors include age, performance status, focal neurologic deficits, mental changes, seizure, symptoms of neoplastic expansion, contrast enhancement, and pathologic grade; however, the value of some of these factors is still unclear.[37] Having an understanding of a patient's prognosis is critical, as this helps guide therapeutic decision making. Although FDG-PET has been tested as a prognostic factor, it has been hampered by FDG's known limitations in the brain as described above, most notably its low specificity.[46,96,97]

In a study by De Witte and colleagues[95] that evaluated MET-PET's role in prognosis, investigators used both a qualitative and quantitative scoring system of MET uptake; the study found that neoplasms with higher MET-PET activity were associated with a statistically significantly shorter survival time.

In a separate study by Kim and colleagues[37] that directly compared MET and FDG uptake as prognostic factors, MET uptake was found to be an independent significant prognostic factor, whereas FDG uptake was not (**Fig. 6**). When both MET-PET and FDG-PET were used in the setting of suspected glioma recurrence, two different studies found that the combination of both radiotracers resulted in the highest prognostic accuracy; however, MET was found to be the preferred single agent because of its increased sensitivity and specificity.[39,94]

MET-PET may also have a niche role in determining the prognosis for patients with gliomas that are suspected or confirmed to be low-grade. Because the outcomes for patients with low-grade gliomas are so variable and there is no consensus on treatment, MET-PET's ability to risk-stratify low-grade gliomas could play a crucial role in management of this subset of gliomas.[98]

Effectiveness of Therapy

In the postradiation or postsurgical brain, the findings of recurrent tumor on contrast-enhanced MR imaging or FDG-PET can be nonspecific, at times indistinguishable from posttreatment inflammatory change or radiation necrosis. Making this distinction is obviously of critical importance, as radiation necrosis may prompt steroid therapy or debulking neurosurgery; alternatively, a finding of neoplastic recurrence may lead to more aggressive therapy or, conversely, palliative care. Although less research has been devoted to this area, several studies have shown that MET-PET is an accurate tool for the evaluation of recurrence in a previously treated brain.[59,94,99–101] In a series of 15 patients suspected of having recurrent brain tumor or radiation injury, Ogawa and colleagues[99] showed that MET-PET was useful in the early detection of recurrent brain neoplasm, whereas FDG-PET was helpful in the detection of radiation necrosis; the investigators concluded that FDG-PET and MET-PET were additive in their accuracy to distinguish radiation necrosis from recurrent or residual neoplasm. In a slightly larger series, Van Laere and colleagues[94] showed that MET-PET had an accuracy, sensitivity, and specificity of 73%, 75%, and 70% respectively, not significantly different than those of FDG-PET (**Fig. 7**). When MET-PET and FDG-PET data were used concurrently, there was slight improvement in accuracy and sensitivity, and a slight decrease in specificity.

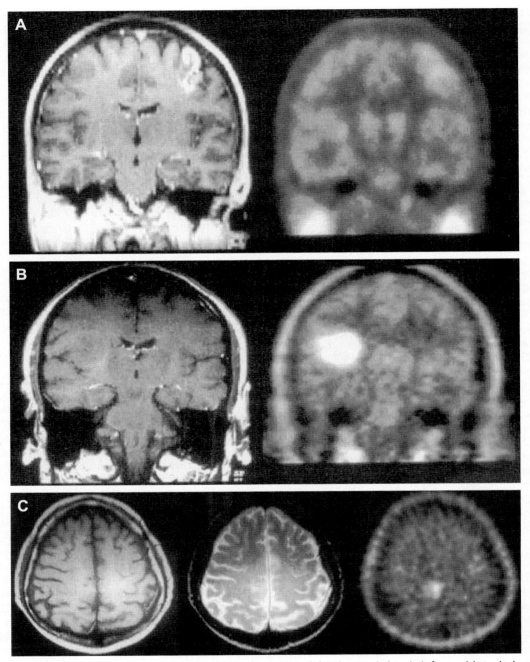

Fig. 5. MET-PET for differential diagnosis of low-grade gliomas. (*A*) Subacute ischemic infarct with typical gyral enhancement on coronal post contrast T1-weighted MR image (*left*) but little MET uptake on coronal PET image (*right*). (*B*) Glioblastoma without enhancement on coronal postcontrast T1-weighted MR image (*left*) but very high MET uptake on coronal PET image (*right*). (*C*) Small parasagittal grade II astrocytoma showing minor signal-intensity alterations on axial T1-weighted (*left*) and T2-weighted (*middle*) MR images, but with intense MET uptake on axial PET image (*right*) with uptake index of 2.43. (*Reproduced from* Herholz K, Holzer T, Bauer B, et al. 11C-methionine PET for differential diagnosis of low-grade gliomas. Neurology 1998;50(5):1316–22; with permission.)

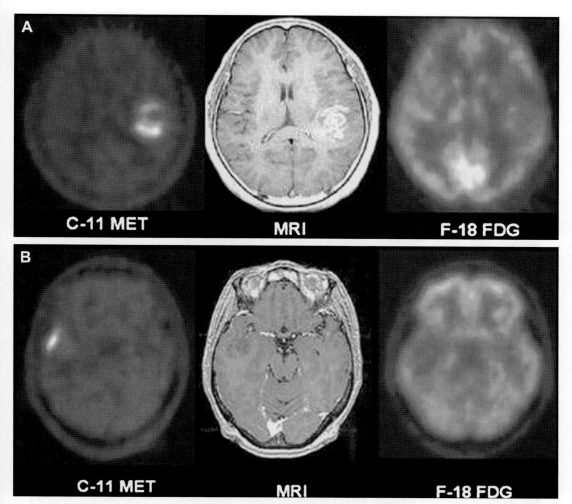

Fig. 6. MET-PET, postcontrast T1-weighted MR image, and FDG-PET of two patients with glioma. (*A*) Axial MET-PET image shows foci of hypermetabolism corresponding to enhancing tumor on axial MR image, whereas axial FDG-PET image shows iso-/hypometabolism in tumor. Pathology was glioblastoma and Ki-67 index of tumor was 40%. Patient died 14 months later, a short survival time. (*B*) A 61-year-old man with history of low-grade glioma treated by local resection and chemotherapy. Axial MET-PET image demonstrates focal area of hypermetabolism in tumor. Axial MR image reveals residual nonenhancing tumor in right insular region, whereas axial FDG-PET image demonstrates hypometabolism similar to that of white matter, consistent with low-grade glioma. Area with MET uptake was confirmed as anaplastic transformation with relatively higher proliferative index (Ki-67 index = 20%) at stereotactic biopsy. (*Reproduced from* Kim S, Chung JK, Im SH, et al. 11C-methionine PET as a prognostic marker in patients with glioma: comparison with 18F-FDG PET. Eur J Nucl Med Mol Imaging 2005;32(1):56; with permission.)

Combined Use of MR Imaging and MET-PET

With the understanding that MET-PET and MR imaging provide different, yet complementary data, investigators have tested the role of combined MET-PET and MR imaging in treatment planning for radiosurgery.[102,103] The addition of metabolic imaging to the anatomic imaging of MR provides valuable information for treatment planning, especially in poorly defined or infiltrative neoplasms.[103]

The next logical step has been to test the role of MET-PET in image-guided surgical resection of brain neoplasms. As described above, MET-PET generally provides a more accurate delineation of neoplastic extent than MR imaging alone. Therefore, Pirotte and colleagues[17] studied whether integration of PET data into neuro-navigational systems for stereotactic tumor resections could lead to improved outcomes. PET scans (some of which used FDG and others that used MET) were performed on 91 patients in whom neoplasm

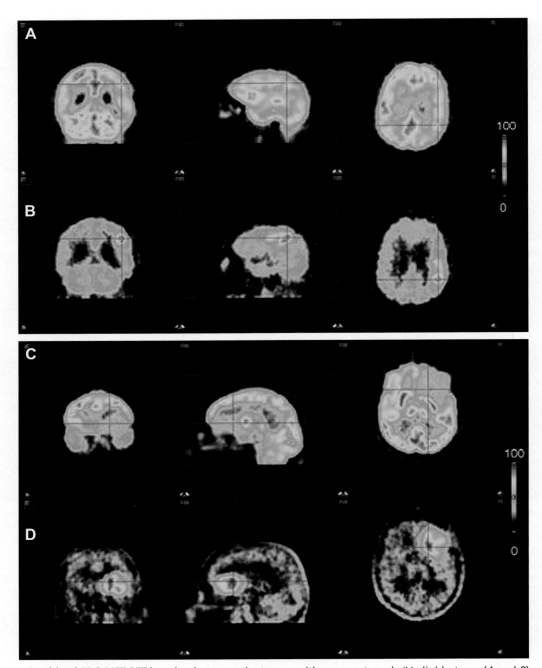

Fig. 7. Combined FDG-MET PET imaging in two patients, one with recurrent grade IV glioblastoma (*A* and *B*) and one without recurrent grade II oligo-astrocytoma tumor (*C* and *D*), the latter patient with disease-free survival of more than 37 months. Images were coregistered by mutual information voxel-based algorithm. (*Reproduced from* Van Laere K, Ceyssens S, Van Calenbergh F, et al. Direct comparison of 18F-FDG and 11C-methionine PET in suspected recurrence of glioma: sensitivity, interobserver variability and prognostic value. Eur J Nucl Med Mol Imaging 2005;32(1):45; with permission.)

boundaries could not be confidently determined on MR imaging for navigation-based resection. These studies were combined with MR imaging for resection navigational planning. Tumor volume based on PET was compared with tumor volume based on MR imaging, and in 80% of cases the difference in volume led to a different final-target volume for surgical resection. For the patients who underwent FDG-PET, the PET data altered surgical planning in 69% of cases. MET-PET, which was used predominantly for the low-grade gliomas, improved the tumor volume definition in 88% of low-grade gliomas and 78% of high-grade gliomas (**Fig. 8**). Total resection of the area of increased metabolic activity (either FDG or MET) was accomplished in 52% of the resections. The investigators concluded that PET provided independent and complementary information about neoplastic extent and resection compared with MR imaging alone.

Additional Radiolabeled Amino Acids

As mentioned above, the study of radiolabeled amino acids in the evaluation of brain tumors has focused primarily on MET-PET. There are other potential radiolabeled amino acids, which, like MET, have lower uptake in normal brain tissue relative to FDG, raising the possibility of their use in the evaluation of brain tumors. FET-, TYR-, and FDOPA-PET, as well as IMT-SPECT, have been studied for this purpose, with sensitivities ranging from approximately 85% to 100%.[104–109] However, to a greater extent than for MET, the exact roles of FET, TYR, FDOPA, and IMT for tumor imaging is unclear and not well established.[106,110]

FET

FET and FDOPA have gained popularity as PET agents because, as opposed to MET and other agents labeled with [11C], such as TYR, the former are labeled with [18F], which has a longer half-life (110 minutes), obviating the need for an on-site cyclotron. Studies have shown that MET-PET and FET-PET have similar accuracies in diagnosing gliomas.[111,112] Furthermore, FET-PET has been shown to have value in the prognosis and evaluation of treatment in patients with gliomas.[113–115]

FDOPA

FDOPA is an amino acid analog taken up by normal brain at the blood-brain barrier by the neutral amino acid transporter. In a relatively large series of 81 patients, Chen and colleagues[109] compared FDOPA-PET to FDG-PET in the evaluation of brain neoplasms. The study found that high-grade and low-grade neoplasms were well visualized with FDOPA-PET, with a significantly higher sensitivity than that of FDG-PET (96% versus 61%), whereas specificities were similar (43%) (**Fig. 9**). FDOPA uptake, however, did not correlate with neoplastic grade, and it did not appear that FDOPA-PET could be used for this purpose. Although only four patients were suspected of having radiation necrosis, FDOPA-PET was able to identify the one patient in this group who had recurrent neoplasm, not radiation necrosis; the investigators suggested that a dedicated study would be helpful to better evaluate FDOPA-PET's potential role in distinguishing recurrent neoplasm from radiation necrosis.

IMT

IMT, an artificial amino acid used in SPECT imaging, is a specific marker for amino acid transport in gliomas.[116] It has been shown to have a potential role in brain neoplasm

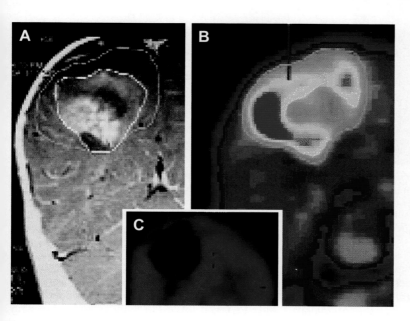

Fig. 8. Coronal postcontrast T1-weighted MR image (*A*) and coronal MET-PET images (*B* and *C*) obtained in a 2-year-old boy with right parietal grade II ganglioglioma showing PET-based contour (*green outline*), which includes MR imaging-based contour defined on fluid-attenuation inversion recovery MR images (*blue outline*). Postoperative coronal MET-PET image (*C*) reveals no residual MET uptake. (*Reproduced from* Pirotte B, Goldman S, Dewitte O, et al. Integrated positron emission tomography and magnetic resonance imaging-guided resection of brain tumors: a report of 103 consecutive procedures. J Neurosurg 2006;104(2):248; with permission.)

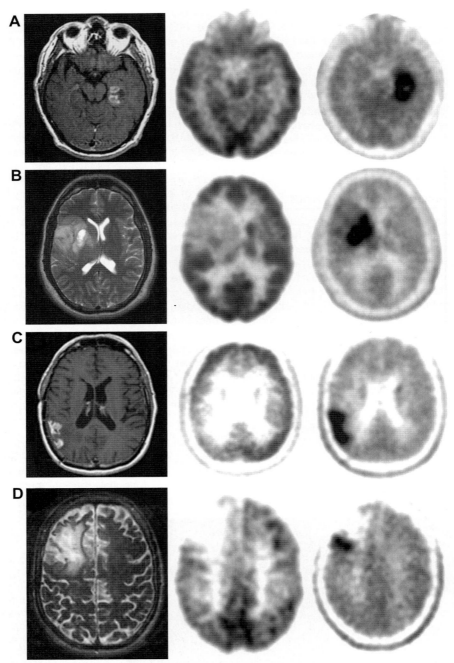

Fig. 9. Axial MR (*left*), FDG-PET (*middle*), and FDOPA-PET (*right*) images of four patients with either newly diagnosed (*A* and *B*) or recurrent (*C* and *D*) brain tumors. (*A*) Glioblastoma. (*B*) Grade II oligodendroglioma. (*C*) Recurrent glioblastoma. (*D*) Recurrent grade II oligodendroglioma. (*Reproduced from* Chen W, Silverman DH, Delaloye S, et al. 18F-FDOPA PET imaging of brain tumors: comparison study with 18F-FDG PET and evaluation of diagnostic accuracy. J Nucl Med 2006;47(6):907; with permission.)

imaging. Numerous studies have found that the IMT-SPECT demonstrates increased uptake in essentially all gliomas, cerebral lymphomas, and metastases.[77,106–108,117] In addition, it might have a niche role in defining neoplasm extent. A study by Grosu and colleagues[118] used MR imaging fusion images, which included both MET-PET and IMT-SPECT for radiation planning purposes. In 100% of cases (n = 30), the region of increased IMT uptake included the entire region of gadolinium enhancement and often extended beyond it. The investigators concluded that use of either IMT-SPECT or MET-PET added value to MR imaging alone for radiation planning and resulted in longer survival times.

One advantage of IMT-SPECT over MET-PET is its lower cost, and despite the reduced spatial resolution of SPECT versus PET (7 mm versus 3 mm, respectively), previous studies have shown similar sensitivities in the identification of gliomas.[119] Another disadvantage of MET-PET, as mentioned above, is the short physical half-life of MET (20 minutes), thus limiting its use to institutions with cyclotrons.

RADIOLABELED CELL MEMBRANE COMPONENTS
CHO

FDG and MET are the two most commonly used PET tracers. More recently, CHO has been targeted as a PET imaging agent because of its ability to image cell membrane turnover, a likely marker of metabolic activity.[11,12,120–122] Choline is a molecule normally found in blood, which enters cell membranes. In tumors, choline is phosphorylated and then, after several biosynthetic steps, is integrated into lecithin, a component of cell membrane phospholipids. Because of a tumor cell's increased proliferation, there is increased cell membrane turnover and, therefore, a greater need for cell membrane components, such as choline.

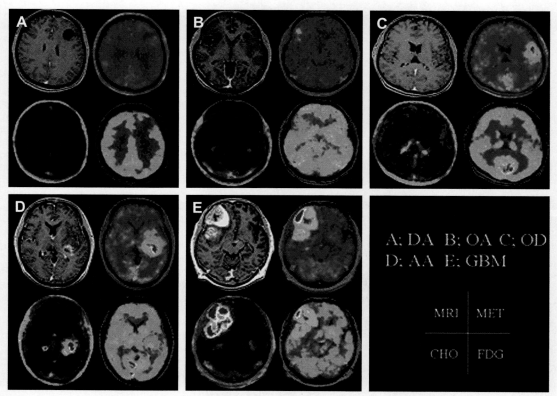

Fig. 10. (*Left top*) Postcontrast T1-weighted MR image. (*Right top*) MET-PET is superimposed on MR image. (*Left bottom*) CHO-PET is superimposed on MR image. (*Right bottom*) FDG-PET is superimposed on MR image. (*A*) A 32-year-old woman with diffuse astrocytoma. MET tumor to normal brain (T/N) ratio = 1.72, CHO T/N ratio = 1.38, and FDG T/N ratio = 0.66. (*B*) A 23-year-old woman with oligoastrocytoma. MET T/N ratio = 2.76, CHO T/N ratio = 1.82, and FDG T/N ratio = 0.92. (*C*) A 44-year-old man with oligodendroglioma. MET T/N ratio = 3.71, CHO T/N ratio = 2.74, and FDG T/N ratio = 1.07. (*D*) A 62-year-old woman with anaplastic astrocytoma. MET T/N ratio = 4.26, CHO T/N ratio = 10.17, and FDG T/N ratio = 1.24. (*E*) A 68-year-old man with glioblastoma multiforme. MET T/N ratio = 6.85, CHO T/N ratio = 33.38, and FDG T/N ratio = 2.55. (*Reproduced from* Kato T, Shinoda J, Nakayama N, et al. Metabolic assessment of gliomas using 11C-methionine, [18F] fluorodeoxyglucose, and 11C-choline positron-emission tomography. AJNR Am J Neuroradiol 2008;29(6):1179; with permission.)

Investigators have evaluated the role, if any, of CHO-PET in comparison to PET with the more established tracers FDG and MET. In a prospective study involving 126 patients with various types of malignancy, including 25 patients with brain neoplasms, Tian and colleagues[12] compared CHO-PET to FDG-PET. For the subset of patients with brain neoplasms, CHO was superior to FDG in delineating the true extent of the tumor. Again, this is likely because of the brain's high baseline uptake of FDG, which likely obscures pathologic

lesions and lowers sensitivity and specificity. In a recent study by Kato and colleagues,[54] PET examinations using FDG, MET, and CHO were used to evaluate 96 gliomas (**Fig. 10**). MR imaging was also performed, and tumor volume and degree of enhancement was assessed. Although PET images were superimposed on the anatomic MR images, it appears that this was done for illustrative purposes rather than to assess the value of combining the two modalities. Again, the study found MET to be a superior tracer compared

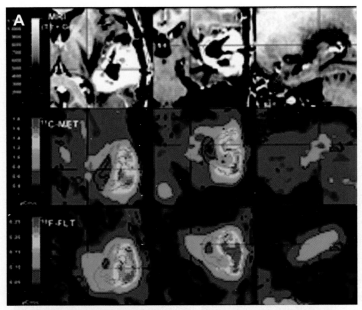

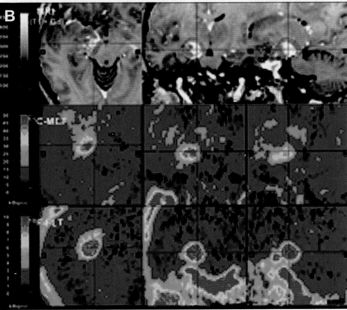

Fig. 11. Two examples of complementary information on activity and extent of tumor as depicted by multimodal imaging. (*A*) A 49-year-old woman with recurrent glioblastoma that had been treated by surgery, radiation, and chemotherapy. FLT-PET images (*bottom row*) seem to depict some extension of tumor toward internal capsule and thalamus not clearly depicted by postcontrast T1-weighted MR (*top row*) and MET-PET (*middle row*) images. Contours on MR images depict tumor extent as measured by FLT-PET, and contours on MET-PET and FLT-PET depict tumor extent as measured by gadolinium enhancement. (*B*) A 58-year-old woman with grade III ganglioglioma. High tumor activity is depicted by high FLT uptake (uptake ratio, 13.0; SUV, 3.0) (*bottom row*), which exceeds involvement shown by gadolinium enhancement on MR imaging (*top row*) to lateral side (volume, 40 cc versus. 14.4 cc). MET-PET images (*middle row*) show even further extension of tumor toward pole of temporal lobe. Contours on MR image depict tumor extent as measured by FLT-PET, and contours on MET-PET and FLT-PET depict tumor extent as measured by gadolinium enhancement. (*Reproduced from* Jacobs AH, Thomas A, Kracht LW, et al. 18F-fluoro-L-thymidine and 11C-methylmethionine as markers of increased transport and proliferation in brain tumors. J Nucl Med 2005;46(12):1952; with permission.)

with FDG and CHO, although the latter may have a role in evaluating oligodendroglial neoplasms.

RADIOLABELED NUCLEOSIDES
FLT

One of the relatively recent developments in the PET evaluation of brain neoplasms involves the study of radiolabeled nucleosides, specifically FLT.[123–126] FLT, phosphorylated by thymidine kinase-1, an enzyme involved in DNA synthesis, is considered a direct marker of tumor proliferation, as opposed to MET and FDG, which reflect increased metabolic activity, a surrogate of tumor proliferation.[127,128] Like MET, FLT has low physiologic uptake in the brain, making it a good candidate for detecting tumors.[125]

Jacobs and colleagues[6] compared MET-PET, FLT-PET, and MR imaging in 23 patients with gliomas (**Fig. 11**). Although FLT-PET's sensitivity was somewhat lower than that of MET-PET (78% versus 91%), the study concluded that FLT-PET provided complementary information on the extent and activity of gliomas. However, the study was confounded by the large number of previously treated patients (15 of 23). Because of these limitations, Hatakeyama and colleagues[126] studied the role of FLT-PET and MET-PET in 41 patients with nontreated newly diagnosed gliomas. The study found that overall, the radiotracers yielded similar findings. There was no significant difference in sensitivity between FLT-PET and MET-PET (83.3% versus 87.8%, respectively). Furthermore, in the patients with low-grade gliomas, both radiotracers performed equally, suggesting that there was no added or complementary role for combined use of the radiotracers. Research into the role FLT-PET is still in its infancy, and future studies will help to clarify its role.

HYPOXIA IMAGING

Hypoxia is a common characteristic of solid neoplasms that results from dysfunctional vascular networks that do not deliver adequate supplies of oxygen to highly metabolically active tumor cells.[129] Hypoxic cells in a solid tumor have been known to be resistant to radiotherapy.[130] The effectiveness of chemotherapy is also modulated by the presence of hypoxic cells.[131] Tumor hypoxia is thought to exert a selective pressure that favors neoplastic progression,[132] metastasis,[133] and a poor clinical outcome.[134]

[18F]-EF5

[18F]-EF5 (2-(2-nitro-1H-imidazol-1-yl)-N-(2,2,3,3,3-pentafluoropropyl)-acetamide) has been employed to measure neoplastic hypoxia in animals and human beings using immunohistochemical methods. [18F]-EF5 is a lipophilic molecule-designed to have a very uniform biodistribution, a feature of obvious benefit for use in PET imaging.

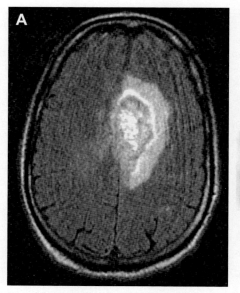
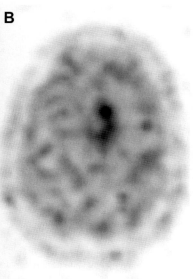

Fig. 12. A 65-year-old man with glioblastoma multiforme underwent radiation therapy and surgery. Axial post-contrast T1-weighted image (A) demonstrates enhancing mass in left frontal lobe. Axial [18F]-EF5-PET image (B) shows focal area of increased tracer uptake in mass indicating intratumoral hypoxia.

[18F]-EF5 is currently in phase II clinical trials using antibody techniques for the detection of hypoxic cells, and predicts radiation response in individual rodent tumors.[135] In human beings, the biologic half-life of [18F]-EF5 is approximately 12 hours, and up to 70% of the administered dose is excreted unchanged in the urine.[136] Preliminary results by Ziemer and colleagues[137] have suggested that [18F]-EF5 is a promising agent for noninvasive assessment of neoplastic hypoxia (**Fig. 12**).

SUMMARY

PET imaging of brain tumors is a rapidly growing field with a promising future. While cross-sectional techniques, especially MR imaging, provide a powerful tool in the evaluation and management of brain neoplasms, they are limited by a lack of molecular information that PET images provide. PET imaging with various radiotracers allows greater insight into tumor type, grade, extent, effectiveness of therapy, and treatment planning. Although more research is needed, the combination of MR imaging with PET will likely lead to more accurate diagnoses, more informed treatment decisions, and improved patient outcomes.

REFERENCES

1. Smirniotopoulos JG. The new WHO classification of brain tumors. Neuroimaging Clin N Am 1999;9(4): 595–613.
2. Kleihues P, Soylemezoglu F, Schauble B, et al. Histopathology, classification, and grading of gliomas. Glia 1995;15(3):211–21.
3. Louis DN, Holland EC, Cairncross JG. Glioma classification: a molecular reappraisal. Am J Pathol 2001;159(3):779–86.
4. Furnari FB, Huang HJ, Cavenee WK. Genetics and malignant progression of human brain tumours. Cancer Surv 1995;25:233–75.
5. Ichimura K, Bolin MB, Goike HM, et al. Deregulation of the p14ARF/MDM2/p53 pathway is a prerequisite for human astrocytic gliomas with G1-S transition control gene abnormalities. Cancer Res 2000; 60(2):417–24.
6. Jacobs AH, Thomas A, Kracht LW, et al. 18F-fluoro-L-thymidine and 11C-methylmethionine as markers of increased transport and proliferation in brain tumors. J Nucl Med 2005;46(12):1948–58.
7. Coleman RE, Hoffman JM, Hanson MW, et al. Clinical application of PET for the evaluation of brain tumors. J Nucl Med 1991;32(4):616–22.
8. Herholz K, Wienhard K, Heiss WD. Validity of PET studies in brain tumors. Cerebrovasc Brain Metab Rev 1990;2(3):240–65.
9. Price P. PET as a potential tool for imaging molecular mechanisms of oncology in man. Trends Mol Med 2001;7(10):442–6.
10. Jacobs AH, Dittmar C, Winkeler A, et al. Molecular imaging of gliomas. Mol Imaging 2002;1(4): 309–35.
11. Utriainen M, Komu M, Vuorinen V, et al. Evaluation of brain tumor metabolism with [11C]choline PET and 1H-MRS. J Neurooncol 2003;62(3):329–38.
12. Tian M, Zhang H, Oriuchi N, et al. Comparison of 11C-choline PET and FDG PET for the differential diagnosis of malignant tumors. Eur J Nucl Med Mol Imaging 2004;31(8):1064–72.
13. Heiss WD, Pawlik G, Herholz K, et al. Regional kinetic constants and cerebral metabolic rate for glucose in normal human volunteers determined by dynamic positron emission tomography of [18F]-2-fluoro-2-deoxy-D-glucose. J Cereb Blood Flow Metab 1984;4(2):212–23.
14. Phelps ME. PET: the merging of biology and imaging into molecular imaging. J Nucl Med 2000;41(4):661–81.
15. Kitajima K, Nakamoto Y, Okizuka H, et al. Accuracy of whole-body FDG-PET/CT for detecting brain metastases from non-central nervous system tumors. Ann Nucl Med 2008;22(7):595–602.
16. Miwa K, Shinoda J, Yano H, et al. Discrepancy between lesion distributions on methionine PET and MR images in patients with glioblastoma multiforme: insight from a PET and MR fusion image study. J Neurol Neurosurg Psychiatr 2004;75(10): 1457–62.
17. Pirotte B, Goldman S, Dewitte O, et al. Integrated positron emission tomography and magnetic resonance imaging-guided resection of brain tumors: a report of 103 consecutive procedures. J Neurosurg 2006;104(2):238–53.
18. Pichler BJ, Judenhofer MS, Wehrl HF. PET/MRI hybrid imaging: devices and initial results. Eur Radiol 2008;18(6):1077–86.
19. Judenhofer MS, Wehrl HF, Newport DF, et al. Simultaneous PET-MRI: a new approach for functional and morphological imaging. Nat Med 2008;14(4): 459–65.
20. Weber G. Enzymology of cancer cells (first of two parts). N Engl J Med 1977;296(9):486–92.
21. Hatanaka M, Augl C, Gilden RV. Evidence for a functional change in the plasma membrane of murine sarcoma virus-infected mouse embryo cells. Transport and transport-associated phosphorylation of 14C-2-deoxy-D-glucose. J Biol Chem 1970;245(4):714–7.
22. Gallagher BM, Fowler JS, Gutterson NI, et al. Metabolic trapping as a principle of radiopharmaceutical design: some factors resposible for the biodistribution of [18F] 2-deoxy-2-fluoro-D-glucose. J Nucl Med 1978;19(10):1154–61.

23. Merrall NW, Plevin R, Gould GW. Growth factors, mitogens, oncogenes and the regulation of glucose transport. Cell Signal 1993;5(6):667–75.

24. Nishioka T, Oda Y, Seino Y, et al. Distribution of the glucose transporters in human brain tumors. Cancer Res 1992;52(14):3972–9.

25. Floeth FW, Pauleit D, Sabel M, et al. 18F-FET PET differentiation of ring-enhancing brain lesions. J Nucl Med 2006;47(5):776–82.

26. Zhuang H, Alavi A. 18-fluorodeoxyglucose positron emission tomographic imaging in the detection and monitoring of infection and inflammation. Semin Nucl Med 2002;32(1):47–59.

27. Kubota R, Yamada S, Kubota K, et al. Intratumoral distribution of fluorine-18-fluorodeoxyglucose in vivo: high accumulation in macrophages and granulation tissues studied by microautoradiography. J Nucl Med 1992;33(11):1972–80.

28. Chakrabarti R, Jung CY, Lee TP, et al. Changes in glucose transport and transporter isoforms during the activation of human peripheral blood lymphocytes by phytohemagglutinin. J Immunol 1994; 152(6):2660–8.

29. Gamelli RL, Liu H, He LK, et al. Augmentations of glucose uptake and glucose transporter-1 in macrophages following thermal injury and sepsis in mice. J Leukoc Biol 1996;59(5):639–47.

30. Sorbara LR, Maldarelli F, Chamoun G, et al. Human immunodeficiency virus type 1 infection of H9 cells induces increased glucose transporter expression. J Virol 1996;70(10):7275–9.

31. Ahmed N, Kansara M, Berridge MV. Acute regulation of glucose transport in a monocyte-macrophage cell line: Glut-3 affinity for glucose is enhanced during the respiratory burst. Biochem J 1997;327(Pt 2):369–75.

32. Janus TJ, Kim EE, Tilbury R, et al. Use of [18F]fluorodeoxyglucose positron emission tomography in patients with primary malignant brain tumors. Ann Neurol 1993;33(5):540–8.

33. Spence AM, Muzi M, Mankoff DA, et al. 18F-FDG PET of gliomas at delayed intervals: improved distinction between tumor and normal gray matter. J Nucl Med 2004;45(10):1653–9.

34. Herholz K, Pietrzyk U, Voges J, et al. Correlation of glucose consumption and tumor cell density in astrocytomas. A stereotactic PET study. J Neurosurg 1993;79(6):853–8.

35. Hustinx R, Smith RJ, Benard F, et al. Can the standardized uptake value characterize primary brain tumors on FDG-PET? Eur J Nucl Med 1999; 26(11):1501–9.

36. Kubota K. From tumor biology to clinical PET: a review of positron emission tomography (PET) in oncology. Ann Nucl Med 2001;15(6):471–86.

37. Kim S, Chung JK, Im SH, et al. 11C-methionine PET as a prognostic marker in patients with glioma comparison with 18F-FDG PET. Eur J Nucl Med Mol Imaging 2005;32(1):52–9.

38. Delbeke D, Meyerowitz C, Lapidus RL, et al. Optimal cutoff levels of F-18 fluorodeoxyglucose uptake in the differentiation of low-grade from high-grade brain tumors with PET. Radiology 1995;195(1):47–52.

39. Kaschten B, Stevenaert A, Sadzot B, et al. Preoperative evaluation of 54 gliomas by PET with fluorine-18-fluorodeoxyglucose and/or carbon-11-methionine. J Nucl Med 1998;39(5):778–85.

40. Ogawa T, Inugami A, Hatazawa J, et al. Clinical positron emission tomography for brain tumors: comparison of fludeoxyglucose F 18 and L-methyl-11C-methionine. AJNR Am J Neuroradiol 1996; 17(2):345–53.

41. Tsuchida T, Takeuchi H, Okazawa H, et al. Grading of brain glioma with 1-11C-acetate PET: comparison with 18F-FDG PET. Nucl Med Biol 2008; 35(2):171–6.

42. Herholz K, Rudolf J, Heiss WD. FDG transport and phosphorylation in human gliomas measured with dynamic PET. J Neurooncol 1992;12(2):159–65.

43. Fischman AJ, Alpert NM. FDG-PET in oncology: there's more to it than looking at pictures. J Nucl Med 1993;34(1):6–11.

44. Stockhammer F, Thomale UW, Plotkin M, et al. Association between fluorine-18-labeled fluorodeoxyglucose uptake and 1p and 19q loss of heterozygosity in World Health Organization Grade II gliomas. J Neurosurg 2007;106(4):633–7.

45. Di Chiro G. Positron emission tomography using [18F] fluorodeoxyglucose in brain tumors. A powerful diagnostic and prognostic tool. Invest Radiol 1987;22(5):360–71.

46. Alavi JB, Alavi A, Chawluk J, et al. Positron emission tomography in patients with glioma. A predictor of prognosis. Cancer 1988;62(6):1074–8.

47. Kim CK, Alavi JB, Alavi A, et al. New grading system of cerebral gliomas using positron emission tomography with F-18 fluorodeoxyglucose. J Neurooncol 1991;10(1):85–91.

48. Barker FG 2nd, Chang SM, Valk PE, et al. 18-Fluorodeoxyglucose uptake and survival of patients with suspected recurrent malignant glioma. Cancer 1997;79(1):115–26.

49. Padma MV, Said S, Jacobs M, et al. Prediction of pathology and survival by FDG PET in gliomas. J Neurooncol 2003;64(3):227–37.

50. Patronas NJ, Di Chiro G, Kufta C, et al. Prediction of survival in glioma patients by means of positron emission tomography. J Neurosurg 1985;62(6): 816–22.

51. Tyler JL, Diksic M, Villemure JG, et al. Metabolic and hemodynamic evaluation of gliomas using positron emission tomography. J Nucl Med 1987; 28(7):1123–33.

52. Rozental JM, Cohen JD, Mehta MP, et al. Acute changes in glucose uptake after treatment: the effects of carmustine (BCNU) on human glioblastoma multiforme. J Neurooncol 1993;15(1):57–66.

53. Kosaka N, Tsuchida T, Uematsu H, et al. 18F-FDG PET of common enhancing malignant brain tumors. Am J Roentgenol 2008;190(6):W365–9.

54. Kato T, Shinoda J, Nakayama N, et al. Metabolic assessment of gliomas using 11C-methionine, [18F] fluorodeoxyglucose, and 11C-choline positron-emission tomography. Am J Neuroradiol 2008;29(6):1176–82.

55. Cremerius U, Striepecke E, Henn W, et al. [18FDG-PET in intracranial meningiomas versus grading, proliferation index, cellular density and cytogenetic analysis]. Nuklearmedizin 1994;33(4):144–9.

56. Henry JM, Heffner RR Jr, Dillard SH, et al. Primary malignant lymphomas of the central nervous system. Cancer 1974;34(4):1293–302.

57. Kracht LW, Bauer A, Herholz K, et al. Positron emission tomography in a case of intracranial hemangiopericytoma. J Comput Assist Tomogr 1999;23(3):365–8.

58. Kim EE, Chung SK, Haynie TP, et al. Differentiation of residual or recurrent tumors from post-treatment changes with F-18 FDG PET. Radiographics 1992; 12(2):269–79.

59. Wurker M, Herholz K, Voges J, et al. Glucose consumption and methionine uptake in low-grade gliomas after iodine-125 brachytherapy. Eur J Nucl Med 1996;23(5):583–6.

60. Brock CS, Young H, O'Reilly SM, et al. Early evaluation of tumour metabolic response using [18F]fluorodeoxyglucose and positron emission tomography: a pilot study following the phase II chemotherapy schedule for temozolomide in recurrent high-grade gliomas. Br J Cancer 2000;82(3):608–15.

61. Reinhardt MJ, Kubota K, Yamada S, et al. Assessment of cancer recurrence in residual tumors after fractionated radiotherapy: a comparison of fluorodeoxyglucose, L-methionine and thymidine. J Nucl Med 1997;38(2):280–7.

62. Yamamoto T, Nishizawa S, Maruyama I, et al. Acute effects of stereotactic radiosurgery on the kinetics of glucose metabolism in metastatic brain tumors: FDG PET study. Ann Nucl Med 2001;15(2):103–9.

63. De Witte O, Levivier M, Violon P, et al. Prognostic value positron emission tomography with [18F]fluoro-2-deoxy-D-glucose in the low-grade glioma. Neurosurgery 1996;39(3):470–6 [discussion: 6–7].

64. Glantz MJ, Hoffman JM, Coleman RE, et al. Identification of early recurrence of primary central nervous system tumors by [18F]fluorodeoxyglucose positron emission tomography. Ann Neurol 1991;29(4):347–55.

65. Langleben DD, Segall GM. PET in differentiation of recurrent brain tumor from radiation injury. J Nucl Med 2000;41(11):1861–7.

66. Ricci PE, Karis JP, Heiserman JE, et al. Differentiating recurrent tumor from radiation necrosis: time for re-evaluation of positron emission tomography? Am J Neuroradiol 1998;19(3):407–13.

67. Henze M, Mohammed A, Schlemmer HP, et al. PET and SPECT for detection of tumor progression in irradiated low-grade astrocytoma: a receiver-operating-characteristic analysis. J Nucl Med 2004; 45(4):579–86.

68. Fulham MJ, Brunetti A, Aloj L, et al. Decreased cerebral glucose metabolism in patients with brain tumors: an effect of corticosteroids. J Neurosurg 1995;83(4):657–64.

69. Wong TZ, Turkington TG, Hawk TC, et al. PET and brain tumor image fusion. Cancer J 2004;10(4): 234–42.

70. Kahn D, Follett KA, Bushnell DL, et al. Diagnosis of recurrent brain tumor: value of 201Tl SPECT vs 18F-fluorodeoxyglucose PET. Am J Roentgenol 1994;163(6):1459–65.

71. Ortega-Lopez N, Mendoza-Vasquez RG, Adame-Ocampo G, et al. [Validation of MRI and 18F-FDG-PET coregistration in patients with primary brain tumors]. Gac Med Mex 2007; 143(4):309–16.

72. Wong TZ, van der Westhuizen GJ, Coleman RE. Positron emission tomography imaging of brain tumors. Neuroimaging Clin N Am 2002;12(4):615–26.

73. Pirotte B, Goldman S, Brucher JM, et al. PET in stereotactic conditions increases the diagnostic yield of brain biopsy. Stereotact Funct Neurosurg 1994;63(1–4):144–9.

74. Levivier M, Goldman S, Pirotte B, et al. Diagnostic yield of stereotactic brain biopsy guided by positron emission tomography with [18F]fluorodeoxyglucose. J Neurosurg 1995;82(3):445–52.

75. Goldman S, Levivier M, Pirotte B, et al. Regional methionine and glucose uptake in high-grade gliomas: a comparative study on PET-guided stereotactic biopsy. J Nucl Med 1997;38(9): 1459–62.

76. Massager N, David P, Goldman S, et al. Combined magnetic resonance imaging- and positron emission tomography-guided stereotactic biopsy in brainstem mass lesions: diagnostic yield in a series of 30 patients. J Neurosurg 2000;93(6):951–7.

77. Jager PL, Vaalburg W, Pruim J, et al. Radiolabeled amino acids: basic aspects and clinical applications in oncology. J Nucl Med 2001;42(3): 432–45.

78. Isselbacher KJ. Sugar and amino acid transport by cells in culture–differences between normal and malignant cells. N Engl J Med 1972;286(17): 929–33.

79. Bergstrom M, Ericson K, Hagenfeldt L, et al. PET study of methionine accumulation in glioma and normal brain tissue: competition with branched

chain amino acids. J Comput Assist Tomogr 1987; 11(2):208–13.

80. Bergstrom M, Lundqvist H, Ericson K, et al. Comparison of the accumulation kinetics of L-(methyl-11C)-methionine and D-(methyl-11C)-methionine in brain tumors studied with positron emission tomography. Acta Radiol 1987;28(3): 225–9.

81. Sato N, Suzuki M, Kuwata N, et al. Evaluation of the malignancy of glioma using 11C-methionine positron emission tomography and proliferating cell nuclear antigen staining. Neurosurg Rev 1999; 22(4):210–4.

82. Lilja A, Bergstrom K, Hartvig P, et al. Dynamic study of supratentorial gliomas with L-methyl-11C-methionine and positron emission tomography. Am J Neuroradiol 1985;6(4):505–14.

83. Derlon JM, Bourdet C, Bustany P, et al. [11C]L-methionine uptake in gliomas. Neurosurgery 1989;25(5):720–8.

84. O'Tuama LA, Phillips PC, Strauss LC, et al. Two-phase [11C]L-methionine PET in childhood brain tumors. Pediatr Neurol 1990;6(3):163–70.

85. Ogawa T, Shishido F, Kanno I, et al. Cerebral glioma: evaluation with methionine PET. Radiology 1993;186(1):45–53.

86. Chung JK, Kim YK, Kim SK, et al. Usefulness of 11C-methionine PET in the evaluation of brain lesions that are hypo- or isometabolic on 18F-FDG PET. Eur J Nucl Med Mol Imaging 2002; 29(2):176–82.

87. Herholz K, Holzer T, Bauer B, et al. 11C-methionine PET for differential diagnosis of low-grade gliomas. Neurology 1998;50(5):1316–22.

88. Bergstrom M, Collins VP, Ehrin E, et al. Discrepancies in brain tumor extent as shown by computed tomography and positron emission tomography using [68Ga]EDTA, [11C]glucose, and [11C]methionine. J Comput Assist Tomogr 1983;7(6):1062–6.

89. Mosskin M, Ericson K, Hindmarsh T, et al. Positron emission tomography compared with magnetic resonance imaging and computed tomography in supratentorial gliomas using multiple stereotactic biopsies as reference. Acta Radiol 1989;30(3): 225–32.

90. Pirotte B, Goldman S, David P, et al. Stereotactic brain biopsy guided by positron emission tomography (PET) with [F-18]fluorodeoxyglucose and [C-11]methionine. Acta Neurochir Suppl 1997;68: 133–8.

91. Kapouleas I, Alavi A, Alves WM, et al. Registration of three-dimensional MR and PET images of the human brain without markers. Radiology 1991; 181(3):731–9.

92. Derlon JM, Petit-Taboue MC, Chapon F, et al. The in vivo metabolic pattern of low-grade brain gliomas: a positron emission tomographic study using 18F-fluorodeoxyglucose and 11C-L-methylmethionine. Neurosurgery 1997;40(2):276–87 [discussion: 87–8].

93. Mosskin M, Bergstrom M, Collins VP, et al. Positron emission tomography with 11C-methionine of intracranial tumours compared with histology of multiple biopsies. Acta Radiol Suppl 1986;369:157–60.

94. Van Laere K, Ceyssens S, Van Calenbergh F, et al. Direct comparison of 18F-FDG and 11C-methionine PET in suspected recurrence of glioma: sensitivity, inter-observer variability and prognostic value. Eur J Nucl Med Mol Imaging 2005;32(1): 39–51.

95. De Witte O, Goldberg I, Wikler D, et al. Positron emission tomography with injection of methionine as a prognostic factor in glioma. J Neurosurg 2001;95(5):746–50.

96. Piepmeier J, Christopher S, Spencer D, et al. Variations in the natural history and survival of patients with supratentorial low-grade astrocytomas. Neurosurgery 1996;38(5):872–8 [discussion: 8–9].

97. Lote K, Egeland T, Hager B, et al. Survival, prognostic factors, and therapeutic efficacy in low-grade glioma: a retrospective study in 379 patients. J Clin Oncol 1997;15(9):3129–40.

98. Ribom D, Eriksson A, Hartman M, et al. Positron emission tomography (11)C-methionine and survival in patients with low-grade gliomas. Cancer 2001; 92(6):1541–9.

99. Ogawa T, Kanno I, Shishido F, et al. Clinical value of PET with 18F-fluorodeoxyglucose and L-methyl-11C-methionine for diagnosis of recurrent brain tumor and radiation injury. Acta Radiol 1991; 32(3):197–202.

100. Lilja A, Lundqvist H, Olsson Y, et al. Positron emission tomography and computed tomography in differential diagnosis between recurrent or residual glioma and treatment-induced brain lesions. Acta Radiol 1989;30(2):121–8.

101. Sonoda Y, Kumabe T, Takahashi T, et al. Clinical usefulness of 11C-MET PET and 201T1 SPECT for differentiation of recurrent glioma from radiation necrosis. Neurol Med Chir (Tokyo) 1998;38(6): 342–7 [discussion: 7–8].

102. Levivier M, Wikler D, Goldman S, et al. Integration of the metabolic data of positron emission tomography in the dosimetry planning of radiosurgery with the gamma knife: early experience with brain tumors. Technical note. J Neurosurg 2000;93(Suppl 3):233–8.

103. Levivier M, Wikler D Jr, Massager N, et al. The integration of metabolic imaging in stereotactic procedures including radiosurgery: a review. J Neurosurg 2002;97(5 Suppl):542–50.

104. Wienhard K, Herholz K, Coenen HH, et al. Increased amino acid transport into brain tumors measured by PET of L-(2-18F)fluorotyrosine. J Nucl Med 1991;32(7):1338–46.

105. Pruim J, Willemsen AT, Molenaar WM, et al. Brain tumors: L-[1-C-11]tyrosine PET for visualization and quantification of protein synthesis rate. Radiology 1995;197(1):221–6.

106. Kuwert T, Morgenroth C, Woesler B, et al. Uptake of iodine-123-alpha-methyl tyrosine by gliomas and non-neoplastic brain lesions. Eur J Nucl Med 1996;23(10):1345–53.

107. Bader JB, Samnick S, Moringlane JR, et al. Evaluation of I-3-[123I]iodo-alpha-methyltyrosine SPET and [18F]fluorodeoxyglucose PET in the detection and grading of recurrences in patients pretreated for gliomas at follow-up: a comparative study with stereotactic biopsy. Eur J Nucl Med 1999;26(2):144–51.

108. Biersack HJ, Coenen HH, Stocklin G, et al. Imaging of brain tumors with L-3-[123I]iodo-alpha-methyl tyrosine and SPECT. J Nucl Med 1989;30(1):110–2.

109. Chen W, Silverman DH, Delaloye S, et al. 18F-FDOPA PET imaging of brain tumors: comparison study with 18F-FDG PET and evaluation of diagnostic accuracy. J Nucl Med 2006;47(6):904–11.

110. de Wolde H, Pruim J, Mastik MF, et al. Proliferative activity in human brain tumors: comparison of histopathology and L-[1-(11)C]tyrosine PET. J Nucl Med 1997;38(9):1369–74.

111. Langen KJ, Jarosch M, Muhlensiepen H, et al. Comparison of fluorotyrosines and methionine uptake in F98 rat gliomas. Nucl Med Biol 2003; 30(5):501–8.

112. Weber WA, Wester HJ, Grosu AL, et al. O-(2-[18F]fluoroethyl)-L-tyrosine and L-[methyl-11C]methionine uptake in brain tumours: initial results of a comparative study. Eur J Nucl Med 2000;27(5):542–9.

113. Floeth FW, Pauleit D, Sabel M, et al. Prognostic value of O-(2-18F-fluoroethyl)-L-tyrosine PET and MRI in low-grade glioma. J Nucl Med 2007;48(4):519–27.

114. Floeth FW, Sabel M, Stoffels G, et al. Prognostic value of 18F-fluoroethyl-L-tyrosine PET and MRI in small nonspecific incidental brain lesions. J Nucl Med 2008;49(5):730–7.

115. Mehrkens JH, Popperl G, Rachinger W, et al. The positive predictive value of O-(2-[18F]fluoroethyl)-L-tyrosine (FET) PET in the diagnosis of a glioma recurrence after multimodal treatment. J Neurooncol 2008;88(1):27–35.

116. Langen KJ, Roosen N, Coenen HH, et al. Brain and brain tumor uptake of L-3-[123I]iodo-alpha-methyl tyrosine: competition with natural L-amino acids. J Nucl Med 1991;32(6):1225–9.

117. Conti PS. Introduction to imaging brain tumor metabolism with positron emission tomography (PET). Cancer Invest 1995;13(2):244–59.

118. Grosu AL, Weber W, Feldmann HJ, et al. First experience with I-123-alpha-methyl-tyrosine spect in the 3-D radiation treatment planning of brain gliomas. Int J Radiat Oncol Biol Phys 2000;47(2):517–26.

119. Langen KJ, Ziemons K, Kiwit JC, et al. 3-[123I]iodo-alpha-methyltyrosine and [methyl-11C]-L-methionine uptake in cerebral gliomas: a comparative study using SPECT and PET. J Nucl Med 1997;38(4):517–22.

120. Shinoura N, Nishijima M, Hara T, et al. Brain tumors: detection with C-11 choline PET. Radiology 1997;202(2):497–503.

121. Ohtani T, Kurihara H, Ishiuchi S, et al. Brain tumour imaging with carbon-11 choline: comparison with FDG PET and gadolinium-enhanced MR imaging. Eur J Nucl Med 2001;28(11):1664–70.

122. Hara T, Kosaka N, Shinoura N, et al. PET imaging of brain tumor with [methyl-11C]choline. J Nucl Med 1997;38(6):842–7.

123. Chen W, Cloughesy T, Kamdar N, et al. Imaging proliferation in brain tumors with 18F-FLT PET: comparison with 18F-FDG. J Nucl Med 2005;46(6):945–52.

124. Choi SJ, Kim JS, Kim JH, et al. [18F]3'-deoxy-3'-fluorothymidine PET for the diagnosis and grading of brain tumors. Eur J Nucl Med Mol Imaging 2005;32(6):653–9.

125. Saga T, Kawashima H, Araki N, et al. Evaluation of primary brain tumors with FLT-PET: usefulness and limitations. Clin Nucl Med 2006;31(12):774–80.

126. Hatakeyama T, Kawai N, Nishiyama Y, et al. (11)C-methionine (MET) and (18)F-fluorothymidine (FLT) PET in patients with newly diagnosed glioma. Eur J Nucl Med Mol Imaging 2008;35(11):2009–17.

127. Shields AF, Grierson JR, Dohmen BM, et al. Imaging proliferation in vivo with [F-18]FLT and positron emission tomography. Nat Med 1998;4(11):1334–6.

128. Hengstschlager M, Knofler M, Mullner EW, et al. Different regulation of thymidine kinase during the cell cycle of normal versus DNA tumor virus-transformed cells. J Biol Chem 1994;269(19):13836–42.

129. Brown JM, Giaccia AJ. Tumour hypoxia: the picture has changed in the 1990s. Int J Radiat Biol 1994;65(1):95–102.

130. Gray LH, Conger AD, Ebert M, et al. The concentration of oxygen dissolved in tissues at the time of irradiation as a factor in radiotherapy. Br J Radiol 1953;26(312):638–48.

131. Janssen HL, Haustermans KM, Balm AJ, et al. Hypoxia in head and neck cancer: how much, how important? Head Neck 2005;27(7):622–38.

132. Hockel M, Schlenger K, Aral B, et al. Association between tumor hypoxia and malignant progression

in advanced cancer of the uterine cervix. Cancer Res 1996;56(19):4509–15.

133. Brizel DM, Scully SP, Harrelson JM, et al. Tumor oxygenation predicts for the likelihood of distant metastases in human soft tissue sarcoma. Cancer Res 1996;56(5):941–3.

134. Brizel DM, Sibley GS, Prosnitz LR, et al. Tumor hypoxia adversely affects the prognosis of carcinoma of the head and neck. Int J Radiat Oncol Biol Phys 1997;38(2):285–9.

135. Evans SM, Jenkins WT, Joiner B, et al. 2-Nitroimidazole (EF5) binding predicts radiation resistance in individual 9L s.c. tumors. Cancer Res 1996;56(2):405–11.

136. Koch CJ, Evans SM, Lord EM. Oxygen dependence of cellular uptake of EF5 [2-(2-nitro-1H-imidazol-1-yl)-N-(2,2,3,3,3-pentafluoropropyl) acetamide]: analysis of drug adducts by fluorescent antibodies vs bound radioactivity. Br J Cancer 1995;72(4):869–74.

137. Ziemer LS, Evans SM, Kachur AV, et al. Noninvasive imaging of tumor hypoxia in rats using the 2-nitroimidazole 18F-EF5. Eur J Nucl Med Mol Imaging 2003;30(2):259–66.

Investigation of Nonneoplastic Neurologic Disorders with PET and MRI

Erik S. Musiek, MD, PhD[a], Drew A. Torigian, MD, MA[b,c,d],
Andrew B. Newberg, MD[e],*

KEYWORDS

- Neurologic • Neurodegenerative • Alzheimer
- Dementia • Brain • Positron emission tomography
- MR imaging • PET/MR imaging

Positron emission tomography (PET) has emerged over the past 30 years as the preeminent method with which to image the biodistribution of radionuclides and has proved to be particularly advantageous for imaging of the brain. Positron emitting radionuclides, such as ^{11}C, ^{18}F, and ^{13}N, can be used to produce a vast number of tracers that are usable for studying body chemistry and function. The emitted positron travels a short distance before collision with an electron, annihilating to produce two 511-keV γ-rays that travel in opposite directions approximately 180° from each other. Because of this phenomenon, modern PET instruments use coincidence detection of photons to minimize background image noise, and thus have approached the theoretic image resolution limit of 3 to 5 mm, resulting in considerable improvement of image quality over other emission tomography methods.[1]

The synthesis of ^{18}F-fluorodeoxyglucose (FDG) was a major development, enabling the study of regional brain metabolism and function using PET.[1,2] FDG, the most commonly employed PET radiotracer, is used to measure the cerebral metabolic rate for glucose (CMRGlc).[1,3] These tracers have been used to investigate a wide variety of neurologic disorders, such as dementia and stroke, but have also been utilized to study the effects of various physiologic stimuli on the human central nervous system. In addition, many other positron emitting compounds, including neurotransmitter analogues, have been synthesized over the past 2 decades for measuring receptor and other chemical activities.[4–7] Recently, the development of novel radiopharmaceutic agents that bind to cerebral amyloid plaques has expanded the role of PET in the diagnosis and investigation of dementia.[8,9] This review discusses the applications of PET in the study and diagnosis

This work was supported, in part, by grants R01-AG028688 and R01 AG-17524.
[a] Department of Neurology, University of Pennsylvania Medical Center, 110 Donner Building, 3400 Spruce Street, Philadelphia, PA 19104, USA
[b] Division of Thoracic Imaging, Department of Radiology, University of Pennsylvania Medical Center, 110 Donner Building, 3400 Spruce Street, Philadelphia, PA 19104, USA
[c] Division of Body Computed Tomography, Department of Radiology, University of Pennsylvania Medical Center, 110 Donner Building, 3400 Spruce Street, Philadelphia, PA 19104, USA
[d] Division of Body MR Imaging, Department of Radiology, University of Pennsylvania Medical Center, 110 Donner Building, 3400 Spruce Street, Philadelphia, PA 19104, USA
[e] Division of Nuclear Medicine, Department of Radiology, University of Pennsylvania Medical Center, 110 Donner Building, 3400 Spruce Street, Philadelphia, PA 19104, USA
* Corresponding author.
E-mail address: andrew.newberg@uphs.upenn.edu (A.B. Newberg).

of neurologic disease and emphasizes the emerging role for combined PET and MR imaging in neuroimaging.

ALZHEIMER DISEASE

Alzheimer disease (AD) is the most common cause of dementia in the United States but remains a clinical diagnosis and requires postmortem pathologic confirmation for definitive diagnosis. Unfortunately, extensive and potentially irreversible damage has often occurred before AD becomes clinically evident, making the development of preventative therapies difficult. Furthermore, although it is possible to make an accurate diagnosis of AD in most patients who have severe disease, it is difficult to differentiate between AD and other dementing disorders in patients who have mild disease.[10–12] Because of its ability to image distinct molecular events, PET has emerged as an extremely promising modality for imaging the brain in AD. Initial efforts in the study of AD using PET centered on the measurement of CMRGlc using FDG-PET, whereas the recent development of amyloid-binding radioligands has sparked extensive new research. Coregistration of functional data from PET with structural data from MR imaging has allowed a greater degree of anatomic resolution and more precise diagnostic accuracy.

Since 1980, numerous studies have used PET in the assessment of patients who have AD.[13–19] Initial FDG-PET studies comparing CMRGlc in patients who had AD with that in age-matched healthy controls (**Fig. 1**) showed that there is a 20% to 30% decrease in whole-brain CMRGlc values in patients who have AD compared with healthy age-matched controls.[20,21] Other studies showed that patients who have AD have decreased whole-brain CMRGlc and that the bilateral parietal and temporal lobes are particularly affected.[22–24] Bilateral parietal hypometabolism is considered a "typical" FDG-PET pattern in AD (**Fig. 2**) and is highly predictive of AD.[15,21,25] This pattern is not pathognomonic for AD, however, and may be seen in patients who have Parkinson disease (PD), bilateral parietal subdural hematomas, bilateral parietal stroke, and bilateral parietal radiation therapy ports.[26]

Importantly, the magnitude and extent of regional hypometabolism on FDG-PET seems to correlate with the severity of the dementia symptoms.[27,28] Moderately affected patients show significantly decreased metabolism in the left midfrontal lobes, bilateral parietal lobes, and superior temporal regions, and these deficits show a similar distribution but of greater degree in advanced AD.

Hypometabolism appears in the cingulate cortex and medial temporal lobe early in the disease course and then involves the temporoparietal, frontal, and subcortical areas at later stages.[29,30] In all patients, the parietal lobes show the greatest change, with a 38% decrease in patients who have moderate AD and a 53% decrease in patients who have severe AD. Haxby and colleagues[22] showed that the premotor cortex had a similar decrease as the parietal association cortex in moderately and severely demented patients. Furthermore, the metabolic ratio between the parietal and premotor cortices and the parietal and prefrontal cortices correlates significantly with the degree of cognitive impairment in patients who have moderate dementia. CMRGlc values decrease more rapidly over time in patients who have AD than in age-matched control subjects.[21] Voxel-based analysis showed a significant decline in metabolism in the parietal, temporal, occipital, frontal, and posterior cingulate cortices in AD after 1 year of disease progression.[31] Studies correlating CMRGlc to Mini-Mental Status Examination scores and other neuropsychologic testing have consistently shown a relation between these measures in patients who have AD, which has been particularly true when parietal and temporal lobe metabolic rates have been compared with neuropsychologic deficits.[16,21,32–34]

Most importantly, FDG-PET imaging seems to increase the accuracy of AD diagnosis. Mosconi and colleagues[35] examined FDG-PET scans from more than 500 patients and used an automated voxel-based method to devise criteria that correctly identified 95% of patients who had AD, 92% of those who had dementia with Lewy bodies, 94% of those who had frontotemporal dementia (FTD), and 94% of normal controls. Silverman and colleagues[36] imaged 284 patients at initial presentation for dementia assessment using FDG-PET and then reimaged these patients at follow-up an average of 2.9 years later. This group identified several patterns of hypometabolism defining patients as PET-positive for AD and found FDG-PET to be 94% sensitive and 73% specific for diagnosing AD and that patients with a negative PET scan have a 0.1 likelihood ratio of developing dementia in the next 3 years. Jagust and colleagues[37] found that imaging patients with FDG-PET provided better diagnostic accuracy than clinical examination for diagnosis of AD and that FDG-PET was indicative of AD an average of 4 years before clinical evaluation. This evidence has led some neurologists to propose revision of the standard National Institute of Neurological and Communicative Disorders and Stroke and Alzheimer's Disease and Related Disorders

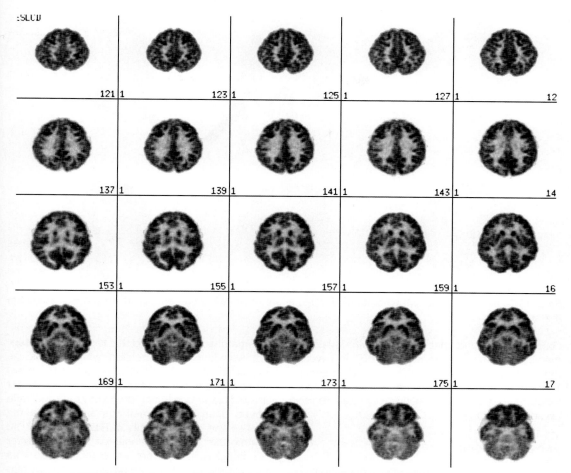

:SLCU

121 1	123 1	125 1	127 1	12
137 1	139 1	141 1	143 1	14
153 1	155 1	157 1	159 1	16
169 1	171 1	173 1	175 1	17

Fig. 1. Normal FDG-PET scan shows uniform and symmetric uptake in cortical and subcortical regions.

Association (NINCDS-ADRDA) AD diagnostic criteria to include FDG-PET imaging.[38]

Studies have also examined the ability of FDG-PET to determine the risk for conversion to AD in patients with mild cognitive impairment (MCI), a condition potentially thought to represent pre-AD.[39] Hypometabolism in expected regions in MCI has been confirmed in numerous studies, and often appears before the development of substantial clinical memory impairment.[40–42] Significant right frontoparietal hypometabolism was reliably identified in patients with MCI who subsequently converted to AD.[43] Significantly greater left parietal, left temporal, and bilateral frontal hypometabolism was identified in patients with MCI who later converted to AD as compared with those who did not.[44] Thus, FDG-PET shows promise in the potential early diagnosis of AD.

Because atrophy and hypometabolism occur in AD, several studies have attempted correction for brain atrophy, because PET scans do not have adequate resolution to separate metabolically inactive ventricular and sulcal cerebrospinal fluid spaces from the rest of the brain.[45,46] MR imaging volumetric determinations have been used to correct the CMRGlc values obtained by PET and have produced conflicting results, because patients who have AD have shown increased[47] or equivalent[48] cerebral metabolism as controls after correction for atrophy. This issue was recently addressed using combined MR imaging and FDG-PET with subsequent image coregistration and voxel-based analysis to compare regional atrophy versus hypometabolism. Interestingly, hypometabolism exceeded atrophy in several AD-affected regions, including the posterior cingulate, precuneus, orbitofrontal cortex, inferior temporoparietal cortex, parahippocampal, angular, and fusiform gyri regions. The hippocampus, a region known to be significantly impaired in AD, showed a similar degree of atrophy and hypometabolism, however.[49] Similarly, Mosconi and

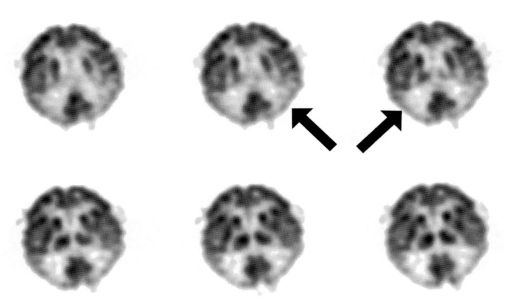

Fig. 2. FDG-PET scan in a patient who has mild to moderate AD shows typical temporoparietal hypometabolism (*arrows*).

colleagues[41] found that patients with MCI had marked hypometabolism on FDG-PET in several regions in the absence of atrophy on MR imaging. Thus, the relation between atrophy and hypometabolism in AD likely depends on brain region and disease stage.

AMYLOID IMAGING

In the past 5 years, significant efforts have focused on development of PET radioligands designed to image the cardinal pathologic hallmark of AD, the amyloid plaque. Amyloid plaques are insoluble extracellular aggregates of β-amyloid protein, and they are invariably found in affected regions of brains of patients who have AD. Amyloid plaques have a high degree of β-pleated sheet conformation and can be targeted with several dyes used in pathologic staining, including Congo red and thioflavin-T. Using these dyes as a model, to date, three distinct positron-emitting radioligands that bind to amyloid have been developed and tested in humans. Among these, N-methyl [^{11}C]2-(4′-methylaminophenyl-6-hydroxybenzathiazole), also known as Pittsburgh Compound B (PiB), has been the most thoroughly studied. PiB is a modified thioflavin-T derivative that readily crosses the blood-brain barrier, and PiB binding has been shown to reflect amyloid plaque content in human brain homogenates in vitro.[50] In 2003, Klunk and colleagues[8] demonstrated that PiB showed significantly increased retention in the disease-affected brain regions in 16 patients who had AD as compared with age-matched controls and that regional PiB retention was inversely correlated with CMRGlc as measured by FDG-PET. Several subsequent studies have confirmed the ability of PiB to detect amyloid plaques in patients who have AD and have refined quantification methods and verified the kinetics and reproducibility of PiB binding.[25,51–55] Postmortem pathologic analysis 3 months after PiB imaging in one patient demonstrated that areas of PiB retention also have high amyloid plaque content.[56] Further studies have demonstrated that in patients who have AD, PiB retention correlates positively with brain atrophy.[57] Controversy exists regarding correlation between PiB binding and disease severity, because some studies show a positive correlation,[58] whereas others do not.[54] A longitudinal analysis of PiB binding in AD showed that although PiB differentiated patients who have AD from controls on initial scanning, there was little increase in PiB binding at 2-year follow-up, despite progression of cognitive decline.[59] This study suggests that PiB intensity may plateau early in the course of the disease and may not be a useful marker of progression, and it also emphasizes the need for additional large long-term longitudinal studies to address this important issue.

Perhaps the most exciting potential application of amyloid imaging is in preclinical diagnosis of AD. Thus, numerous studies have used amyloid imaging techniques in patients with MCI, in the hope of predicting progression to fulminant AD. In a small study, 21 patients with MCI showed an intermediate degree of PiB binding, and those who converted to AD within 3 years showed the highest PiB uptake on initial scanning.[60] Kemppainen and colleagues[61] found that 8 of 13 patients with MCI had significantly higher PiB uptake in several disease-affected regions and that, as a group, patients with MCI had significantly higher PiB uptake than control patients. Several other studies have shown some overlap between AD and MCI and between MCI and normal aging.[62,63] For example, Pike and colleagues[64] showed that 97% of patients who had AD, 61% of patients with MCI, and 22% of control patients had significant PiB uptake, whereas 60% of patients with MCI showed "AD-like" PiB uptake in a second study.[54] It remains to be seen whether these presumed cognitively normal patients with positive PiB scans have early preclinical AD and progress to dementia. The "cognitive reserve" hypothesis may play a role in interpreting these studies, because a recent study shows that patients with higher education have significantly more amyloid deposition on PiB scans than less educated patients with a similar degree of cognitive impairment, suggesting that high-functioning patients remain cognitively intact further into the pathologic course of AD.[65] A study by Fotenos and colleagues[66] showed similar results when comparing high versus low socioeconomic status patients and analyzing PiB PET and volumetric MR imaging. Thus, further research is needed to develop methods to distinguish MCI fully from normal aging using PiB.

A shortcoming of currently available PiB is that it uses ^{11}C labeling, which has a short half-life, thus limiting its use to facilities with an on-site cyclotron. Three other molecularly distinct amyloid imaging PET ligands, which are labeled with ^{18}F, have been independently developed. The first, 2-(1-(6-[(2-[^{18}F]fluoroethyl)(methyl)amino]-2-naphthyl)ethylidene)malononitrile (FDDNP), binds with high affinity and specificity to amyloid plaques and neurofibrillary tangles.[67,68] FDDNP-PET imaging was performed in 25 patients with a clinical diagnosis of AD, 28 with MCI, and 28 normal controls, in conjunction with FDG-PET and volumetric MR imaging. FDDNP retention was greatest in disease-affected brain regions, correlated inversely with FDG-PET and brain volume, and was more accurate in distinguishing patients who had AD from controls than FDG-PET or volumetric MR imaging.[69] FDDNP also showed significantly increased binding in MCI, and is thus a promising candidate ligand for early AD diagnosis.

The second ^{18}F-labeled amyloid imaging agent is ^{18}F-BAY94-9172. Like PiB and FDDNP, ^{18}F-BAY94-9172 labeled disease-associated regions, including the frontal cortex, posterior cingulate,

and precuneus regions, in patients who had AD and showed significantly greater uptake in 15 patients who had AD than in 15 controls.[70] The investigators reported 100% sensitivity and 90% specificity for detection of AD, but no patients with MCI were included. Of note, an ^{18}F-labeled PiB is currently in development. FDDNP and ^{18}F-BAY94-9172 show promise for diagnosis of AD and would increase availability to more remote PET centers because of the extended half-life of ^{18}F; however, as is the case with PiB, larger studies are needed to define their utility.

Finally, the compound (E)-4-(2-(6-(2-(2-(2-[^{18}F]fluoroethoxy)ethoxy)ethoxy)pyridin-3-yl)vinyl)-N-methylbenzenamine ([^{18}F]-AV-45) has shown promise as another potential ^{18}F-labeled amyloid PET imaging agent (Fig. 3). Similar to the other agents, this compound has shown good sensitivity for differentiating patients who have AD from controls, and it is currently being evaluated and used in several clinical trials.

The combination of PiB PET with structural MR imaging allows for improved anatomic delineation and detection of regional changes in amyloid deposition, which is important for diagnosis of AD and differentiation from other dementing diseases. Mikhno and colleagues[71] found that voxel based-quantification involving MR imaging coregistration improved PiB quantification and allowed for automation of scan analysis. Jack and colleagues[63] examined the relation between volumetric MR imaging and PiB-PET in the diagnosis of AD. PiB retention was quantified using a combined score evaluating six regions of interest compared with the cerebellum (an uninvolved brain region that serves as a control in most studies). Frontal lobes showed increased PiB retention with minimal atrophy, whereas medial temporal lobes had an opposite profile. Ultimately, the combination of PiB-PET with MR imaging showed stronger correlation with cognitive performance than either modality alone, demonstrating that PiB and MR imaging provide complementary information and increase the accuracy of PiB imaging.[63]

In summary, the diagnosis of AD has proved quite difficult in early disease, and FDG-PET and amyloid-binding ligands show great promise not only for the radiologic premorbid diagnosis of AD but potentially for early or even presymptomatic diagnosis, thus opening the door for the development of a new generation of neuroprotective therapies.

FRONTOTEMPORAL DEMENTIA

FTD is a highly heterogeneous neurodegenerative dementia with a predilection for the frontal and

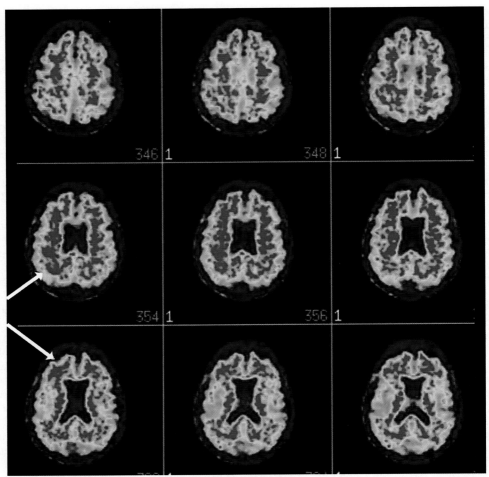

Fig. 3. ^{18}F-AV-45 amyloid PET scan in a patient who has AD shows extensive uptake throughout the cortex (*arrows*), particularly in the frontal cortices.

temporal lobes. FTD is called Pick disease when Pick bodies (argyrophilic inclusions) are present. FTD is associated with cognitive and language dysfunction, in addition to prominent behavioral changes, but can often be difficult to distinguish from AD in early stages. The most common finding in PET images is hypometabolism in the frontal and anterior temporal lobes bilaterally.[72–76] Hypometabolism appears first in the frontal lobes and then moves into the temporal and parietal lobes as the disease progresses.[77] This pattern of anterior hypometabolism is consistent with the findings on histopathologic examination, in addition to frontal and temporal lobe atrophy on CT and MR imaging.[73,78] Several studies have shown that addition of FDG-PET imaging to the diagnostic battery improved diagnostic accuracy, sensitivity, and specificity of FTD and aided in differentiation from AD.[79,80] The combination of volumetric MR imaging and FDG-PET has revealed that unlike AD, atrophy and hypometabolism occur concurrently in FTD.[81] Amyloid deposition is not a pathogenic feature of FTD. Thus, PiB-PET has shown excellent utility in differentiation of AD from FTD based on the absence of cortical PiB retention in FTD in two small studies,[54,82] although a third study described 4 of 12 patients who had FTD with a positive PiB scan.[83] Thus, FDG and PiB-PET are useful tools for the diagnosis of FTD and its differentiation from AD.

PARKINSON'S DISEASE

PD is caused by loss of the pigmented dopaminergic neurons in the substantia nigra and the locus coeruleus, and is characterized clinically by bradykinesia, resting tremor, and rigidity. The loss of pigmented neurons is associated with decreased production and storage of dopamine and nigrostriatal system dysfunction. It is believed that, initially, there is an "up-regulation" of dopamine receptors, followed by a down-regulation that occurs as the disease progresses.[84] A decrease in size of the substantia nigra pars compacta (SNpc), the site of dopaminergic cell bodies that project to the striatum, is a pathologic hallmark of PD and can be observed on MR imaging.[85] CT and MR imaging are used in the diagnosis of PD primarily to rule out other intracranial disorders, however. PET offers the ability to study not only cerebral metabolism but several aspects of dopaminergic neurotransmission, including dopamine synthesis, storage, and receptor expression, which may prove extremely useful in the diagnosis of PD and in the exploration of the pathophysiology of this disease.[86–88]

Several studies using FDG-PET have reported hypermetabolism in the basal ganglia in early untreated PD.[89,90] Other studies found no significant striatal changes in FDG metabolism in patients who had PD.[91,92] Another group reported decreases in glucose metabolism in the basal ganglia contralateral to the side of the symptoms in patients who had hemiparkinsonism-hemiatrophy syndrome.[93] More recently, FDG-PET has been used to identify metabolic changes in basal ganglia nuclei associated with PD, such as subthalamic nucleus and internal globus pallidus hyperactivity,[94,95] in addition to network changes that occur after deep brain stimulation.[96,97]

Dopaminergic dysfunction plays a primary role in PD, and a variety of radiotracers that can specifically measure the dopamine system have been developed. PET imaging in PD has also been performed with ^{18}F-fluoro-L-phenylalanine (DOPA) (Fig. 4), which is taken up by dopaminergic

neurons and converted to ^{18}F-dopamine by aromatic amino acid decarboxylase. ^{18}F-DOPA can be used to image dopaminergic cell mass in the SNpc and has revealed abnormalities in the nigrostriatal dopaminergic projections,[98–101] in addition to reduced basal ganglia activity in PD.[102,103] Reduced ^{18}F-DOPA uptake in the posterior putamen was observed in patients who had early untreated PD as compared with normal controls.[104] Garnett and colleagues[105] showed that in hemiparkinsonism, there is a marked decrease in ^{18}F-DOPA uptake in the contralateral basal ganglia. There is also decreased activity, although to a lesser extent, in the ipsilateral basal ganglia, however. ^{18}F-DOPA studies have also detected lesions in the dopaminergic pathway in patients who have parkinsonism caused by the parkinsonian toxin 1-methyl-4-phenyl-1,2,3,6-tetrahydropyridine (MPTP).[106] Decreased ^{18}F-DOPA uptake has also been described in asymptomatic members of a kindred who had familial PD, suggesting a role for ^{18}F-DOPA imaging in the presymptomatic diagnosis of PD.[107]

PET ligands have been developed that bind specifically to the presynaptic dopamine transporter, and they have revealed significant declines in dopamine transporter activity in PD.[108–111] Ligands with affinity for the presynaptic vesicular monoamine transporter VMAT2, which stores dopamine in the presynaptic terminal, have also been developed. One such ligand, ^{11}C-DTZB, showed decreased signal in the caudate and putamen of patients who had PD.[112] The relation between ^{18}F-DOPA, the dopamine transporter ligand ^{11}C-methyphenidate, and ^{11}C-DTZB in patients who have PD was explored by Lee and colleagues,[109] who demonstrated a compensatory up-regulation of ^{18}F-DOPA accumulation and dopamine

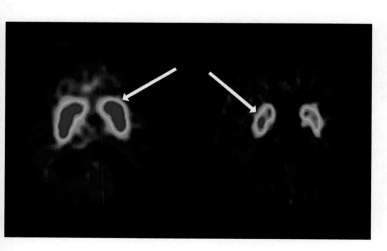

Fig. 4. ^{18}F-DOPA PET scans of a control subject (left) and a patient who has PD (right) show significantly decreased binding in the striatum in the patient who has PD (arrows).

transporter down-regulation as PD progresses. Another study showed decreased ^{11}C-methyl-phenidate binding, which preceded PD, in patients who had familial PD caused by mutations in leucine-rich repeat kinase 2.[113]

Radioligands that bind to dopamine receptors have provided more insight into nigrostriatal signaling changes in PD. The D2 ligand, ^{11}C-raclopride, has been used in patients who have PD. An increase in ^{11}C-raclopride activity (receptor up-regulation) has been observed in the striatum contralateral to hemiparkinsonian symptoms in early disease.[114,115] This corroborates the theory of initial up-regulation of dopamine receptors followed by subsequent down-regulation as the disease progresses.[116] A third D2 ligand, ^{18}F-des-methoxyfallypride, has shown utility in differentiating idiopathic PD from atypical Parkinson syndromes.[117] The abundance and diversity of PET imaging agents targeted at dopaminergic neurotransmission have allowed for detailed analysis and novel insights into the nigrostriatal pathologic findings in PD.

PARKINSON'S DISEASE DEMENTIA

Dementia occurs late in the course of PD in up to 40% of cases, although other forms of dementia, such as AD, can also affect patients who have PD. Peppard and colleagues[118] showed that patients who had PD with dementia differed from patients who had PD without dementia in that the former had hypometabolic perirolandic and angular gyrus regions. Patients who had PD with dementia did not have significantly different CMRGlc values than patients who had AD, however. Amyloid imaging with PiB has been used to address this issue and has revealed an absence of cortical amyloid signal in 8 of 10 patients who had PD with dementia, with some PiB retention in the pons and mesencephalon attributable to binding to Lewy bodies.[119]

"PARKINSON PLUS" SYNDROMES: PROGRESSIVE SUPRANUCLEAR PALSY, MULTISYSTEM ATROPHY, AND CORTICOBASILAR GANGLIONIC DEGENERATION

"Parkinson-plus" syndromes are a heterogeneous family of progressive neurodegenerative diseases that have atypical parkinsonism (characterized by prominent rigidity and postural instability and less tremor) as a unifying feature. The diagnosis of these diseases is notoriously difficult, and PET imaging has been extensively investigated as a means of distinguishing them.

Progressive supranuclear palsy (PSP) is a progressive neurodegenerative disease characterized by a supranuclear gaze palsy, atypical parkinsonism (with dystonia and axial rigidity), and, eventually, dementia. FDG-PET studies have demonstrated that PSP is associated with hypometabolism of the basal ganglia, thalamus, pons, and cerebral cortex but not of the cerebellum.[120,121] Foster and colleagues[120] found that the superior frontal cortex has the most significant involvement. D'Antona and colleagues[122] also reported frontal hypometabolism in patients who had PSP. Goffinet and colleagues[121] used FDG-PET to show that the motor and premotor areas were severely hypometabolic. Other studies have demonstrated more globally decreased cerebral metabolism in PSP with or without a predilection for the frontal lobes.[123,124] Juh and colleagues[125] described a pattern of hypometabolism in the caudate nucleus, thalamus, midbrain, and cingulate gyrus in PSP that differentiates it from PD. Leenders and colleagues[124] also found significantly decreased ^{18}F-DOPA uptake in the striatum in patients who had PSP. This decrease correlated with the degree of reduced frontal blood flow. FDG and ^{18}F-DOPA imaging of three patients who had familial PSP showed decreased ^{18}F-DOPA uptake in the caudate and putamen and decreased FDG metabolism in the prefrontal and premotor cortex.[126] Interestingly, several asymptomatic relatives of these patients also showed similar deficits. A second study of familial PSP showed FDG deficits in the striatum, orbitofrontal cortex, and amygdala.[127] A study of nine patients who had PSP using the D2 receptor ligand ^{11}C-raclopride reported reductions in striatal receptor density. Furthermore, the same patients had decreased relative cerebral blood flow in the frontal cortex and striatum, in contrast to patients who had PD and patients with striatonigral degeneration. Combined PET and MR imaging analysis demonstrated that corpus callosum atrophy is present in PSP and is associated with cognitive impairment and frontal cortical hypometabolism.[128] A pattern of hypometabolism in the brain stem and medial frontal cortex was found to discriminate PSP from multiple system atrophy (MSA) and controls.[129]

MSA is a complex set of atypical parkinsonian syndromes with prominent autonomic symptoms that are divided into MSA-P (Parkinson type, including striatonigral degeneration) and MSA-C (cerebellar type, including olivopontocerebellar atrophy). Although rare, this entity is believed to account for 5% to 11% of patients diagnosed with PD. The results of PET imaging using ^{18}F-DOPA and FDG-PET have shown that patients who have MSA have decreased striatal, brain stem, and cerebellar glucose metabolism (although perhaps within the normal range), in addition to decreased ^{18}F-DOPA uptake in the putamen and caudate compared with controls.[76,125,130,131] Cerebellar hypometabolism is notably present in MSA but is absent in PD and PSP. Corticobasilar ganglionic degeneration (CBD) is another Parkinson-spectrum disorder characterized by asymmetric, often unilateral, parkinsonism with prominent rigidity, limb apraxias, and cortical sensory abnormalities. Marked asymmetric cortical hypometabolism in the frontoparietal region, in addition to striatal deficits, was described in the hemisphere contralateral to clinical symptoms.[76,132] Unilateral parietal lobe hypometabolism on FDG-PET was noted as a distinguishing factor between CBD and PSP.[133,134]

HUNTINGTON'S DISEASE

Huntington's disease (HD) is an autosomal dominant trinucleotide repeat disease characterized by adult onset of psychiatric disturbances, chorea, and, ultimately, dementia and death. The pathologic hallmark of HD is atrophy of the neostriatum, particularly the caudate and putamen, which is readily apparent on CT or MR imaging late in the disease course. Studies using FDG-PET have shown bilateral hypometabolism in the caudate and putamen, which precedes caudate atrophy on CT.[92,135,136] Further, the degree of basal ganglia hypometabolism correlates with the degree of disability.[120,137] Caudate hypometabolism was found to precede significant psychiatric or neurologic symptoms in patients who have HD, suggesting that FDG-PET could be used in the early or even presymptomatic diagnosis of HD.[138,139] Young and colleagues[140] found that caudate hypometabolism was insufficient to distinguish asymptomatic patients at risk for HD from normal controls reliably, however. Subsequent studies in genetically confirmed chorea-free patients who had HD supported the observation of caudate hypometabolism that precedes frank neurologic symptoms and caudate atrophy.[141–143] Cortical hypometabolism has also been described in patients who have HD with severe cognitive involvement.[143] Studies using dopamine receptor ligands have demonstrated progressive loss of striatal D2 receptors and have found that decreased binding of the D2-selective ligands ^{11}C-N-methylspiperone and ^{11}C-raclopride occurs early in HD.[144–147] One study showed decreased striatal dopamine D1 and D2 receptor density in asymptomatic patients who had HD, suggesting that dopamine receptor

imaging may be useful for presymptomatic HD diagnosis.[148] Feigin and colleagues[149] combined MR imaging structural imaging with FDG-PET to demonstrate compensatory hypermetabolism in the thalamus, which occurs concurrently with worsening basal ganglia hypometabolism and brain volume loss as HD progresses. In summary, PET imaging with FDG and dopamine receptor ligands shows promise in the diagnosis and monitoring of HD.

EPILEPSY

One of the most common and successful uses of PET in clinical neurology and neurosurgery has been in the evaluation of epilepsy. The focus of partial seizures can be identified using FDG-PET, because these areas have increased metabolism during the seizure and decreased metabolism in the interictal period (**Fig. 5**).[150–153] It has been shown that single hypometabolic regions can be identified in 55% to 80% of patients with focal electroencephalography (EEG) abnormalities.[154] Performing ictal PET studies is somewhat impractical, however, because of the short half-life of the positron emitters and other logistic reasons, but it is effective for detecting seizure foci in patients with partial seizures as hypermetabolic areas.[155] High-resolution interictal PET imaging is routinely used in the planning of epilepsy surgery for localizing epileptogenic foci.[156] FDG-PET is also useful in predicting postoperative outcome after epilepsy surgery. Studies have shown that patients with a higher degree of temporal lobe hypometabolism (ie, more distinct asymmetry) benefit more from surgery than those with less distinct temporal asymmetry.[157,158] Other studies have shown that patients with hypometabolism isolated to the affected temporal lobe have a higher likelihood of a successful surgical outcome.[159–161] A study using statistical parametric mapping (SPM) compared hemispheric asymmetry on FDG-PET images in patients who had mesial temporal lobe epilepsy (TLE) with controls.[162] When the SPM program was used to detect temporal interhemispheric asymmetry, hypometabolism was identified on the side chosen for resection in most cases (71% sensitivity, 100% specificity) and was predictive of a favorable postsurgical outcome in 90% of the patients. Another study of 180 surgical specimens from patients who had frontal lobe epilepsy (FLE) found a high correlation between hypometabolic regions on PET images and histopathologic changes in the surgical specimens, again demonstrating the value of PET in detecting seizure foci.[163]

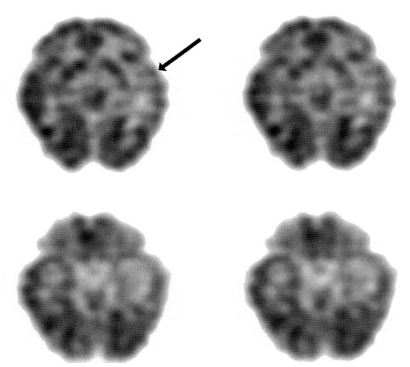

Fig. 5. FDG-PET scan shows decreased metabolism in the left temporal lobe (*arrow*) consistent with the site of seizure focus.

PET can also be used in the diagnosis of epilepsy. Studies show that the sensitivity of FDG-PET in detecting TLE foci is greater than 70% in patients with complex partial seizures.[164–167] The other major site of seizure focus in partial epilepsy is the frontal lobe. Because many of these seizures begin in the medial or inferior aspect of the frontal lobe, scalp EEG readings often do not provide adequate localization of foci.[168] Franck and colleagues[169] used FDG-PET to study 13 patients presumed to have FLE and found PET to be the best modality for localizing seizure foci in this location.

PET studies using ^{11}C-flumazenil, a benzodiazepine receptor ligand, in TLE showed decreased benzodiazepine receptor activity in the medial temporal lobe[170] and thalami.[171] This reduction in benzodiazepine receptor activity may correlate with the frequency of seizures, because ^{11}C-flumazenil binding is thought to serve as a surrogate marker for γ-aminobutyric acid receptor density.[172] Several other studies of benzodiazepine receptors showed that the areas of abnormal benzodiazepine receptor binding were more extensive than anatomic abnormalities observed on MR imaging, or even than the hypometabolic areas observed on interictal FDG-PET.[173,174]

TRAUMATIC BRAIN INJURY

FDG-PET has been used in the study of traumatic brain injury (TBI) (**Fig. 6**), and combined PET/MRI approaches have proved most valuable in distinguishing hypometabolism attributable to cerebral dysfunction from that caused by structural damage.[175] Lesions like cortical contusions, intracranial hematoma, and resultant encephalomalacia have metabolic effects that are confined primarily to the site of injury. Subdural and epidural hematomas often cause widespread hypometabolism, however, and may even affect the contralateral hemisphere.[176] Diffuse axonal injury has been found to cause diffuse cortical hypometabolism that is particularly marked in the parietal and occipital cortices.[177] Furthermore, crossed cerebellar diaschisis, in addition to ipsilateral cerebellar hypometabolism, has been found in patients who have head injury with supratentorial lesions.[178]

Alavi[177] found a good correlation between the severity of head trauma as measured by the Glasgow Coma Scale and the extent of whole-brain hypometabolism. Another study demonstrated that regionally decreased glucose metabolism was observed in 88% of patients.[179] Up to half of patients who have TBI may also have increased glucose metabolism as early as 1 week after

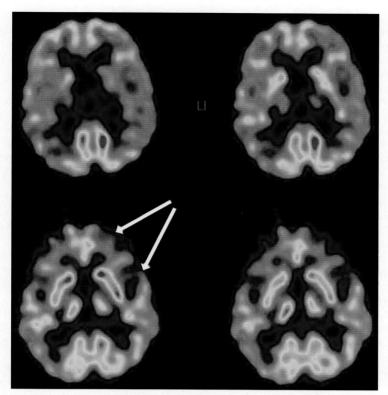

Fig. 6. FDG-PET scan of patient who has a head injury shows decreased metabolism in the frontal and temporal lobes (*arrows*) compared with the basal ganglia.

injury.[180] FDG-PET studies in patients with persistent neuropsychiatric deficits after TBI have shown regional hypometabolism in the cingulate gyrus, lingual gyrus, cuneus, and medial prefrontal cortex.[181,182] PET imaging may not be as helpful in determining the overall prognosis in patients who have head injury, however, particularly children and adolescents, with respect to rehabilitation.[183]

SUMMARY

Neuroimaging with PET provides metabolic and molecular information that cannot be obtained from other imaging modalities and provides novel insights into the pathogenesis and diagnosis of a diverse array of neurologic diseases. As the library of novel PET ligands expands, so does the potential role for PET in the study of neurologic disease. The emergence of PET amyloid imaging reveals the incredible potential for PET neuroimaging. Recent technical advances in our ability to combine structural MR imaging data with functional and molecular PET data have enhanced the power of PET for the study of the brain. Thus, PET and MR imaging should continue to play an

expanding role in the diagnosis and investigation of neurologic disease conditions.

REFERENCES

1. Alavi A, Hirsch LJ. Studies of central nervous system disorders with single photon emission computed tomography and positron emission tomography: evolution over the past 2 decades. Semin Nucl Med 1991;21(1):58–81.
2. Tewson TJ, Welch MJ, Raichle ME. [18F]-labeled 3-deoxy-3-fluoro-D-glucose: synthesis and preliminary biodistribution data. J Nucl Med 1978; 19(12):1339–45.
3. Phelps ME, Huang SC, Hoffman EJ, et al. Tomographic measurement of local cerebral glucose metabolic rate in humans with (F-18)2-fluoro-2-deoxy-D-glucose: validation of method. Ann Neurol 1979;6(5):371–88.
4. Kessler RM. Imaging methods for evaluating brain function in man. Neurobiol Aging 2003;24(Suppl 1):S21–35 [discussion: S7–9].
5. Kung HF. Overview of radiopharmaceuticals for diagnosis of central nervous disorders. Crit Rev Clin Lab Sci 1991;28(4):269–86.
6. Maziere B, Maziere M. Positron emission tomography studies of brain receptors. Fundam Clin Pharmacol 1991;5(1):61–91.

7. Herholz K, Carter SF, Jones M. Positron emission tomography imaging in dementia. Br J Radiol 2007;80(Spec No 2):S160–7.

8. Klunk WE, Engler H, Nordberg A, et al. Imaging brain amyloid in Alzheimer's disease with Pittsburgh Compound-B. Ann Neurol 2004;55(3):306–19.

9. Villemagne VL, Fodero-Tavoletti MT, Pike KE, et al. The ART of loss: abeta imaging in the evaluation of Alzheimer's disease and other dementias. Mol Neurobiol 2008;38(1):1–15.

10. Tierney MC, Fisher RH, Lewis AJ, et al. The NINCDS-ADRDA Work Group criteria for the clinical diagnosis of probable Alzheimer's disease: a clinicopathologic study of 57 cases. Neurology 1988;38(3):359–64.

11. Joachim CL, Morris JH, Selkoe DJ. Clinically diagnosed Alzheimer's disease: autopsy results in 150 cases. Ann Neurol 1988;24(1):50–6.

12. Cummings JL, Vinters HV, Cole GM, et al. Alzheimer's disease: etiologies, pathophysiology, cognitive reserve, and treatment opportunities. Neurology 1998;51(1 Suppl 1):S2–17 [discussion: S65–7].

13. Friedland RP, Budinger TF, Brant-Zawadzki M, et al. The diagnosis of Alzheimer-type dementia. A preliminary comparison of positron emission tomography and proton magnetic resonance. JAMA 1984;252(19):2750–2.

14. Frackowiak RS. PET: studies in dementia. Psychiatry Res 1989;29(3):353–5.

15. Friedland RP, Jagust WJ, Huesman RH, et al. Regional cerebral glucose transport and utilization in Alzheimer's disease. Neurology 1989;39(11):1427–34.

16. Foster NL, Chase TN, Mansi L, et al. Cortical abnormalities in Alzheimer's disease. Ann Neurol 1984;16(6):649–54.

17. Duara R, Grady C, Haxby J, et al. Positron emission tomography in Alzheimer's disease. Neurology 1986;36(7):879–87.

18. Loewenstein DA, Barker WW, Chang JY, et al. Predominant left hemisphere metabolic dysfunction in dementia. Arch Neurol 1989;46(2):146–52.

19. Jagust WJ, Friedland RP, Budinger TF, et al. Longitudinal studies of regional cerebral metabolism in Alzheimer's disease. Neurology 1988;38(6):909–12.

20. Farkas T, Ferris SH, Wolf AP, et al. 18F-2-deoxy-2-fluoro-D-glucose as a tracer in the positron emission tomographic study of senile dementia. Am J Psychiatry 1982;139(3):352–3.

21. Chase TN, Foster NL, Fedio P, et al. Regional cortical dysfunction in Alzheimer's disease as determined by positron emission tomography. Ann Neurol 1984;15(Suppl):S170–4.

22. Haxby JV, Duara R, Grady CL, et al. Relations between neuropsychological and cerebral metabolic asymmetries in early Alzheimer's disease. J Cereb Blood Flow Metab 1985;5(2):193–200.

23. Kumar A, Schapiro MB, Grady CL, et al. Anatomic, metabolic, neuropsychological, and molecular genetic studies of three pairs of identical twins discordant for dementia of the Alzheimer's type. Arch Neurol 1991;48(2):160–8.

24. Rapoport SI, Horwitz B, Grady CL, et al. Abnormal brain glucose metabolism in Alzheimer's disease, as measured by position emission tomography. Adv Exp Med Biol 1991;291:231–48.

25. Li Y, Rinne JO, Mosconi L, et al. Regional analysis of FDG and PIB-PET images in normal aging, mild cognitive impairment, and Alzheimer's disease. Eur J Nucl Med Mol Imaging 2008;35(12):2169–81.

26. Mazziotta JC, Frackowiak RS, Phelps ME. The use of positron emission tomography in the clinical assessment of dementia. Semin Nucl Med 1992;22(4):233–46.

27. Cutler NR, Haxby JV, Duara R, et al. Clinical history, brain metabolism, and neuropsychological function in Alzheimer's disease. Ann Neurol 1985;18(3):298–309.

28. Newberg A, Cotter A, Udeshi M, et al. A metabolic imaging severity rating scale for the assessment of cognitive impairment. Clin Nucl Med 2003;28(7):565–70.

29. Choo IH, Lee DY, Youn JC, et al. Topographic patterns of brain functional impairment progression according to clinical severity staging in 116 Alzheimer disease patients: FDG-PET study. Alzheimer Dis Assoc Disord 2007;21(2):77–84.

30. Mosconi L, Tsui WH, Rusinek H, et al. Quantitation, regional vulnerability, and kinetic modeling of brain glucose metabolism in mild Alzheimer's disease. Eur J Nucl Med Mol Imaging 2007;34(9):1467–79.

31. Alexander GE, Chen K, Pietrini P, et al. Longitudinal PET evaluation of cerebral metabolic decline in dementia: a potential outcome measure in Alzheimer's disease treatment studies. Am J Psychiatry 2002;159(5):738–45.

32. Eberling JL, Nordahl TE, Kusubov N, et al. Reduced temporal lobe glucose metabolism in aging. J Neuroimaging 1995;5(3):178–82.

33. Sheridan PH, Sato S, Foster N, et al. Relation of EEG alpha background to parietal lobe function in Alzheimer's disease as measured by positron emission tomography and psychometry. Neurology 1988;38(5):747–50.

34. McGeer PL, Kamo H, Harrop R, et al. Comparison of PET, MRI, and CT with pathology in a proven case of Alzheimer's disease. Neurology 1986;36(12):1569–74.

35. Mosconi L, Tsui WH, Herholz K, et al. Multicenter standardized 18F-FDG PET diagnosis of mild

cognitive impairment, Alzheimer's disease, and other dementias. J Nucl Med 2008;49(3):390–8.

36. Silverman DHS, Small GW, Chang CY, et al. Positron emission tomography in evaluation of dementia: regional brain metabolism and long-term outcome. JAMA 2001;286(17):2120–7.

37. Jagust W, Reed B, Mungas D, et al. What does flurodeoxyglucose PET imaging add to a clinical diagnosis of dementia? Neurology 2007;69(9): 871–7.

38. Dubois B, Feldman HH, Jacova C, et al. Research criteria for the diagnosis of Alzheimer's disease: revising the NINCDS-ADRDA criteria. Lancet Neurol 2007;6(8):734–46.

39. Nestor PJ, Scheltens P, Hodges JR. Advances in the early detection of Alzheimer's disease. Nat Med 2004;10(Suppl):S34–41.

40. Mosconi L, Tsui WH, De Santi S, et al. Reduced hippocampal metabolism in MCI and AD: automated FDG-PET image analysis. Neurology 2005; 64(11):1860–7.

41. Mosconi L, Sorbi S, de Leon MJ, et al. Hypometabolism exceeds atrophy in presymptomatic early-onset familial Alzheimer's disease. J Nucl Med 2006;47(11):1778–86.

42. Drzezga A, Grimmer T, Riemenschneider M, et al. Prediction of individual clinical outcome in MCI by means of genetic assessment and (18)F-FDG PET. J Nucl Med 2005;46(10):1625–32.

43. Chetelat G, Desgranges B, de la Sayette V, et al. Mild cognitive impairment: can FDG-PET predict who is to rapidly convert to Alzheimer's disease? Neurology 2003;60(8):1374–7.

44. Caselli RJ, Chen K, Lee W, et al. Correlating cerebral hypometabolism with future memory decline in subsequent converters to amnestic pre-mild cognitive impairment. Arch Neurol 2008;65(9): 1231–6.

45. Labbe C, Froment JC, Kennedy A, et al. Positron emission tomography metabolic data corrected for cortical atrophy using magnetic resonance imaging. Alzheimer Dis Assoc Disord 1996;10(3): 141–70.

46. Clark C, Hayden M, Hollenberg S, et al. Controlling for cerebral atrophy in positron emission tomography data. J Cereb Blood Flow Metab 1987;7(4): 510–2.

47. Schlageter NL, Horwitz B, Creasey H, et al. Relation of measured brain glucose utilisation and cerebral atrophy in man. J Neurol Neurosurg Psychiatry 1987;50(6):779–85.

48. Alavi A, Newberg AB, Souder E, et al. Quantitative analysis of PET and MRI data in normal aging and Alzheimer's disease: atrophy weighted total brain metabolism and absolute whole brain metabolism as reliable discriminators. J Nucl Med 1993; 34(10):1681–7.

49. Chetelat G, Desgranges B, Landeau B, et al. Direct voxel-based comparison between grey matter hypometabolism and atrophy in Alzheimer's disease. Brain 2008;131(Pt 1):60–71.

50. Klunk WE, Lopresti BJ, Ikonomovic MD, et al. Binding of the positron emission tomography tracer Pittsburgh compound-B reflects the amount of amyloid-beta in Alzheimer's disease brain but not in transgenic mouse brain. J Neurosci 2005; 25(46):10598–606.

51. Lopresti BJ, Klunk WE, Mathis CA, et al. Simplified quantification of Pittsburgh Compound B amyloid imaging PET studies: a comparative analysis. J Nucl Med 2005;46(12):1959–72.

52. Ziolko SK, Weissfeld LA, Klunk WE, et al. Evaluation of voxel-based methods for the statistical analysis of PIB PET amyloid imaging studies in Alzheimer's disease. Neuroimage 2006;33(1): 94–102.

53. Price JC, Klunk WE, Lopresti BJ, et al. Kinetic modeling of amyloid binding in humans using PET imaging and Pittsburgh Compound-B. J Cereb Blood Flow Metab 2005;25(11):1528–47.

54. Rowe CC, Ng S, Ackermann U, et al. Imaging beta-amyloid burden in aging and dementia. Neurology 2007;68(20):1718–25.

55. Yaqub M, Tolboom N, Boellaard R, et al. Simplified parametric methods for [11C]PIB studies. Neuroimage 2008;42(1):76–86.

56. Bacskai BJ, Frosch MP, Freeman SH, et al. Molecular imaging with Pittsburgh Compound B confirmed at autopsy: a case report. Arch Neurol 2007;64(3):431–4.

57. Archer HA, Edison P, Brooks DJ, et al. Amyloid load and cerebral atrophy in Alzheimer's disease: an 11C-PIB positron emission tomography study. Ann Neurol 2006;60(1):145–7.

58. Grimmer T, Henriksen G, Wester HJ, et al. Clinical severity of Alzheimer's disease is associated with PIB uptake in PET. Neurobiol Aging 2008, in press.

59. Engler H, Forsberg A, Almkvist O, et al. Two-year follow-up of amyloid deposition in patients with Alzheimer's disease. Brain 2006;129(Pt 11): 2856–66.

60. Forsberg A, Engler H, Almkvist O, et al. PET imaging of amyloid deposition in patients with mild cognitive impairment. Neurobiol Aging 2008; 29(10):1456–65.

61. Kemppainen NM, Aalto S, Wilson IA, et al. PET amyloid ligand [11C]PIB uptake is increased in mild cognitive impairment. Neurology 2007; 68(19):1603–6.

62. Fripp J, Bourgeat P, Acosta O, et al. Appearance modeling of (11)C PiB PET images: characterizing amyloid deposition in Alzheimer's disease, mild cognitive impairment and healthy aging. Neuroimage 2008;43(3):430–9.

63. Jack CR Jr, Lowe VJ, Senjem ML, et al. 11C PiB and structural MRI provide complementary information in imaging of Alzheimer's disease and amnestic mild cognitive impairment. Brain 2008; 131(Pt 3):665–80.

64. Pike KE, Savage G, Villemagne VL, et al. Beta-amyloid imaging and memory in non-demented individuals: evidence for preclinical Alzheimer's disease. Brain 2007;130(Pt 11):2837–44.

65. Kemppainen NM, Aalto S, Karrasch M, et al. Cognitive reserve hypothesis: Pittsburgh Compound B and fluorodeoxyglucose positron emission tomography in relation to education in mild Alzheimer's disease. Ann Neurol 2008;63(1):112–8.

66. Fotenos AF, Mintun MA, Snyder AZ, et al. Brain volume decline in aging: evidence for a relation between socioeconomic status, preclinical Alzheimer disease, and reserve. Arch Neurol 2008;65(1):113–20.

67. Agdeppa ED, Kepe V, Liu J, et al. Binding characteristics of radiofluorinated 6-dialkylamino-2-naphthylethylidene derivatives as positron emission tomography imaging probes for beta-amyloid plaques in Alzheimer's disease. J Neurosci 2001; 21(24):RC189.

68. Shoghi-Jadid K, Small GW, Agdeppa ED, et al. Localization of neurofibrillary tangles and beta-amyloid plaques in the brains of living patients with Alzheimer disease. Am J Geriatr Psychiatry 2002;10(1):24–35.

69. Small GW, Kepe V, Ercoli LM, et al. PET of brain amyloid and tau in mild cognitive impairment. N Engl J Med 2006;355(25):2652–63.

70. Rowe CC, Ackerman U, Browne W, et al. Imaging of amyloid beta in Alzheimer's disease with 18F-BAY94-9172, a novel PET tracer: proof of mechanism. Lancet Neurol 2008;7(2):129–35.

71. Mikhno A, Devanand D, Pelton G, et al. Voxel-based analysis of 11C-PIB scans for diagnosing Alzheimer's disease. J Nucl Med 2008;49(8): 1262–9.

72. Kamo H, McGeer PL, Harrop R, et al. Positron emission tomography and histopathology in Pick's disease. Neurology 1987;37(3):439–45.

73. Lieberman AP, Trojanowski JQ, Lee VM, et al. Cognitive, neuroimaging, and pathological studies in a patient with Pick's disease. Ann Neurol 1998; 43(2):259–65.

74. Heiss WD, Kessler J, Szelies B, et al. Positron emission tomography in the differential diagnosis of organic dementias. J Neural Transm Suppl 1991; 33:13–9.

75. Salmon E, Sadzot B, Maquet P, et al. Differential diagnosis of Alzheimer's disease with PET. J Nucl Med 1994;35(3):391–8.

76. Goto I, Taniwaki T, Hosokawa S, et al. Positron emission tomographic (PET) studies in dementia. J Neurol Sci 1993;114(1):1–6.

77. Diehl-Schmid J, Grimmer T, Drzezga A, et al. Decline of cerebral glucose metabolism in frontotemporal dementia: a longitudinal 18F-FDG-PET-study. Neurobiol Aging 2007;28(1):42–50.

78. Wechsler AF, Verity MA, Rosenschein S, et al. Pick's disease. A clinical, computed tomographic, and histologic study with Golgi impregnation observations. Arch Neurol 1982;39(5):287–90.

79. Mendez MF, Shapira JS, McMurtray A, et al. Accuracy of the clinical evaluation for frontotemporal dementia. Arch Neurol 2007;64(6):830–5.

80. Foster NL, Heidebrink JL, Clark CM, et al. FDG-PET improves accuracy in distinguishing frontotemporal dementia and Alzheimer's disease. Brain 2007; 130(10):2616–35.

81. Kanda T, Ishii K, Uemura T, et al. Comparison of grey matter and metabolic reductions in frontotemporal dementia using FDG-PET and voxel-based morphometric MR studies. Eur J Nucl Med Mol Imaging 2008;35(12):2227–34.

82. Engler H, Santillo AF, Wang SX, et al. In vivo amyloid imaging with PET in frontotemporal dementia. Eur J Nucl Med Mol Imaging 2008;35(1):100–6.

83. Rabinovici GD, Furst AJ, O'Neil JP, et al. 11C-PIB PET imaging in Alzheimer disease and frontotemporal lobar degeneration. Neurology 2007;68(15): 1205–12.

84. Marsden CD. Basal ganglia disease. Lancet 1982; 2(8308):1141–7.

85. Braffman BH, Grossman RI, Goldberg HI, et al. MR imaging of Parkinson disease with spin-echo and gradient-echo sequences. AJR Am J Roentgenol 1989;152(1):159–65.

86. Calne DB, Snow BJ. PET imaging in Parkinsonism. Adv Neurol 1993;60:484–7.

87. Eidelberg D. Positron emission tomography studies in Parkinsonism. Neurol Clin 1992;10(2): 421–33.

88. Ravina B, Eidelberg D, Ahlskog JE, et al. The role of radiotracer imaging in Parkinson disease. Neurology 2005;64(2):208–15.

89. Rougemont D, Baron JC, Collard P, et al. Local cerebral glucose utilisation in treated and untreated patients with Parkinson's disease. J Neurol Neurosurg Psychiatry 1984;47(8):824–30.

90. Eidelberg D, Moeller JR, Dhawan V, et al. The metabolic anatomy of Parkinson's disease: complementary [18F]fluorodeoxyglucose and [18F]fluorodopa positron emission tomographic studies. Mov Disord 1990;5(3):203–13.

91. Kuhl DE, Metter EJ, Riege WH. Patterns of local cerebral glucose utilization determined in Parkin-

son's disease by the [18F]fluorodeoxyglucose method. Ann Neurol 1984;15(5):419–24.

92. Kuhl DE, Metter EJ, Riege WH, et al. Patterns of cerebral glucose utilization in Parkinson's disease and Huntington's disease. Ann Neurol 1984; 15(Suppl):S119–25.

93. Przedborski S, Goldman S, Giladi N, et al. Positron emission tomography in hemiparkinsonism-hemiatrophy syndrome. Adv Neurol 1993;60:501–5.

94. Lin TP, Carbon M, Tang C, et al. Metabolic correlates of subthalamic nucleus activity in Parkinson's disease. Brain 2008;131(Pt 5):1373–80.

95. Huang C, Tang C, Feigin A, et al. Changes in network activity with the progression of Parkinson's disease. Brain 2007;130(Pt 7):1834–46.

96. Hilker R, Voges J, Weber T, et al. STN-DBS activates the target area in Parkinson disease: an FDG-PET study. Neurology 2008;71(10):708–13.

97. Asanuma K, Tang C, Ma Y, et al. Network modulation in the treatment of Parkinson's disease. Brain 2006;129(Pt 10):2667–78.

98. Brooks DJ, Ibanez V, Sawle GV, et al. Differing patterns of striatal 18F-dopa uptake in Parkinson's disease, multiple system atrophy, and progressive supranuclear palsy. Ann Neurol 1990;28(4):547–55.

99. Martin WR, Palmer MR, Patlak CS, et al. Nigrostriatal function in humans studied with positron emission tomography. Ann Neurol 1989;26(4):535–42.

100. Martin WR. Parkinson's disease: positron emission tomographic studies. Semin Neurol 1989;9(4): 345–50.

101. Nahmias C, Garnett ES, Firnau G, et al. Striatal dopamine distribution in parkinsonian patients during life. J Neurol Sci 1985;69(3):223–30.

102. Leenders KL, Palmer AJ, Quinn N, et al. Brain dopamine metabolism in patients with Parkinson's disease measured with positron emission tomography. J Neurol Neurosurg Psychiatry 1986;49(8): 853–60.

103. Leenders KL, Salmon EP, Tyrrell P, et al. The nigrostriatal dopaminergic system assessed in vivo by positron emission tomography in healthy volunteer subjects and patients with Parkinson's disease. Arch Neurol 1990;47(12):1290–8.

104. Rinne OJ, Nurmi E, Ruottinen HM, et al. [(18)F]FDOPA and [(18)F]CFT are both sensitive PET markers to detect presynaptic dopaminergic hypofunction in early Parkinson's disease. Synapse 2001;40(3):193–200.

105. Garnett ES, Nahmias C, Firnau G. Central dopaminergic pathways in hemiparkinsonism examined by positron emission tomography. Can J Neurol Sci 1984;11(1 Suppl):174–9.

106. Calne DB, Langston JW, Martin WR, et al. Positron emission tomography after MPTP: observations relating to the cause of Parkinson's disease. Nature 1985;317(6034):246–8.

107. Sawle GV, Wroe SJ, Lees AJ, et al. The identification of presymptomatic parkinsonism: clinical and [18F]dopa positron emission tomography studies in an Irish kindred. Ann Neurol 1992;32(5):609–17.

108. Nurmi E, Ruottinen HM, Kaasinen V, et al. Progression in Parkinson's disease: a positron emission tomography study with a dopamine transporter ligand [18F]CFT. Ann Neurol 2000;47(6):804–8.

109. Lee CS, Samii A, Sossi V, et al. In vivo positron emission tomographic evidence for compensatory changes in presynaptic dopaminergic nerve terminals in Parkinson's disease. Ann Neurol 2000;47(4): 493–503.

110. Ouchi Y, Yoshikawa E, Okada H, et al. Alterations in binding site density of dopamine transporter in the striatum, orbitofrontal cortex, and amygdala in early Parkinson's disease: compartment analysis for beta-CFT binding with positron emission tomography. Ann Neurol 1999;45(5):601–10.

111. Ouchi Y, Kanno T, Okada H, et al. Presynaptic and postsynaptic dopaminergic binding densities in the nigrostriatal and mesocortical systems in early Parkinson's disease: a double-tracer positron emission tomography study. Ann Neurol 1999; 46(5):723–31.

112. Frey KA, Koeppe RA, Kilbourn MR, et al. Presynaptic monoaminergic vesicles in Parkinson's disease and normal aging. Ann Neurol 1996;40(6):873–84.

113. Adams JR, van Netten H, Schulzer M, et al. PET in LRRK2 mutations: comparison to sporadic Parkinson's disease and evidence for presymptomatic compensation. Brain 2005;128(Pt 12):2777–85.

114. Rinne JO, Laihinen A, Rinne UK, et al. PET study on striatal dopamine D2 receptor changes during the progression of early Parkinson's disease. Mov Disord 1993;8(2):134–8.

115. Sawle GV, Playford ED, Brooks DJ, et al. Asymmetrical pre-synaptic and post-synaptic changes in the striatal dopamine projection in dopa naive parkinsonism. Diagnostic implications of the D2 receptor status. Brain 1993;116(Pt 4):853–67.

116. Antonini A, Schwarz J, Oertel WH, et al. Long-term changes of striatal dopamine D2 receptors in patients with Parkinson's disease: a study with positron emission tomography and [11C]raclopride. Mov Disord 1997;12(1):33–8.

117. Schreckenberger M, Hagele S, Siessmeier T, et al. The dopamine D2 receptor ligand 18F-desmethoxyfallypride: an appropriate fluorinated PET tracer for the differential diagnosis of parkinsonism. Eur J Nucl Med Mol Imaging 2004;31(8):1128–35.

118. Peppard RF, Martin WR, Clark CM, et al. Cortical glucose metabolism in Parkinson's and Alzheimer's disease. J Neurosci Res 1990;27(4):561–8.

119. Maetzler W, Reimold M, Liepelt I, et al. [11C]PIB binding in Parkinson's disease dementia. Neuroimage 2008;39(3):1027–33.

120. Foster NL, Gilman S, Berent S, et al. Cerebral hypometabolism in progressive supranuclear palsy studied with positron emission tomography. Ann Neurol 1988;24(3):399–406.

121. Goffinet AM, De Volder AG, Gillain C, et al. Positron tomography demonstrates frontal lobe hypometabolism in progressive supranuclear palsy. Ann Neurol 1989;25(2):131–9.

122. D'Antona R, Baron JC, Samson Y, et al. Subcortical dementia. Frontal cortex hypometabolism detected by positron tomography in patients with progressive supranuclear palsy. Brain 1985;108(Pt 3):785–99.

123. Santens P, De Reuck J, Crevits L, et al. Cerebral oxygen metabolism in patients with progressive supranuclear palsy: a positron emission tomography study. Eur Neurol 1997;37(1):18–22.

124. Leenders KL, Frackowiak RS, Lees AJ. Steele-Richardson-Olszewski syndrome. Brain energy metabolism, blood flow and fluorodopa uptake measured by positron emission tomography. Brain 1988;111(Pt 3):615–30.

125. Juh R, Kim J, Moon D, et al. Different metabolic patterns analysis of Parkinsonism on the 18F-FDG PET. Eur J Radiol 2004;51(3):223–33.

126. Piccini P, de Yebenez J, Lees AJ, et al. Familial progressive supranuclear palsy: detection of subclinical cases using 18F-dopa and 18fluorodeoxyglucose positron emission tomography. Arch Neurol 2001;58(11):1846–51.

127. Tai YF, Ahsan RL, de Yebenes JG, et al. Characterization of dopaminergic dysfunction in familial progressive supranuclear palsy: an 18F-dopa PET study. J Neural Transm 2007;114(3):337–40.

128. Yamauchi H, Fukuyama H, Nagahama Y, et al. Atrophy of the corpus callosum, cognitive impairment, and cortical hypometabolism in progressive supranuclear palsy. Ann Neurol 1997;41(5):606–14.

129. Eckert T, Tang C, Ma Y, et al. Abnormal metabolic networks in atypical parkinsonism. Mov Disord 2008;23(5):727–33.

130. Otsuka M, Kuwabara Y, Ichiya Y, et al. Differentiating between multiple system atrophy and Parkinson's disease by positron emission tomography with 18F-dopa and 18F-FDG. Ann Nucl Med 1997;11(3):251–7.

131. Gilman S, Koeppe RA, Junck L, et al. Patterns of cerebral glucose metabolism detected with positron emission tomography differ in multiple system atrophy and olivopontocerebellar atrophy. Ann Neurol 1994;36(2):166–75.

132. Nagahama Y, Fukuyama H, Turjanski N, et al. Cerebral glucose metabolism in corticobasal degeneration: comparison with progressive supranuclear palsy and normal controls. Mov Disord 1997;12(5):691–6.

133. Hosaka K, Ishii K, Sakamoto S, et al. Voxel-based comparison of regional cerebral glucose metabolism between PSP and corticobasal degeneration. J Neurol Sci 2002;199(1–2):67–71.

134. Juh R, Pae CU, Kim TS, et al. Cerebral glucose metabolism in corticobasal degeneration comparison with progressive supranuclear palsy using statistical mapping analysis. Neurosci Lett 2005;383(1–2):22–7.

135. Kuhl DE, Phelps ME, Markham CH, et al. Cerebral metabolism and atrophy in Huntington's disease determined by 18FDG and computed tomographic scan. Ann Neurol 1982;12(5):425–34.

136. Garnett ES, Firnau G, Nahmias C, et al. Reduced striatal glucose consumption and prolonged reaction time are early features in Huntington's disease. J Neurol Sci 1984;65(2):231–7.

137. Young AB, Penney JB, Starosta-Rubinstein S, et al. PET scan investigations of Huntington's disease: cerebral metabolic correlates of neurological features and functional decline. Ann Neurol 1986;20(3):296–303.

138. Hayden MR, Martin WR, Stoessl AJ, et al. Positron emission tomography in the early diagnosis of Huntington's disease. Neurology 1986;36(7):888–94.

139. Mazziotta JC, Phelps ME, Pahl JJ, et al. Reduced cerebral glucose metabolism in asymptomatic subjects at risk for Huntington's disease. N Engl J Med 1987;316(7):357–62.

140. Young AB, Penney JB, Starosta-Rubinstein S, et al. Normal caudate glucose metabolism in persons at risk for Huntington's disease. Arch Neurol 1987;44(3):254–7.

141. Grafton ST, Mazziotta JC, Pahl JJ, et al. A comparison of neurological, metabolic, structural, and genetic evaluations in persons at risk for Huntington's disease. Ann Neurol 1990;28(5):614–21.

142. Grafton ST, Mazziotta JC, Pahl JJ, et al. Serial changes of cerebral glucose metabolism and caudate size in persons at risk for Huntington's disease. Arch Neurol 1992;49(11):1161–7.

143. Kuwert T, Lange HW, Langen KJ, et al. Cortical and subcortical glucose consumption measured by PET in patients with Huntington's disease. Brain 1990;113(Pt 5):1405–23.

144. Leenders KL, Frackowiak RS, Quinn N, et al. Brain energy metabolism and dopaminergic function in Huntington's disease measured in vivo using positron emission tomography. Mov Disord 1986;1(1):69–77.

145. Antonini A, Leenders KL, Eidelberg D. [11C]-raclopride-PET studies of the Huntington's disease rate of progression: relevance of the trinucleotide repeat length. Ann Neurol 1998;43(2):253–5.

146. van Oostrom JC, Maguire RP, Verschuuren-Bemelmans CC, et al. Striatal dopamine D2

receptors, metabolism, and volume in preclinical Huntington disease. Neurology 2005;65(6):941–3.

147. Brandt J, Folstein SE, Wong DF, et al. D2 receptors in Huntington's disease: positron emission tomography findings and clinical correlates. J Neuropsychiatry Clin Neurosci 1990;2(1):20–7.

148. Weeks RA, Piccini P, Harding AE, et al. Striatal D1 and D2 dopamine receptor loss in asymptomatic mutation carriers of Huntington's disease. Ann Neurol 1996;40(1):49–54.

149. Feigin A, Tang C, Ma Y, et al. Thalamic metabolism and symptom onset in preclinical Huntington's disease. Brain 2007;130(Pt 11):2858–67.

150. Abou-Khalil BW, Siegel GJ, Sackellares JC, et al. Positron emission tomography studies of cerebral glucose metabolism in chronic partial epilepsy. Ann Neurol 1987;22(4):480–6.

151. Engel J Jr, Brown WJ, Kuhl DE, et al. Pathological findings underlying focal temporal lobe hypometabolism in partial epilepsy. Ann Neurol 1982;12(6):518–28.

152. Engel J Jr, Kuhl DE, Phelps ME, et al. Comparative localization of epileptic foci in partial epilepsy by PCT and EEG. Ann Neurol 1982;12(6):529–37.

153. Theodore WH, Newmark ME, Sato S, et al. [18F]fluorodeoxyglucose positron emission tomography in refractory complex partial seizures. Ann Neurol 1983;14(4):429–37.

154. Duncan R. Epilepsy, cerebral blood flow, and cerebral metabolic rate. Cerebrovasc Brain Metab Rev 1992;4(2):105–21.

155. Chugani HT, Rintahaka PJ, Shewmon DA. Ictal patterns of cerebral glucose utilization in children with epilepsy. Epilepsia 1994;35(4):813–22.

156. Schramm J, Clusmann H. The surgery of epilepsy. Neurosurgery 2008;62(Suppl 2):463–81 [discussion: 81].

157. Theodore WH, Sato S, Kufta C, et al. Temporal lobectomy for uncontrolled seizures: the role of positron emission tomography. Ann Neurol 1992;32(6):789–94.

158. Delbeke D, Lawrence SK, Abou-Khalil BW, et al. Postsurgical outcome of patients with uncontrolled complex partial seizures and temporal lobe hypometabolism on 18FDG-positron emission tomography. Invest Radiol 1996;31(5):261–6.

159. Manno EM, Sperling MR, Ding X, et al. Predictors of outcome after anterior temporal lobectomy: positron emission tomography. Neurology 1994;44(12):2331–6.

160. Radtke RA, Hanson MW, Hoffman JM, et al. Temporal lobe hypometabolism on PET: predictor of seizure control after temporal lobectomy. Neurology 1993;43(6):1088–92.

161. Wong CY, Geller EB, Chen EQ, et al. Outcome of temporal lobe epilepsy surgery predicted by statistical parametric PET imaging. J Nucl Med 1996;37(7):1094–100.

162. Van Bogaert P, Massager N, Tugendhaft P, et al. Statistical parametric mapping of regional glucose metabolism in mesial temporal lobe epilepsy. Neuroimage 2000;12(2):129–38.

163. Robitaille Y, Rasmussen T, Dubeau F, et al. Histopathology of nonneoplastic lesions in frontal lobe epilepsy. Review of 180 cases with recent MRI and PET correlations. Adv Neurol 1992;57:499–513.

164. Engel J Jr, Kuhl DE, Phelps ME. Patterns of human local cerebral glucose metabolism during epileptic seizures. Science 1982;218(4567):64–6.

165. Theodore WH, Fishbein D, Dubinsky R. Patterns of cerebral glucose metabolism in patients with partial seizures. Neurology 1988;38(8):1201–6.

166. Markand ON, Salanova V, Worth R, et al. Comparative study of interictal PET and ictal SPECT in complex partial seizures. Acta Neurol Scand 1997;95(3):129–36.

167. Knowlton RC, Laxer KD, Ende G, et al. Presurgical multimodality neuroimaging in electroencephalographic lateralized temporal lobe epilepsy. Ann Neurol 1997;42(6):829–37.

168. Sammaritano M, de Lotbiniere A, Andermann F, et al. False lateralization by surface EEG of seizure onset in patients with temporal lobe epilepsy and gross focal cerebral lesions. Ann Neurol 1987;21(4):361–9.

169. Franck G, Maquet P, Sadzot B, et al. Contribution of positron emission tomography to the investigation of epilepsies of frontal lobe origin. Adv Neurol 1992;57:471–85.

170. Savic I, Persson A, Roland P, et al. In-vivo demonstration of reduced benzodiazepine receptor binding in human epileptic foci. Lancet 1988;2(8616):863–6.

171. Juhasz C, Nagy F, Watson C, et al. Glucose and [11C]flumazenil positron emission tomography abnormalities of thalamic nuclei in temporal lobe epilepsy. Neurology 1999;53(9):2037–45.

172. Savic I, Svanborg E, Thorell JO. Cortical benzodiazepine receptor changes are related to frequency of partial seizures: a positron emission tomography study. Epilepsia 1996;37(3):236–44.

173. Arnold S, Berthele A, Drzezga A, et al. Reduction of benzodiazepine receptor binding is related to the seizure onset zone in extratemporal focal cortical dysplasia. Epilepsia 2000;41(7):818–24.

174. Richardson MP, Koepp MJ, Brooks DJ, et al. Benzodiazepine receptors in focal epilepsy with cortical dysgenesis: an 11C-flumazenil PET study. Ann Neurol 1996;40(2):188–98.

175. Dubroff JG, Newberg A. Neuroimaging of traumatic brain injury. Semin Neurol 2008;28(4):548–57.

176. Garada B, Klufas RA, Schwartz RB. Neuroimaging in closed head injury. Semin Clin Neuropsychiatry 1997;2(3):188–95.

177. Alavi A. Functional and anatomic studies of head injury. J Neuropsychiatry Clin Neurosci 1989;1(1):S45–50.

178. Alavi A, Mirot A, Newberg A, et al. Fluorine 18-FDG evaluation of crossed cerebellar diaschisis in head injury. J Nucl Med 1997;38(11):1717–20.

179. Bergsneider M, Hovda DA, Lee SM, et al. Dissociation of cerebral glucose metabolism and level of consciousness during the period of metabolic depression following human traumatic brain injury. J Neurotrauma 2000;17(5):389–401.

180. Bergsneider M, Hovda DA, Shalmon E, et al. Cerebral hyperglycolysis following severe traumatic brain injury in humans: a positron emission tomography study. J Neurosurg 1997;86(2):241–51.

181. Nakashima T, Nakayama N, Miwa K, et al. Focal brain glucose hypometabolism in patients with neuropsychologic deficits after diffuse axonal injury. AJNR Am J Neuroradiol 2007;28(2):236–42.

182. Kato T, Nakayama N, Yasokawa Y, et al. Statistical image analysis of cerebral glucose metabolism in patients with cognitive impairment following diffuse traumatic brain injury. J Neurotrauma 2007;24(6):919–26.

183. Worley G, Hoffman JM, Paine SS, et al. 18-Fluorodeoxyglucose positron emission tomography in children and adolescents with traumatic brain injury. Dev Med Child Neurol 1995;37(3):213–20.

PET/CT-MR Imaging in Head and Neck Cancer Including Pitfalls and Physiologic Variations

Laurie A. Loevner, MD*, Ann K. Kim, MD, Igor Mikityansky, MD

KEYWORDS

- PET-CT • PET-MR imaging • Cancer
- Head and neck • Larynx • Pitfalls • Pharynx
- Physiologic variations

This article emphasizes the strengths and potential pitfalls of functional and anatomic imaging in patients who have head and neck cancer with an emphasis on the treated neck, including patients who have undergone surgery and/or radiation therapy. Functional imaging with PET typically is performed with the radiopharmaceutical ^{18}F-2-fluoro-2-deoxy-D-glucose (^{18}F-FDG), a D-glucose analogue. Increased vascularity of tumors and glucose metabolism by malignant cells result in preferential increase in uptake of FDG by the tumor cells. The inability to process the metabolites of the modified glucose molecule causes intracellular accumulation of ^{18}F-containing radioisotopes. This phenomenon allows diagnosis and staging of oncology patients. The ability to assess the metabolic status of the tissues is the main advantage of FDG-PET and is a limitation of cross-sectional imaging (ie, CT and MR imaging). The converse is also true: the spatial resolution and the ability to visualize the relationship of adjacent structures on CT and MR imaging in assessing patients who have head and neck cancer usually are limitations of FDG-PET. Through a careful review of pertinent anatomy, of the physiologic variations seen in PET imaging with particular attention to those seen in the treated neck, and an analysis of both PET and cross-sectional images, this article emphasizes the complementary roles that PET and cross-sectional imaging play in assessing patients who have head and

neck cancer. Many questions unanswered; large multicenter trials and long-term follow-up will be needed to determine the exact roles that functional and anatomic imaging may play in monitoring therapy, surveillance, and patient outcomes, including long-term survival.

NORMAL ANATOMY

The nasopharynx is located behind and above the hard palate. The nasopharynx is bounded superiorly by the floor of the sphenoid sinus and the clivus, anteriorly by the nasal choana, inferiorly by the superior surface of the soft palate, posteriorly by the prevertebral musculature and clivus; and laterally by the parapharyngeal space.

The lateral wall of the nasopharynx, the fossa of Rosenmüller located superior and posterior to the torus tubarius, is the most common site of nasopharyngeal cancer. The eustachian tube enters the nasopharynx through the sinus of Morgagni, an opening in the pharyngobasilar fascia. This opening is a potential route for the spread of tumor from the nasopharynx to the parapharyngeal space and to other extra-mucosal spaces of the head and neck. Nasopharyngeal cancer may spread from the parapharyngeal space into the masticator space with infiltration of the muscles of mastication and potential spread along the mandibular nerve. The pharyngobasilar fascia is the cranial extension of the superior constrictor

Division of Neuroradiology, Department of Radiology, Hospital of the University of Pennsylvania, 3400 Spruce Street, Philadelphia, PA 19104, USA
* Corresponding author.
E-mail address: laurie.loevner@uphs.upenn.edu (L.A. Loevner).

PET Clin 3 (2009) 335–353
doi:10.1016/j.cpet.2009.04.008

muscle from the soft palate to the base of the skull. The foramen lacerum and foramen ovale, located superior and lateral to the nasopharynx, respectively, are additional potential pathways for tumor extension into the intracranial cavity. The retrostyloid parapharyngeal space, also referred to as the "carotid space," is the most posterior lateral space of the nasopharynx.

Between the nasopharynx and the vertebral bodies are the retropharyngeal and prevertebral spaces. The retropharynx contains the lateral nodes of Rouviere. These nodes are the first-echelon nodes in the lymphatic drainage of the nasopharynx.

The larynx comprises three subdivisions: the supraglottis, the glottis, and the subglottis. The supraglottis comprises the epiglottis, the aryepiglottic folds, the false vocal cords, and the arytenoid cartilages. The glottis includes the true vocal cords, the vocal ligament, which extends from the arytenoid cartilage to the thyroid cartilage, and the anterior and posterior commissures. The glottis extends from the level of the mid-laryngeal ventricle to 1 cm below the apex of the laryngeal ventricle. The subglottic region extends from this lower border of the glottis to the inferior aspect of the cricoid cartilage. Lesions arising below the cricoid cartilage are considered tracheal in nature.

The larynx is secured on an osseous and cartilaginous framework that includes the hyoid bone, the epiglottis, the thyroid cartilage, the cricoid cartilage, and the arytenoids. The cricoid cartilage is the only one of these cartilages that is required to maintain airway patency. The epiglottis protects the airway during swallowing. The vocal ligament provides support for the true vocal cord. The lower cricoarytenoid joint identifies the level of the true vocal cords. The true vocal cords predominantly comprise the thyroarytenoid muscle. The cricoarytenoid muscle moves the arytenoids, allowing glottic speech.

The vagus nerve and specifically the recurrent and the superior laryngeal nerves innervate the larynx. The superior laryngeal nerve innervates the cricothyroid muscle. It is important to understand the course of the vagus and recurrent laryngeal nerve. The vagus nerve descends through the jugular foramen into the carotid sheath and follows the carotid sheath inferiorly. The recurrent laryngeal nerves loop around the aortic arch on the left and the subclavian artery on the right before ascending in the tracheoesophageal groove. The recurrent laryngeal nerve penetrates the thyrohyoid membrane and innervates the larynx. The lymphatics of the supraglottis are abundant, whereas those at the glottic level are sparse.

The larynx is bordered anteriorly by the pre-epiglottic space and laterally by the paraglottic space. The pre-epiglottic space is triangular and contains predominantly adipose tissue, as well as collagen fibers and fibrous tissue. There is a rich lymphatic network within the pre-epiglottic fat, but no lymph nodes are located within this space. The pre-epiglottic space is bounded superiorly by the hyoepiglottic ligament, inferiorly by the conus elasticus, posteriorly by the epiglottis and quadrangular membrane, and anteriorly by the thyroid cartilage and the thyrohyoid membrane. The paraglottic space contains fat, lymphatics, and small muscles. It is medial to the thyroid

---

Box 1
American Joint Committee on Cancer classification of cervical lymph nodes based on level and location

Level I

    Ia: Submental

    Ib: Submandibular

Level II: Anterior cervical lymph node chain: lymph nodes in the internal jugular chain from the skull base to the level of the hyoid bone

    IIa: Nodes anterior, medial, or lateral to the internal jugular vein

    IIb: Nodes posterior to the internal jugular vein with a fat plane between the node and the vessel

Level III: Nodes along the internal jugular chain between the hyoid bone and the cricoid cartilage

Level IV: Nodes along the internal jugular chain between the cricoid cartilage and the clavicle

Level V: Nodes along the spinal accessory chain, posterior to the sternocleidomastoid muscle

    Va: Level V nodes from the skull base to lower border of cricoid cartilage

    Vb: Level V nodes from lower border of cricoid cartilage to the clavicle

Level VI: Nodes in the visceral compartment from the hyoid bone superiorly to the suprasternal notch inferiorly. On each side, the lateral border is formed by the medial border of carotid sheath.

Level VII: Nodes in the superior mediastinum

Data from American Joint Committee on Cancer Staging manual. 6th edition. New York: Springer-Verlag; 2002.

lamina throughout its craniocaudad extent. The pre-epiglottic and paraglottic spaces are not clearly delineated at the posterosuperior aspect of the larynx, but posteroinferiorly the pre-epiglottic and paraglottic spaces are distinct anatomically, separated by a thin membrane composed of fibrous tissue. Spread of tumor into these submucosal spaces allows the transglottic spread of cancer.

The cervical lymph nodes are the first echelon in assessing metastatic disease in a patient who has head and neck cancer. Knowledge of the nodal classification system,[1] namely the anatomic levels of the cervical lymph nodes used by clinical colleagues, is essential. Radiologic reports of pathologic nodes should use this classification of cervical lymph nodes. Level I lymph nodes are those in the submandibular and submental region. Levels II through IV are nodes along the anterior cervical lymph chain. Level V nodes are those in the posterior compartment along the spinal accessory chain, and level VI nodes are medial to the carotid arteries in the visceral compartment between the hyoid bone and manubrium (**Box 1**).

The Larynx: Head and Neck Cancer

Direct visualization combined with endoscopy is sensitive in evaluating the mucosa of the aerodigestive tract, but even extensive neoplastic infiltration of the deep spaces surrounding the larynx often is difficult to detect on physical and endoscopic examination. As a result, patients often are clinically understaged. Radiologic imaging has played an increasingly important role in the staging of head and neck cancer. The major role of CT and MR imaging of the larynx is in evaluating tumor extent. The choice of treatment, including the need for and the type of surgery selected, are guided by the site of origin of the primary tumor and staging at the time of clinical presentation. Staging is determined by the following factors: (1) submucosal tumor spread into the pre-epiglottic and paraglottic spaces; (2) cartilage invasion; (3) lymphadenopathy; and (4) distant metastases. Aggressive treatment at initial presentation based on accurate clinical staging provides the best chance of cure. When possible, radiation therapy and/or speech-conserving surgery are desired. Radiation is an excellent treatment modality but must be used with careful consideration, particularly in young patients who have a significant risk of a second primary cancer of the aerodigestive tract (15%–20%) during their lifetime.[2–4] Recurrent cancers are difficult to treat and have a poor prognosis.[4,5]

LIMITATIONS OF CT AND MR IMAGING IN THE TREATED NECK

In all patients who have cancer, one of the major limiting factors of conventional cross-sectional imaging is that it is a morphologic study that looks at the structural aspects of the solid organs but does not necessarily address regions of biologically active tumor, either within the primary site or within lymph nodes or distant metastatic sites. Most cancers arising in the head and neck are squamous cell carcinomas.[6] The

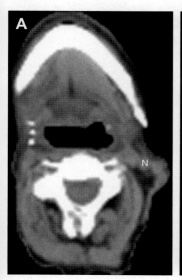
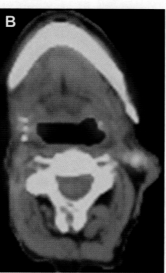

Fig. 1. Contralateral nodal metastasis detected by PET in a patient previously treated for right oropharyngeal cancer. (*A*) Axial CT image from PET-CT scan shows treatment for prior cancer including right neck dissection. There is a left IIA lymph node (N) that is not abnormal by CT criteria. (*B*) Corresponding fused PET-CT image shows intense uptake in this node, which on subsequent biopsy revealed recurrent squamous cell carcinoma.

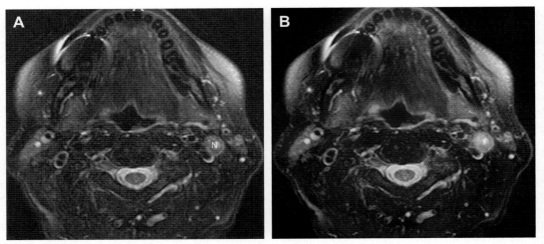

Fig. 2. FDG uptake in a metastatic lymph node that was equivocal on MR imaging. (*A*) Axial T2-weighted MR image shows an equivocal left IIA lymph node (N). (*B*) Corresponding fused PET-MR image shows uptake in this node.

regional cervical nodal metastases that are commonly seen with these malignant tumors frequently are necrotic.[7] In the neck treated with irradiation (and increasingly with adjuvant chemotherapy), both the primary tumor and the cervical nodal metastases may undergo further necrosis during treatment. Frequently, there is uncertainty whether the residual mass visualized

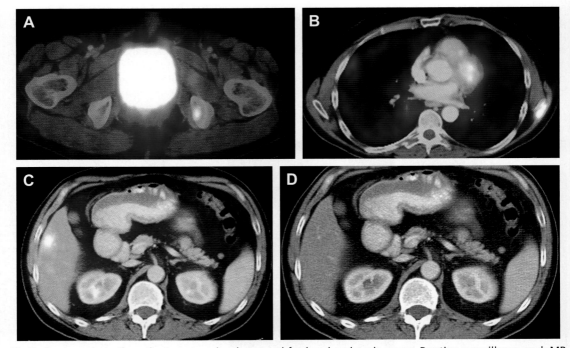

Fig. 3. An asymptomatic patient was previously treated for head and neck cancer. Routine surveillance neck MR imaging (not shown) was negative. (*A*) PET-CT showed a metastatic focus with increased FDG avidity in the left ischium. (*B*) An FDG-avid left scapular tip metastasis. These bone marrow metastases were difficult to detect on CT images alone. (*C*) Also noted is an FDG-avid metastasis in the right lobe of the liver. (*D*) The liver metastasis is not detectable on the enhanced CT alone.

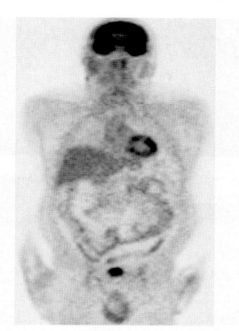

Fig. 4. Normal distribution of FDG. There is high uptake in the gray matter of brain. The myocardium has variable uptake. There should be relatively low uptake in lungs, mediastinum, and liver. There is variable activity in gastrointestinal tract (esophagus, stomach, colon). The skeletal muscles should have relatively low uptake if patient is calm and appropriately at rest before imaging. The collecting systems of the urinary tract excrete FDG and therefore are normally FDG avid.

on CT and MR imaging represents viable tumor or treated tissue.

One of the most important issues in determining prognosis in patients who have head and neck cancer is the identification of regional cervical nodal metastases, which affect long-term survival.[8–10] In newly diagnosed head and neck squamous cell carcinoma, necrosis within cervical lymph nodes is a very strong indicator of the presence of metastatic disease.[7] Necrosis within a cervical lymph node should be considered tumor until proven otherwise. Enlargement of lymph nodes also is an indicator of the possible presence of metastatic disease. At least 10% of cervical lymph nodes harboring cancer are normal by CT and MR imaging criteria, however.[11] Specifically, CT and MR imaging may show lymph nodes that are normal in size and have normal architectural features, rendering an interpretation of "no pathologic nodes by imaging criteria" despite the presence of metabolically active neoplasm. One of the key strengths of functional imaging is the ability to detect metabolic activity caused by the presence of neoplasm within these lymph nodes that appear normal on CT and MR imaging (Figs. 1 and 2).[12,13] The detection of regional nodal metastases on FDG-PET affects patient prognosis and management.[14–16] Poor ability to identify small osseous and solid-organ metastasis in the treated neck is another limitation of CT and MR imaging (Fig. 3).[17–19] The detection of distant metastases may determine that a patient is no longer a surgical candidate. It is well known that surgery and irradiation therapy in the head and neck result in distorted anatomy as well as inflammatory changes both in the site of the primary tumor and in the lateral neck. Because of the overlapping attenuations of muscle, tumor, and edema on CT imaging, it can be difficult even for an experienced radiologist to distinguish reliably posttreatment changes and complications of treatment from tumor.[20]

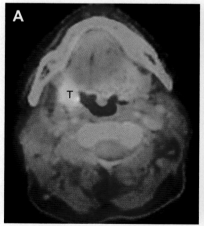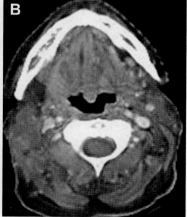

Fig. 5. Routine follow-up imaging in a 54-year-old patient after left tonsillectomy for squamous cell carcinoma. (A) Fused PET-CT image shows intense physiologic uptake in the remaining right palatine tonsil (T). (B) Corresponding CT image shows no mass in the right tonsil.

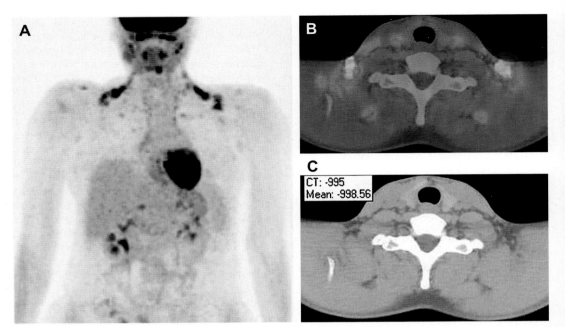

Fig. 6. Physiologic uptake in brown fat in a 24-year-old woman treated for Hodgkin's disease. (*A*) Coronal FDG image shows bilaterally symmetric uptake in the supraclavicular fossa. Note the symmetry and linear nature of FDG uptake, which is typical of brown fat in this location. (*B*) Axial fused PET-CT shows bilateral uptake in the supraclavicular fossa. (*C*) Corresponding axial CT scan shows uptake is within fat.

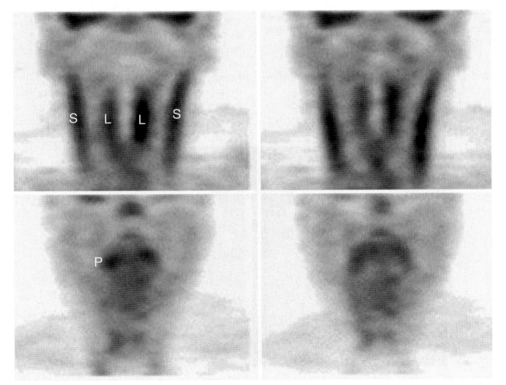

Fig. 7. Coronal PET images show physiologic uptake in paired bilateral sternocleidomastoid muscles (S), longus colli/capitis muscle complex (L), and in palatine tonsils (P).

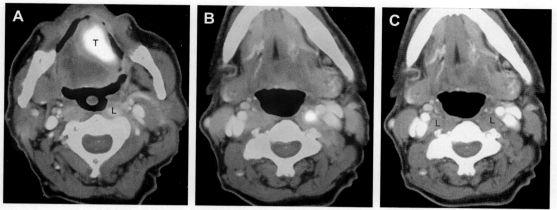

Fig. 8. Physiologic uptake in the left prevertebral muscles was misinterpreted as a retropharyngeal node in a patient who had newly diagnosed advanced tongue carcinoma. (*A*) Fused PET-CT image shows intense uptake in the left tongue carcinoma (T). Focal uptake is seen in the left prevertebral longus muscle complex initially misinterpreted as a retropharyngeal node. Note similar but asymmetric uptake in right prevertebral muscles. (*B*) Fused PET-CT image inferior to *A* again shows asymmetric bilateral uptake in the prevertebral muscles (L). (*C*) Corresponding CT image clearly shows that FDG uptake corresponds to muscles. In interpreting the scan, it is important to understand that metastases to retropharyngeal nodes are unusual in primary tongue cancers.

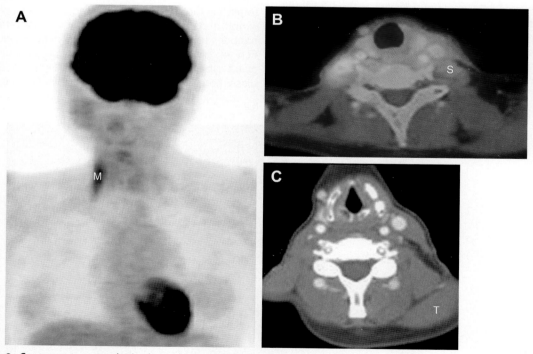

Fig. 9. Compensatory uptake in the scalenius muscle caused by injury to the spinal accessory nerve (cranial nerve 11). (*A*) Coronal PET image shows FDG uptake in the right neck (M). The linear nature of uptake should suggest this uptake is in muscle. (*B*) Axial fused PET-CT image shows uptake in the right scalenius muscle. S, left scalenius muscle complex. (*C*) Axial CT scan shows atrophy of the right trapezius muscle related to spinal accessory nerve injury. T, normal left trapezius muscle.

LIMITATIONS OF FDG-PET IN IMAGING THE TREATED NECK

PET typically is performed with the radiopharmaceutical ^{18}F-FDG, a D-glucose analogue. Increased vascularity and glucose metabolism of malignant cells result in preferential increase of FDG uptake by the tumor cells. The inability to process the metabolites of the modified glucose molecule causes intracellular accumulation of ^{18}F-containing radioisotopes. This phenomenon allows the diagnosis and staging of oncology patients. FDG-PET alone has the limitations of reduced spatial resolution as well as anatomic localization.[16,21] Perhaps the most significant contribution that CT has added to combined PET-CT modality is the ability to localize precisely regions of FDG uptake anatomically. A major pitfall of FDG-PET is the physiologic variation in the distribution of FDG radiotracer, especially in the head and neck.[22,23] The variations in FDG distribution become even more complex in patients who have been treated for head and neck cancer. The altered anatomy caused by surgery results in functional differences in the way patients use their necks, changing the pattern of radioisotope uptake on FDG-PET images. Further interpretative errors arise from poor understanding of both the posttreatment anatomy and the biology of head and neck cancer. Therefore, knowledge of head and neck cancers based on their anatomic site of occurrence, their typical patterns of lymph node metastases, and their patterns of recurrence is important in providing accurate interpretation of PET scans.

The normal distribution pattern of FDG (**Fig. 4**) includes high uptake in the gray matter of the brain and relatively low uptake in the lungs, mediastinum, and liver.[24] The myocardium has variable uptake that depends on several factors, including cardiac function, blood sugar levels, and physical activity before imaging.[24–26] The variable activity in the gastrointestinal tract (esophagus, stomach, colon) is a result of a variety of factors, most importantly persistent peristalsis and bowel activity. The skeletal muscles are expected to demonstrate relatively low uptake if the patient is calm and appropriately rested before imaging. The collecting systems of the urinary tract (calyces in the kidneys, and the ureters) excrete the FDG and therefore normally are FDG avid. It is important not to mistake the ureters for metastatic lymph nodes in the abdomen.

Physiologic variations of FDG uptake and distribution in the treated neck may occur in lymphoid tissue,[22,23,27] the salivary glands,[22,23,27] muscles (including the true vocal cords, the skeletal muscles, and oral cavity tongue),[22,23,27] and within brown fat.[28,29] Physiologic uptake may occur in the salivary glands (parotid and submandibular glands) as a sequela of radiation therapy and may be unilateral or bilateral depending on the therapy regimen. A common pitfall in PET is misinterpreting the submandibular gland as a malignant lymph node.[30] This misinterpretation most often happens in the setting of a unilateral neck dissection in which the contralateral submandibular gland typically is resected with the lymph node dissection. The remaining submandibular gland

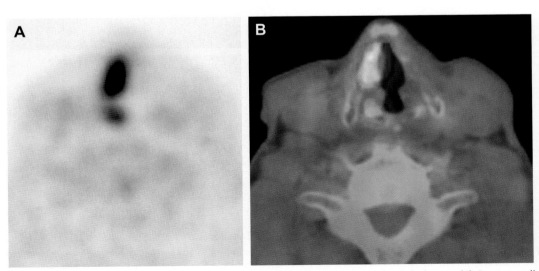

Fig. 10. Left vocal cord paralysis. (*A*) Axial PET scan shows physiologic uptake in the right larynx. (*B*) Corresponding axial fused PET-CT image shows uptake is in the right true vocal cord and arytenoid. Physiologic uptake in the contralateral cord is typical in the setting of vocal cord paralysis.

is mistaken for a neoplastic lymph node. In the pharynx, Waldeyer's ring consists of lymphoid tissue that includes the adenoids in the nasopharynx and paired palatine and lingual tonsils at the base of the tongue in the oropharynx. When these lymphoid tissue structures are resected to treat an underlying neoplasm, asymmetric physiologic uptake in the corresponding contralateral structure is common (Fig. 5).[31–34]

The uptake of FDG in brown adipose tissue (fat) may serve as another potential source of false-positive FDG-PET interpretations.[28,29,35] Brown fat plays an important role in cold-induced and weight-loss–induced thermogenesis. It frequently is formed in patients who have had rapid weight loss, such as patients being treated for cancer, and is more common in the winter. It also is more common in children and in women. The brown color of the fat probably is related to vascularity and increased mitochondrial density. FDG uptake in metabolic brown fat is explained by the presence of glucose transporters in brown adipose tissue. Brown fat commonly is bilaterally symmetric and occurs in the mediastinum, but it may be present in the paravertebral, cervical, axillary, and abdominal regions and in the

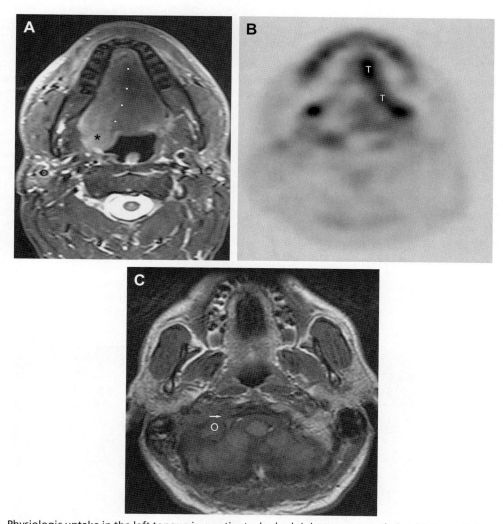

Fig. 11. Physiologic uptake in the left tongue in a patient who had right tongue paralysis misinterpreted as cancer. (A) Axial T2-weighted MR image with enlargement of the right base of tongue (*) initially interpreted as carcinoma. Closer evaluation showed the geographic nature of the signal abnormality (dots) consistent with right tongue paralysis rather than carcinoma. (B) Axial PET scan shows asymmetric uptake in the left tongue (T) misinterpreted as left tongue carcinoma. (C) Axial T1-weighted MR image at the base of the skull shows replacement of the right occipital condyle with tumor (O) and extension into the right hypoglossal canal that caused the patient's 12th (hypoglossal) nerve palsy. Biopsy revealed metastatic prostate carcinoma.

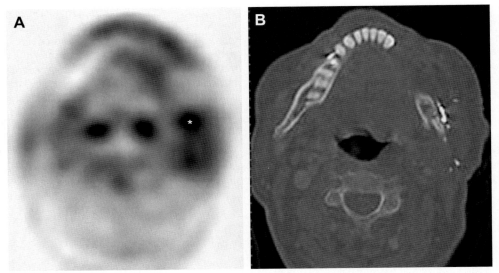

Fig. 12. Physiologic FDG uptake in reparative bone around a left mandibular graft. (*A*) Axial FDG-PET scan shows increased uptake in reparative bone at the graft site (*). (*B*) Corresponding axial CT scan in bone detail shows graft and reparative bone. (*Courtesy of* Barton F. Branstetter, MD, University of Pittsburg Medical Center, Pittsburg, PA.)

supraclavicular fossa (**Fig. 6**). In these regions, focal FDG uptake can be misinterpreted as primary malignancy or nodal metastases. Fusion PET/CT images are useful in avoiding this pitfall by localizing the focal FDG uptake precisely to regions of fat.

Some muscles in the neck that commonly may have physiologic uptake include the spinal cervicalis and splenius capitis muscles, the prevertebral muscles (longus colli and longus capitis), and the scalenius muscles.[28,36,37] This uptake may be symmetric or asymmetric. To minimize skeletal muscle uptake, it is important that the patient be at rest before imaging. Bilaterally symmetric muscle uptake usually is elongated in appearance and hence less often is misinterpreted as pathology (**Fig. 7**).[36]

In the treated neck, physiologic muscle uptake often is unilateral because of surgical absence of the contralateral muscles. Irradiated necks and untreated necks may show symmetric or asymmetric muscle uptake. Asymmetric uptake in the prevertebral muscles may be misinterpreted as retropharyngeal lymph nodes or a primary nasopharyngeal cancer (**Fig. 8**). In addition, in patients treated with surgery and/or irradiation, injury to the

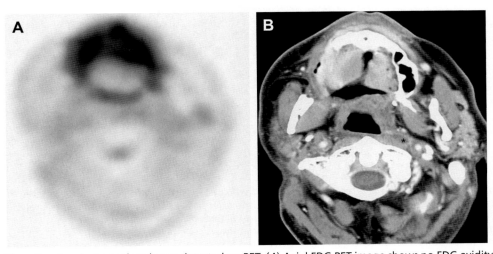

Fig. 13. Necrotic retropharyngeal node not detected on PET. (*A*) Axial FDG PET image shows no FDG avidity in the neck. (*B*) Corresponding axial CT image at same level as *A* shows necrotic left retropharyngeal node (*).

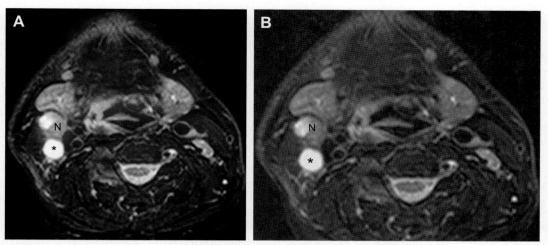

Fig. 14. Cystic cervical lymph node negative on FDG PET. (*A*) Fused PET-MR image shows a complex cystic and solid right level II node (N). Note the uptake of FDG only in the solid portion of the node. (*B*) The purely cystic right II lymph node (*) posterior to the complex lymph node (N) has no FDG uptake.

spinal accessory nerve (cranial nerve 11) may result in compensatory uptake in the ipsilateral anterior scalenius muscle (**Fig. 9**). One also should see associated atrophy of the ipsilateral trapezius muscle. If the patient has been talking, chewing gum, or eating before FDG imaging, there will be uptake in the muscles of mastication in the tongue. A vocal cord paralysis may result in normal physiologic uptake in the contralateral vocal cord that frequently is misinterpreted as a glottis cancer (**Fig. 10**).[38,39] Review of cross-sectional imaging

frequently shows the secondary findings of vocal cord paralysis, including dilation of the ipsilateral piriform sinus, vallecula, and laryngeal ventricle. These findings and the patient history will help avoid this false-positive pitfall. Tongue motion and swallowing are essential to clear secretions accumulating in the mouth. After partial glossectomy or irradiation and chemotherapy, patients usually have mucositis, sometimes have functional loss, and often have difficulty holding the tongue still both before and during the examination. This

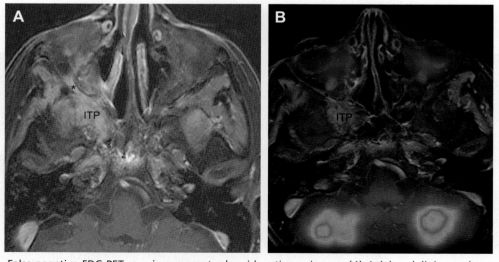

Fig. 15. False-negative FDG-PET scan in recurrent adenoid cystic carcinoma. (*A*) Axial gadolinium-enhanced fat-suppressed T1-weighted MR image shows enhancing tissue in the right inferior orbital fissure (*) and in the right infra-temporal fossa (ITP). Although this enhancement could reflect posttreatment granulation tissue, the appearance is concerning for neoplasm. (*B*) Axial fused PET-MR image shows enhancing tissue is not FDG avid. This finding was interpreted indicating that no tumor was present. Biopsy confirmed adenoid cystic carcinoma.

motion results in uptake in the residual anatomic or functioning tongue; this uptake should not be misinterpreted as residual or recurrent carcinoma (**Fig. 11**). Frequently, clinical correlation and manual palpation are necessary to confirm that uptake in the tongue represents muscular activity rather than neoplasm.

Sequelae of treatment and its complications also may result in false-positive interpretations on PET imaging. Specifically, inflammation (frequently seen with radiation therapy), radiation necrosis, and infection-abscess formation may result in FDG uptake that can be mistaken for recurrent or residual neoplasm. The presence of air in the involved soft tissues on the CT scan is an important associated finding and should raise concern for infection or radiation necrosis. In patients who have undergone surgical placement

of reconstructive grafts, such as positioning of a mandibular implant following a partial mandibulectomy, reparative bone formation can result in physiologic uptake of FDG (**Fig. 12**). Unrelated FDG uptake may occur outside of the head and neck in patients treated medically for head and neck cancer. Patients receiving systemic chemotherapy may experience gastritis or colitis, resulting in diffuse or focal regions of FDG uptake in the stomach or colon, respectively.

Other pitfalls of FDG PET in the treated neck include the inability to detect hypermetabolic activity in the cancer-harboring nodes. Lack of FDG avidity within cancer-containing nodes may be related to multiple factors including low cellularity,[40] the presence of cystic adenopathy,[41] or lymph nodes that are primarily necrotic (**Figs. 13** and **14**).[42,43] On close observation of FDG images,

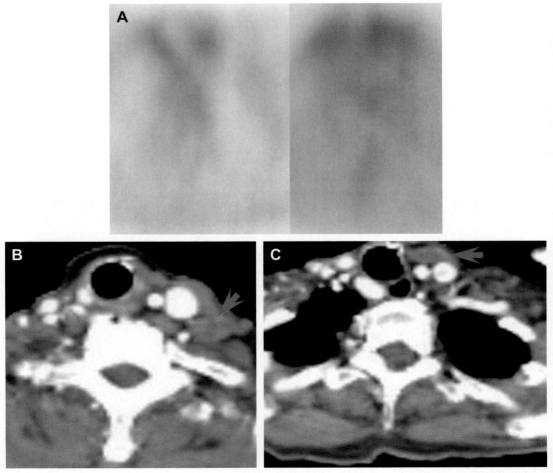

Fig. 16. Recurrent medullary thyroid cancer in cervical lymph nodes not detected on PET. (*A*) Axial FDG-PET images show no areas of FDG uptake. (*B, C*) Axial contrast-enhanced CT scans show metastatic lymph nodes posterior (*B*) and anterior (*C*) to the left carotid sheath. Medullary cancer was confirmed on fine-needle aspiration.

one may see a faint halo of FDG uptake in the residual surrounding lymphatic tissue, with predominant central photopenia related to necrosis and/or cystic change.

Malignant neoplasms sometimes do not show FDG avidity. Neoplasms that may not always demonstrate FDG avidity include mucinous adenocarcinomas,[40] salivary tumors (especially adenoid cystic carcinoma (**Fig. 15**) and mucoepidermoid carcinoma),[44] and thyroid cancers (iodine avid differentiated cancers and some medullary cancers) (**Fig. 16**). In contrast, not all areas of increased FDG uptake on a PET scan are malignant. Many FDG-avid neoplasms in the head and neck are benign, such as partially transformed pleomorphic adenomas, oncocytomas, Warthin's tumors, and schwannomas.[45–50] When evaluating a treated neck, it is important to localize the anatomic areas of FDG uptake in the neck correctly so that potentially benign lesions are not mistaken for malignant lymphadenopathy. For instance, incidental benign FDG-avid parotid tumors commonly are misinterpreted as metastatic nodes (**Fig. 17**).

APPLICATIONS OF PET-CT IN THE TREATED NECK

One may perform FDG PET imaging in head and neck cancer for several reasons. These reasons include initial staging of patients who present with advanced tumors, restaging in known or suspected recurrences, monitoring response to therapy (to determine if a therapy is working),

and evaluation of the patient who has an unknown primary site of tumor. In patients who have advanced tumors of the aerodigestive tract or sinonasal cavity at presentation, PET-CT may be indicated to evaluate for distant metastases. The presence of distant metastases will alter the patient's therapeutic management, prognosis, and long-term outcome significantly. In certain instances, the presence of distant disease will render the patient a non-surgical candidate.

PET-CT also is performed frequently for surveillance and follow-up imaging in patients at risk for developing loco-regional recurrence or distant metastatic disease. In patients who do not have clinical or radiologic evidence of recurrent disease on routine cross-sectional imaging, PET may detect a subclinical recurrence. Whether detection of these subclinical recurrences affects long-term survival, and what effect this impact has on quality-of-life measures remains to be determined. In patients who have suspected or known recurrent or residual disease, PET-CT plays a critical role in restaging, especially if surgical resection is being contemplated. If distant metastatic disease is identified on PET, it is unlikely that a large radical surgical procedure would be performed, because such surgery often causes significant losses in social and functional as well as cosmetic deformity and will not improve survival. In addition, in patients undergoing restaging, specific findings isolated to the head and neck may alter patient management. The role of the radiologist is to evaluate the primary site for recurrence and, if recurrence is present, to

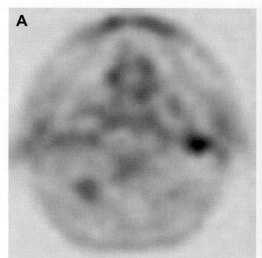 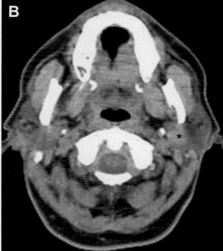

Fig. 17. Benign parotid tumor misinterpreted as metastatic lymph node in a patient treated for left oropharyngeal cancer. (*A*) Axial FDG-PET image shows the focal area of FDG uptake in the upper left neck initially interpreted as metastatic disease to level II lymph node. (*B*) Axial CT scan shows that the area of FDG uptake is in a benign oncocytoma (*) in the deep lobe of the left parotid gland.

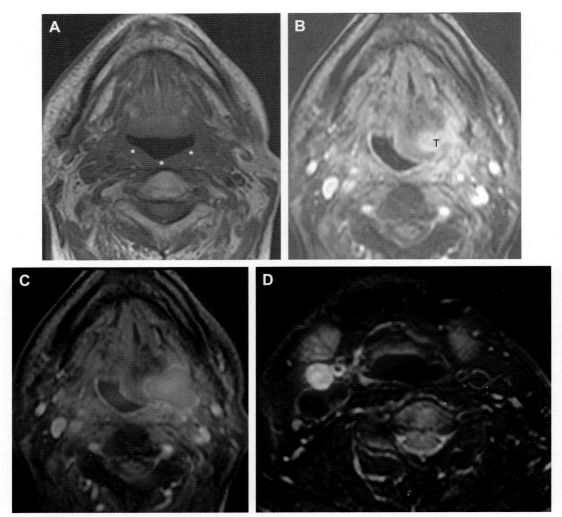

Fig. 18. PET-MR fusion performed to restage recurrent base of tongue carcinoma. The patient was treated with chemo-irradiation. (*A*) Axial T1-weighted MR image 1 year after treatment shows normal-appearing base of tongue. There are sequelae of radiation therapy including reticulation of subcutaneous fat and mucosal thickening in pharynx (*). (*B*) Axial gadolinium-enhanced fat-suppressed T1-weighted MR image shows enhancing recurrent tumor at the left base of the tongue (T). (*C*) Fused PET-MR image shows FDG-avid left base of tongue tumor. (*D*) Fused PET-MR scan shows a small, subcentimeter metastatic lymph node in the contralateral right neck detected by PET but found not to be pathologic by cross-sectional imaging criteria. This finding altered patient management, necessitating right neck dissection. There were no distant metastases.

assess the extent of tumor so that the surgeon can determine operative candidacy. Close evaluation of the contralateral and ipsilateral sides for nodal recurrence is essential for planning neck dissection (**Fig. 18**). Among the many pitfalls of PET in the assessment of the lungs in these patients are the presence of small lung metastases that may not be FDG avid (**Fig. 19**), inflammatory nodules[51–55] or lung infarctions[56] that may be FDG avid and mistaken for metastatic disease, and the frequent misidentification of aspirates or pneumonitis for

metastatic disease or a primary lung carcinoma (**Fig. 20**).[57]

PET-CT also is indicated in patients who have a history of a treated and presumptively cured head and neck cancer presenting with a neck mass (lymphadenopathy). This presentation would be atypical for the recurrence of the initial tumor. If such a patient has been treated previously for a head and neck cancer, it always is important to consider the possibility of a new, second primary cancer (**Fig. 21**).

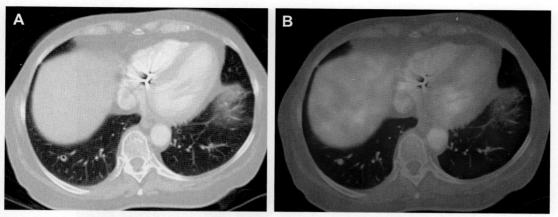

Fig. 19. Lung metastases not detected on PET. (*A*) Axial CT image shows small, bilateral new pulmonary nodules (*). (*B*) Corresponding fused PET-CT shows these nodules are not FDG avid.

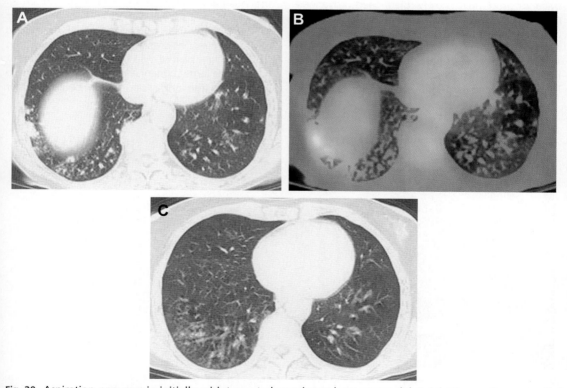

Fig. 20. Aspiration pneumonia initially misinterpreted as primary lung cancer. (*A*) Axial CT scan shows opacity/airspace disease in the right lower lobe. (*B*) Axial fused PET-CT shows this airspace disease is markedly FDG avid. (*C*) Follow-up chest CT scan 6 weeks later shows nearly total resolution of airspace disease following antibiotic therapy.

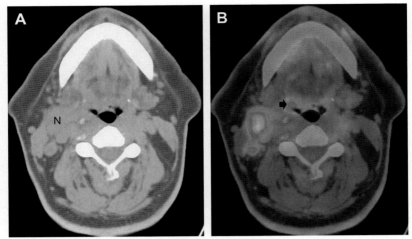

Fig. 21. A 67-year-old man treated 4 years ago for T1N0 glottic cancer presented with a new right neck mass. (*A*) Axial CT image shows multiple right IIA lymph nodes (N). (*B*) Fused axial PET-CT scan shows FDG-avid malignant lymphadenopathy in the right neck. Also detected is a new primary right base of tongue cancer (*arrow*) not detected on conventional cross-sectional imaging or physical examination with direct visualization.

Finally, an important pitfall of PET imaging is the possible failure to identify metastatic disease.[12,58–63] This pitfall is especially important in patients who have newly diagnosed advanced head and neck cancers in whom extensive therapy including a radical resection is being contemplated and has been observed at the authors' institution in a particular subset of patients, namely those who have advanced sinonasal carcinomas. Their initial PET-CT imaging is negative for distant disease; however, a subsequent surveillance PET-CT scan after completion of therapy reveals widely metastatic distant disease (**Fig. 22**). This situation raises the questions: Were these metastases there at presentation? If so, why were they not detected on PET imaging? One reason potential metastatic disease present at presentation is not detected on FDG-PET may be that the FDG is taken up preferentially by the large primary neoplasm, leaving little to circulate in the remainder of the body; another

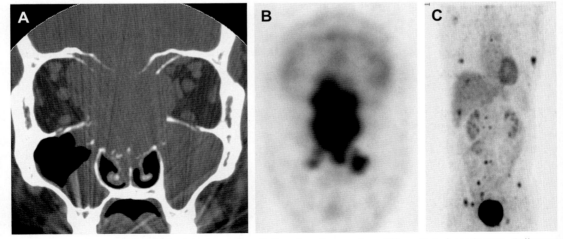

Fig. 22. The patient was treated with chemo-irradiation for sinonasal undifferentiated carcinoma. Follow-up surveillance PET-CT imaging shows widespread metastatic disease. (*A*) Coronal CT image at presentation shows a large neoplasm replacing the sinonasal cavity with orbital and intracranial extension. (*B*) PET scan obtained at presentation shows intense FDG uptake in sinonasal tumor. (*C*) Follow-up PET-CT obtained 6 months after chemo-irradiation shows lung, liver, and bone marrow metastases.

explanation is that the metastases may net be dense enough or large enough to be detected. It also is possible that in patients receiving systemic chemotherapy, inflammation incited around the metastatic foci may be responsible, in part, for the subsequent increase in FDG uptake in these lesions.

SUMMARY

The limitations of CT after therapy, most notably the overlapping attenuations of normal structures, tumor, and edema, and the limitations of PET after therapy, most notably spatial resolution, accurate localization of abnormalities, and physiologic variations of FDG distribution, are overcome by the targeted use of anatomic and molecular imaging that are complementary. Anatomic and molecular imaging together allow optimal evaluation and interpretation of a patient who has cancer. Effective assessment of patients who have head and neck cancer can be achieved through a careful review of pertinent anatomy, with awareness of the physiologic variations (especially those in the treated head and neck) seen in PET imaging, and analysis of both the PET and cross-sectional images.

REFERENCES

1. Greene FL, Page DL, Fritz AG, et al. AJCC cancer staging manual. 6th edition. New York: Springer-Verlag; 2002.
2. Day GL, Blot WJ. Second primary tumors in patients with oral cancer. Cancer 1992;70:14–9.
3. Narayana A, Vaughan AT, Fisher SG, et al. Second primary tumors in laryngeal cancer: results of long-term follow-up. Int J Radiat Oncol Biol Phys 1998; 42:557–62.
4. Rennemo E, Zatterstrom U, Boysen M. Impact of second primary tumors on survival in head and neck cancer: an analysis of 2,063 cases. Laryngoscope 2008;118:1350–6.
5. Di ME, Sellhaus B, Hausmann R, et al. Survival in second primary malignancies of patients with head and neck cancer. J Laryngol Otol 2002;116:831–8.
6. Vokes EE, Weichselbaum RR, Lippman SM, et al. Head and neck cancer. N Engl J Med 1993;328: 184–94.
7. van den Brekel MW, Stel HV, Castelijns JA, et al. Cervical lymph node metastasis: assessment of radiologic criteria. Radiology 1990;177:379–84.
8. Cerezo L, Millan I, Torre A, et al. Prognostic factors for survival and tumor control in cervical lymph node metastases from head and neck cancer. A multivariate study of 492 cases. Cancer 1992;69: 1224–34.
9. Schuller DE, McGuirt WF, McCabe BF, et al. The prognostic significance of metastatic cervical lymph nodes. Laryngoscope 1980;90:557–70.
10. Snow GB, Annyas AA, van Slooten EA, et al. Prognostic factors of neck node metastasis. Clin Otolaryngol Allied Sci 1982;7:185–92.
11. de Bondt RB, Nelemans PJ, Hofman PA, et al. Detection of lymph node metastases in head and neck cancer: a meta-analysis comparing US, USgFNAC, CT and MR imaging. Eur J Radiol 2007;64: 266–72.
12. Yamazaki Y, Saitoh M, Notani K, et al. Assessment of cervical lymph node metastases using FDG-PET in patients with head and neck cancer. Ann Nucl Med 2008;22:177–84.
13. Hannah A, Scott AM, Tochon-Danguy H, et al. Evaluation of 18 F-fluorodeoxyglucose positron emission tomography and computed tomography with histopathologic correlation in the initial staging of head and neck cancer. Ann Surg 2002;236:208–17.
14. Fleming AJ Jr, Smith SP Jr, Paul CM, et al. Impact of [18F]-2-fluorodeoxyglucose-positron emission tomography/computed tomography on previously untreated head and neck cancer patients. Laryngoscope 2007;117:1173–9.
15. Zanation AM, Sutton DK, Couch ME, et al. Use, accuracy, and implications for patient management of [18F]-2-fluorodeoxyglucose-positron emission/computerized tomography for head and neck tumors. Laryngoscope 2005;115:1186–90.
16. Schoder H, Yeung HW, Gonen M, et al. Head and neck cancer: clinical usefulness and accuracy of PET/CT image fusion. Radiology 2004;231:65–72.
17. Teknos TN, Rosenthal EL, Lee D, et al. Positron emission tomography in the evaluation of stage III and IV head and neck cancer. Head Neck 2001; 23:1056–60.
18. Hafidh MA, Lacy PD, Hughes JP, et al. Evaluation of the impact of addition of PET to CT and MR scanning in the staging of patients with head and neck carcinomas. Eur Arch Otorhinolaryngol 2006;263:853–9.
19. Nakamoto Y, Cohade C, Tatsumi M, et al. CT appearance of bone metastases detected with FDG PET as part of the same PET/CT examination. Radiology 2005;237:627–34.
20. Lell M, Baum U, Greess H, et al. Head and neck tumors: imaging recurrent tumor and post-therapeutic changes with CT and MRI. Eur J Radiol 2000;33:239–47.
21. Fukui MB, Blodgett TM, Snyderman CH, et al. Combined PET-CT in the head and neck: part 2. Diagnostic uses and pitfalls of oncologic imaging. Radiographics 2005;25:913–30.
22. Blodgett TM, Fukui MB, Snyderman CH, et al. Combined PET-CT in the head and neck: part 1. Physiologic, altered physiologic, and artifactual FDG uptake. Radiographics 2005;25:897–912.

23. Goerres GW, von Schulthess GK, Hany TF. Positron emission tomography and PET CT of the head and neck: FDG uptake in normal anatomy, in benign lesions, and in changes resulting from treatment. AJR Am J Roentgenol 2002;179:1337–43.

24. Shreve PD, Anzai Y, Wahl RL. Pitfalls in oncologic diagnosis with FDG PET imaging: physiologic and benign variants. Radiographics 1999;19: 61–77.

25. de GM, Meeuwis AP, Kok PJ, et al. Influence of blood glucose level, age and fasting period on non-pathological FDG uptake in heart and gut. Eur J Nucl Med Mol Imaging 2005;32:98–101.

26. Israel O, Weiler-Sagie M, Rispler S, et al. PET/CT quantitation of the effect of patient-related factors on cardiac 18F-FDG uptake. J Nucl Med 2007;48: 234–9.

27. Jabour BA, Choi Y, Hoh CK, et al. Extracranial head and neck: PET imaging with 2-[F-18]fluoro-2-deoxy-D-glucose and MR imaging correlation. Radiology 1993;186:27–35.

28. Cohade C, Osman M, Pannu HK, et al. Uptake in supraclavicular area fat ("USA-Fat"): description on 18F-FDG PET/CT. J Nucl Med 2003;44:170–6.

29. Hany TF, Gharehpapagh E, Kamel EM, et al. Brown adipose tissue: a factor to consider in symmetrical tracer uptake in the neck and upper chest region. Eur J Nucl Med Mol Imaging 2002;29:1393–8.

30. Shipchandler TZ, Lorenz RR. Unilateral submandibular gland aplasia masquerading as cancer nodal metastasis. Am J Otolaryngol 2008;29:432–4.

31. Davis E, Solis V, Rosenberg RJ, et al. Asymmetric tongue muscle uptake of F-18 FDG: possible marker for cranial nerve XII paralysis. Clin Nucl Med 2004; 29:531–3.

32. Wong WL, Gibson D, Sanghera B, et al. Evaluation of normal FDG uptake in palatine tonsil and its potential value for detecting occult head and neck cancers: a PET CT study. Nucl Med Commun 2007;28:675–80.

33. Nakamoto Y, Tatsumi M, Hammoud D, et al. Normal FDG distribution patterns in the head and neck: PET/CT evaluation. Radiology 2005;234:879–85.

34. Chen YK, Su CT, Chi KH, et al. Utility of 18F-FDG PET/CT uptake patterns in Waldeyer's ring for differentiating benign from malignant lesions in lateral pharyngeal recess of nasopharynx. J Nucl Med 2007;48:8–14.

35. Nedergaard J, Bengtsson T, Cannon B. Unexpected evidence for active brown adipose tissue in adult humans. Am J Physiol Endocrinol Metab 2007;293: E444–52.

36. Jacene HA, Goudarzi B, Wahl RL. Scalene muscle uptake: a potential pitfall in head and neck PET/CT. Eur J Nucl Med Mol Imaging 2008;35:89–94.

37. Jackson RS, Schlarman TC, Hubble WL, et al. Prevalence and patterns of physiologic muscle uptake detected with whole-body 18F-FDG PET. J Nucl Med Technol 2006;34:29–33.

38. Lee M, Ramaswamy MR, Lilien DL, et al. Unilateral vocal cord paralysis causes contralateral false-positive positron emission tomography scans of the larynx. Ann Otol Rhinol Laryngol 2005;114: 202–6.

39. Heller MT, Meltzer CC, Fukui MB, et al. Superphysiologic FDG uptake in the non-paralyzed vocal cord. Resolution of a false-positive PET result with combined PET-CT imaging. Clin Positron Imaging 2000;3:207–11.

40. Berger KL, Nicholson SA, Dehdashti F, et al. FDG PET evaluation of mucinous neoplasms: correlation of FDG uptake with histopathologic features. AJR Am J Roentgenol 2000;174:1005–8.

41. Goldenberg D, Sciubba J, Koch WM. Cystic metastasis from head and neck squamous cell cancer: a distinct disease variant? Head Neck 2006;28:633–8.

42. Inohara H, Enomoto K, Tomiyama Y, et al. The role of CT and (18) F-FDG PET in managing the neck in node-positive head and neck cancer after chemoradiotherapy. Acta Otolaryngol 2008;1–7 [Epub ahead of print].

43. Zhang GY, Hu WH, Liu LZ, et al. [Comparison between PET/CT and MRI in diagnosing lymph node metastasis and N staging of nasopharyngeal carcinoma]. Zhonghua Zhong Liu Za Zhi 2006;28:381–4 [In Chinese].

44. Ishizumi T, Tateishi U, Watanabe S, et al. F-18 FDG PET/CT imaging of low-grade mucoepidermoid carcinoma of the bronchus. Ann Nucl Med 2007; 21:299–302.

45. Chang CY, Fan YM, Bai CY, et al. Schwannoma mimicking lung cancer metastases demonstrated by PET/CT. Clin Nucl Med 2006;31:644–5.

46. Hamada K, Ueda T, Higuchi I, et al. Peripheral nerve schwannoma: two cases exhibiting increased FDG uptake in early and delayed PET imaging. Skeletal Radiol 2005;34:52–7.

47. Otsuka H, Graham MM, Kogame M, et al. The impact of FDG-PET in the management of patients with salivary gland malignancy. Ann Nucl Med 2005;19:691–4.

48. Subramaniam RM, Durnick DK, Peller PJ. F-18 FDG PET/CT imaging of submandibular gland oncocytoma. Clin Nucl Med 2008;33:472–4.

49. Shah VN, Branstetter BF. Oncocytoma of the parotid gland: a potential false-positive finding on 18F-FDG PET. AJR Am J Roentgenol 2007;189:W212–4.

50. Schwarz E, Hurlimann S, Soyka JD, et al. FDG-positive Warthin's tumors in cervical lymph nodes mimicking metastases in tongue cancer staging with PET/CT. Otolaryngol Head Neck Surg 2009; 140:134–5.

51. Ohtsuka T, Nomori H, Watanabe K, et al. False-positive findings on [18F] FDG-PET caused by non-neoplastic cellular elements after neoadjuvant

chemoradiotherapy for non-small cell lung cancer. Jpn J Clin Oncol 2005;35:271–3.

52. Tomita M, Ichinari H, Tomita Y, et al. A case of non-small cell lung cancer with false-positive staging by positron emission tomography. Ann Thorac Cardiovasc Surg 2003;9:397–400.

53. Yang SN, Liang JA, Lin FJ, et al. Differentiating benign and malignant pulmonary lesions with FDG-PET. Anticancer Res 2001;21:4153–7.

54. Mackie GC, Pohlen JM. Mediastinal histoplasmosis: F-18 FDG PET and CT findings simulating malignant disease. Clin Nucl Med 2005;30:633–5.

55. Ahmadzadehfar H, Palmedo H, Strunk H, et al. False positive 18F-FDG-PET/CT in a patient after talc pleurodesis. Lung Cancer 2007;58:418–21.

56. Kamel EM, McKee TA, Calcagni ML, et al. Occult lung infarction may induce false interpretation of 18F-FDG PET in primary staging of pulmonary malignancies. Eur J Nucl Med Mol Imaging 2005;32:641–6.

57. Tahon F, Berthezene Y, Hominal S, et al. Exogenous lipoid pneumonia with unusual CT pattern and FDG positron emission tomography scan findings. Eur Radiol 2002;12(Suppl 3):S171–3 [Epub 2002 Oct 1:S171–3].

58. Schroeder U, Dietlein M, Wittekindt C, et al. Is there a need for positron emission tomography imaging to stage the N0 neck in T1-T2 squamous cell carcinoma of the oral cavity or oropharynx? Ann Otol Rhinol Laryngol 2008;117:854–63.

59. Nahmias C, Carlson ER, Duncan LD, et al. Positron emission tomography/computerized tomography (PET/CT) scanning for preoperative staging of patients with oral/head and neck cancer. J Oral Maxillofac Surg 2007;65:2524–35.

60. Tan A, Adelstein DJ, Rybicki LA, et al. Ability of positron emission tomography to detect residual neck node disease in patients with head and neck squamous cell carcinoma after definitive chemoradiotherapy. Arch Otolaryngol Head Neck Surg 2007;133:435–40.

61. Ng SH, Yen TC, Chang JT, et al. Prospective study of [18F]fluorodeoxyglucose positron emission tomography and computed tomography and magnetic resonance imaging in oral cavity squamous cell carcinoma with palpably negative neck. J Clin Oncol 2006;24:4371–6.

62. Stoeckli SJ, Steinert H, Pfaltz M, et al. Is there a role for positron emission tomography with 18F-fluorodeoxyglucose in the initial staging of nodal negative oral and oropharyngeal squamous cell carcinoma. Head Neck 2002;24:345–9.

63. Isles MG, McConkey C, Mehanna HM. A systematic review and meta-analysis of the role of positron emission tomography in the follow up of head and neck squamous cell carcinoma following radiotherapy or chemoradiotherapy. Clin Otolaryngol 2008;33:210–22.

PET/CT in Neuroendocrine Tumors: Evaluation of Receptor Status and Metabolism

Vikas Prasad, MD[a], Valentina Ambrosini, MD, PhD[b],
Abass Alavi, MD, PhD (Hon), DSc (Hon)[c], Stefano Fanti, MD[b],
Richard P. Baum, MD, PhD[a],*

KEYWORDS
- Neuroendocrine tumors • PET/CT
- Somatostatin receptor imaging • Ga-68 • F-18 DOPA

Neuroendocrine tumors (NETs) include a diverse group of neoplasms characterized by their endocrine function and specific histologic characteristics. Previously known as carcinoid tumors, the term coined by Oberndorfer[1] in 1907 for small intestinal lesions, most NET neoplasms were wrongly thought to originate from the neural crest. Recently, the origin of these tumors has been traced to pluripotent stem cells or differentiated neuroendocrine cells.[2] APUD-oma (amine precursor uptake and decarboxylation), gastroenteropancreatic (GEP) tumor, islet cell tumor, neuroendocrine carcinoma, and other names have been suggested to cover the wide variety of tumor types that belong to the NET group.[2]

The most common sites from which NETs originate are the bronchus/lungs and GEP tract and, less often, the skin, adrenal glands, thyroid, and genital tract.[3] NETs that have a common origin from the foregut, midgut, or hindgut share similar functional manifestations, histochemistry, and secretory granules.[3] Histologically, NETs can be classified based on the degree of differentiation (**Box 1**).[4,5] A new tumor, node, and metastasis staging scheme has been proposed for foregut NETs, and it has been shown by some groups to have good correlation with prognosis.

The presence or absence of symptoms because of biogenic amines and hormones has been the basis for classifying NETs as functional or nonfunctional tumors. Nearly 33% to 50% of all NETs are nonfunctional, whereas the rest are associated with various symptoms.

Numerous factors are known to have an influence on survival and prognosis of patients, among which the presence of liver metastases is the single most important factor. A correlation has been found between the size of the primary tumor and the probability of metastases for small intestinal carcinoids. Metastases to the liver can be found in 15% to 25% of tumors if the tumor diameter is in less than 1 cm, 58% to 80% if it is 1 to 2 cm, and more than 75% if the tumor size is more than 2 cm.[3] These prognostic factors make it essential to use reliable diagnostic indicators before treating patients with a particular treatment regimen.

This article originally appeared in *PET Clinics* 2007;2:351–375
[a] Department of Nuclear Medicine and Center for PET/CT, Zentralklinik Bad Berka GmbH, Robert Koch Allee-9, 99437 Bad Berka, Germany
[b] Department of Nuclear Medicine, University of Bologna, Policlinico S. Orsola-Malpighi, via Massarenti 9, 40138 Bologna, Italy
[c] Department of Radiology, Hospital of the University of Pennsylvania, 3400 Spruce Street, 110 Donner Building, Philadelphia, PA 19104, USA
* Corresponding author.
E-mail address: info@rpbaum.de (R.P. Baum).

PET Clin 3 (2009) 355–379
doi:10.1016/j.cpet.2009.04.010
1556-8598/09/$ – see front matter © 2009 Elsevier Inc. All rights reserved.

DIAGNOSIS OF NEUROENDOCRINE TUMORS: HISTOPATHOLOGY, BIOCHEMICAL INVESTIGATION, STRUCTURAL IMAGING

Biochemical Investigations

The most validated markers for the diagnosis and the follow-up of carcinoid tumors include[2]

1. Chromogranin A (CGA)
2. 5-Hydroxyindoleacetic acid (urinary metabolite of serotonin)
3. Gastrin
4. Serotonin
5. Pancreastatin
6. Neurokinin A (substance K)

For follow-up, serial measurements of these markers are made every 3 to 6 months. The absolute value of CGA is not a determinate of tumor burden; nor can it rule out or confirm metastases. Changes in CGA level by 25% over the baseline are considered significant. There has been a concordance between the CGA levels and the findings on ^{131}I-metaiodobenzylguanidine (MIBG) scintigraphy. A CGA level in the reference range has been found to be highly predictive of normal scintigraphy results. Several other conditions lead to elevated levels of CGA, however, such as hypergastrinemia caused by electrochromaffin-like cell hyperplasia secondary to proton pump inhibitors, renal insufficiency, and severe hypertension. Circadian rhythm of CGA warrants the need for blood sampling at approximately the same time at every visit for follow-up purposes.

In cases in which gastrinoma is suspected (history of abdominal pain, diarrhea, and gastroesophageal reflux disease) a fasting gastrin level-should be measured. For insulinoma, an elevated insulin level should be demonstrated in fasting state. C-peptide and serum glucose levels are also measured. For pheochromocytoma, metanephrines, catecholamines, and their metabolites should be measured in the blood and urine.[2,3]

Histopathology

In the past, NETs were lumped together as a single entity because they were characterized by their propensity to stain with silver and have abnormal levels of neuroendocrine tissue markers, such as chromogranin, neuron-specific enolase, and synaptophysin, when immunohistochemical methods were used. The recent World Health Organization classification and the new tumor, node, and metastasis staging[6] scheme have taken into consideration the different histopathologic behavior of these tumors in characterizing them further. These classifications have been shown to have good correlation with prognosis.

Structural Diagnostic Imaging

Surgical resection remains the mainstay of treatment of NET; after biochemical confirmation, the next step in the diagnostic algorithm is to stage the disease. Although CT and MR imaging are accurate in providing correct anatomic location of the lesions, structural imaging methodologies are of limited use in diagnosing an unknown tumor and defining its prognosis of NETs. The extent of the tumor, in terms of metastases, often can be underestimated based on morphologic criteria because molecular changes precede structural alterations with most disorders. Likewise, in therapy monitoring, the size criteria are often inadequate for detecting early response. The role of ultrasound (US) in the diagnosis of NET is also limited and depends largely on the site of disease. For the detection of liver metastases, US has a high diagnostic accuracy. In cases in which a gastric or pancreatic primary tumor is suspected, endoscopic US is of diagnostic value.

Molecular/Metabolic Imaging

Positron emission tomography (PET) is increasingly being used for detecting disease at the molecular/metabolic level. The feasibility of fusing functional imaging (PET or single photon emission CT [SPECT]) with structural imaging (CT/MR imaging) overcomes certain shortcomings of purely functional imaging alone for diagnostic and therapeutic purposes. This article covers only the role of PET and PET/CT in the management of patients with NETs. It includes potential PET radiopharmaceuticals used for this purpose, imaging protocols, and the various indications for PET or PET/CT in NETs.

Table 1
Positron emission tomography radiopharmaceuticals for the diagnosis of neuroendocrine tumors

	Radiopharmaceutical	Receptor/Metabolic Target	Indication and Comments
PET	^{18}F-FDG	Glycolytic pathway	All NETs. Sensitivity in NET is low compared with other radiopharmaceuticals. Useful for undifferentiated NET. Observation of flip-flop mechanism with SMS-R PET
	^{68}Ga-DOTA-NOC	Somatostatin receptor (pansomatostatin, high affinity for SSTR2, 3, and 5)	All SSTR + VE NETs
	^{68}Ga-DOTA-TOC	Somatostatin receptor (highest affinity for SSTR2)	All SSTR + VE NETs
	^{11}C-5-HTP	Serotonin production pathway	All serotonin-producing NETs
	^{11}C-DOPA	Dopamine production pathway	Pheochromocytoma, paraganglioma, neuroblastoma. Short half-life, cost of production, and difficulty in obtaining[11] C-labeled compounds pose limitations for this compound
	^{18}F-DOPA	Dopamine production pathway	Pheochromocytoma, paraganglioma, neuroblastoma, glomus tumor
	^{18}F-FDA	Catecholamine precursor	Pheochromocytoma, paraganglioma, neuroblastoma
	^{64}Cu-TETA-octretoide	Somatostatin receptor	All SSTR + VE NETs
	^{18}F-FP-Gluc-TOCA	Somatostatin receptor	All SSTR + VE NETs
	^{11}C-ephedrine	Catecholamine transporter	Pheochromocytoma, neuroblastoma, study of sympathetic nervous system
	^{11}C-hydroxyephidrine	Catecholamine transporter	Pheochromocytoma, neuroblastoma, study of sympathetic nervous system

Abbreviation: VE; positive.

POSITRON EMISSION TOMOGRAPHY RADIOPHARMACEUTICALS

PET radiopharmaceuticals can be directed toward assessing receptor expression or characterizing the intratumoral metabolic processes. The metabolic events and receptor targets that are currently being examined by PET are as follows (**Table 1**):

Receptor targets:
1. Somatostatin receptor expression
2. Miscellaneous other peptide receptors

Metabolic processes:
1. Serotonin production pathway
2. Biogenic amine storage
3. Catecholamine transport
4. Glucose metabolism

Receptor-Targeting Radiopharmaceuticals

Somatostatin receptor-based radiopharmaceuticals

The abundance of somatostatin receptor (SSTR) expression on NETs (**Table 2**) has resulted in the development of several radiopharmaceuticals that are directed toward these sites. Among the five different SSTR types, most NETs express SSTR2, with a low percentage expressing SSTR1 and SSTR5.[7–9]

The currently used somatostatin radiopharmaceuticals (**Table 3**) are derivatives of octreotide, lanreotide, or vapreotide and show variable binding to SSTR.[8,10–12] ^{68}Ga-DOTA-TOC was the first radiopharmaceutical used for PET imaging of NETs. Wild and colleagues[11,12] have shown that the compound ^{68}Ga-DOTA-NOC has three to four times higher binding affinity to SSTR2, 3, and 5 than ^{68}Ga-DOTA-TOC, which results in detection of a wide range of SSTR-positive tumors (pansomatostatin analog) and has a significant effect on diagnosis, staging, and therapy of NETs and various other somatostatin-receptor expressing tumors. Other somatostatin analogs, such as DOTA-NOC-ATE [(DOTA-1Nal[3], Thr8)-octreotide] and DOTA-BOC-ATE [(DOTA, BzThi[3], Thr[8])-octreotide], are in the preclinical stages of development. SSTR antagonists, (NH(2)-CO-c(DCys-Phe-Tyr-DAgl(8)Me,2-naphthoyl)-Lys-Thr-Phe-Cys)-OH (sst(3)-ODN-8) and (sst(2)-ANT), also have been labeled with [111]In. They have been shown to be superior to SSTR agonists (in mice model) for in vivo targeting of SSTR2- and SSTR3-rich tumors.[13,14]

[68]Ga is eluted from a ^{68}Ga/68Ge generator. Currently, several vendors supply Ga-68/Ge-68 generators, making it widely accessible around the globe. [68]Ga ($t_{1/2}$ = 68 min) is a positron emitter with an 89% positron emission rate and a negligible gamma emission (1077 keV) of only 3.2%. The long half-life of the mother radionuclide [68]Ge (270.8 days) makes it possible to use the generator for approximately 9 to 12 months, depending on the requirement.

Table 2
Somatostatin receptor expression on different tumors

Tumor Types	Receptor Subtypes
Gastroenteropancreatic NET	SSTR1, SSTR2, SSTR5
Neuroblastoma	SSTR2
Meningioma	SSTR2
Breast carcinoma	SSTR2
Medulloblastoma	SSTR2
Lymphoma	SSTR2, SSTR5
Renal cell carcinoma	SSTR2
Paraganglioma	SSTR1, SSTR2, SSTR3
Small-cell lung cancer	SSTR2
Hepatoma	SSTR2
Prostate carcinoma	SSTR1
Sarcoma	SSTR1, SSTR2, SSTR4
Inactive pituitary adenoma	SSTR1, SSTR2, SSTR3, SSTR5
Growth hormone–producing pituitary adenoma	SSTR2, SSTR3, SSTR5
Gastric carcinomas	SSTR1, SSTR2, SSTR5
Ependydomas	SSTR1
Pheochromocytoma	SSTR1, SSTR2, SSTR5

Table 3
Affinity profiles (IC_{50}) of somatostatin receptor subtypes for different somatostatin analogs used in diagnostic imaging with positron emission tomography/CT or single photon emission CT

Somatostatin Analogs	SSTR1	SSTR2	SSTR3	SSTR4	SSTR5
Native somatostatin (S28)	5.2	2.7	7.7	5.6	4.0
In-DTPA-octreotide	> 10,000	22	182	> 1000	237
In-DOTA-[Tyr3]octreotide (DOTA-TOC)	> 10,000	4.6	120	230	130
DOTA-lanreotide (DOTA-LAN)	> 10,000	26	771	> 10,000	73
DOTA-[Tyr3]octreotate (DOTA-TATE)	> 10,000	1.5	> 1000	453	547
Y-DOTA-TOC	> 10,000	11	389	> 10,000	114
Ga-DOTA-TOC	> 10,000	2.5	613	> 1000	73
In-DOTA[1-Nal3]octreotide (DOTA-NOC)	> 10,000	2.9	8	227	11.2
Y-DOTA[1-Nal3]octreotide (DOTA-NOC)	> 1000	3.3	26	> 1000	10.4
In-DOTA-NOC-ATE	> 10,000	2	13	160	4.3
In-DOTA-BOC-ATE	> 1000	1.4	5.5	135	3.9

IC50 is expressed in nanomoles (lower value represent higher receptor affinity).

For labeling purposes, the ^{68}Ga eluate is first concentrated and purified using a micro chromatography method as described by Rösch and colleagues.[15,16] After preconcentration and purification of the initial generator eluates, ^{68}Ga(III) is re-eluted with 400 μL 98% acetone/0.05 N HCl solution (2×10^{-5} mol HCl). This fraction is used for labeling of DOTA-octreotide derivatives, such as DOTA-TOC, DOTA-NOC, or DOTA-TATE. For the production of ^{68}Ga-DOTA-NOC, 1 GBq ^{68}Ga is put into a vial containing 30 to 50 μg of the peptide. Subsequently, ^{68}Ga-DOTA-NOC is purified and finally eluted using 0.5 mL ethanol into 4.5 mL of isotonic saline. Radiolabeling yields of more than 95% can usually be achieved within 15 minutes. Overall, 370 to 700 MBq of ^{68}Ga-DOTA-NOC are obtained within 20 minutes.

For DOTA-TOC, the processed eluate containing ^{68}Ga (up to 700 MBq) is added to 4 to 4.5 mL pure H_2O in the reagent vial containing 7 to 14 nmol DOTA-TOC with addition of HERPES buffer. ^{68}Ga-labeled DOTA-derived octreotides are purified from unreacted ^{68}Ga species by reversed phase chromatography. The reaction mixture is then passed through a small C18 cartridge; after washing the cartridge with 5 mL H_2O, the ^{68}Ga-labeled peptide is recovered with 200 to 400 μL of pure ethanol. A radiolabeling yield of 88% at approximately 99°C is achieved within 10 minutes with specific activities of up to 450 MBq/μmol of peptide.[17]

Miscellaneous peptides

Several other peptides have been developed by radiopharmacists for imaging NETs. Bombesin labeled with ^{68}Ga is one such peptide that is being investigated in undifferentiated prostate cancers, breast carcinomas, small-cell lung cancer, and renal cell carcinomas and some NETs. VIP, a 28 amino acid peptide that was initially isolated from porcine intestine, has been studied for imaging of neuroendocrine GEP tumors, especially VIPomas.[18–22] Other peptides that have been used for receptor scintigraphy of NETs include cholecystokinin (CCK-B), gastrin, minigastrin and others. Work is ongoing to determine the best peptide for targeting these tumors.[23–28]

Metabolism-Targeted Radiopharmaceuticals

Pharmaceuticals that target the serotonin production pathway

Most of the clinical symptoms of a NET are caused by excessive production of serotonin.

Table 4
Drugs that interfere with vesicular monoamine transporters, leading to wrong interpretation of ^{123}I/^{131}I-MIBG single photon emission CT, ^{11}C-E/^{11}C-HED/^{18}F-FDA positron emission tomography scans

Mechanism	Drugs
Uptake-1 inhibition	Sympathomimetics (eg, cocaine, opioids) Tricyclic antidepressants (eg, amitryptaline, imipramine, ioxapine) Antipsychotic/antiemetics (eg, phenithiazines, thioxanthenes, butyrophenones) Antihypertensive/cardiovascular agents Tetracyclic antidepressants (eg, Maprotiline, mirtazapine)
Inhibition of granular uptake	Antihypertensive/cardiovascular agents (eg, Reserpine) For movement disorders (eg, tetrabenazine)
Competitive inhibition of granular uptake	Sympathomimetic (eg, norepinephrine) Antidepressants (eg, serotonin) Antihypertensives (eg, guanethidine)
Depletion of storage granules	Antihypertensive/cardiovascular agents (eg, Reserpine, guanethidine, labetolol, bethanidine) Sympathomemtics (eg, phenylephrine, phenylpropanolamine, ephedrine, pseudoephedrine, amphetamine, dobutamine, dopamine, metarminol)
Increased uptake and retention	Antihypertensives/calcium channel blockers (eg, angiotensin-converting enzyme inhibitors)

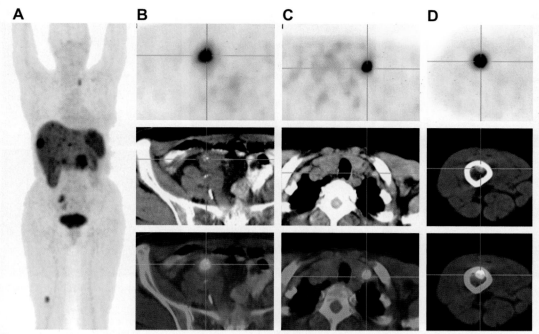

Fig. 1. Ga-68 DOTA-TATE PET/CT: Whole-body diagnosis ("one stop shop"). Maximum intensity projection image (*A*) showing an abdominal lesion, liver metastases, a left supraclaviular lesion and a hot spot in the right thigh. Transversal PET/CT slices reveal the primary tumor (previously unknown) in the ileum (*B*), a left parathyroidal lymph node metastasis (*C*) and a bone marrow metastasis (also previously unknown) in the right distal femur (*D*).

5-Hydroxytryptophan is one of the intermediates in the production pathway that has been labeled successfully with [11]C.[29,30] A phase 1 clinical trial is underway to ascertain the role of ^{11}C-labeled-5-hydroxytryptophan in functional, serotonin-producing NETs.

Pharmaceuticals that target biogenic amine production and storage mechanism

NETs are characterized by the production and storage of several biogenic amines. One tracer with a design based on this observation is [11]C- or ^{18}F-labeled L-dihydroxyphenylalanine (DOPA).

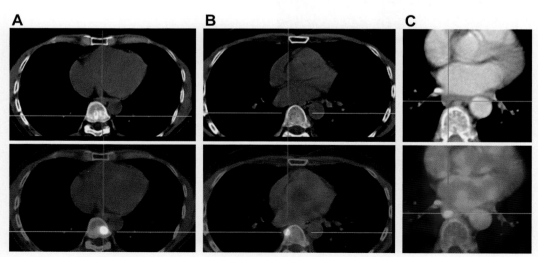

Fig. 2. Ga-68 DOTA-NOC PET/CT: Accuracy and sensitivity of disease localization. Osteoblastic metastases in thoracic vertebra (*A*), bone marrow metastasis (*B*) without anatomical alteration on CT (in MRI size 3 mm in diameter), and small prevertebral/paracardiac metastasis of neuroendocrine tumor (*C*).

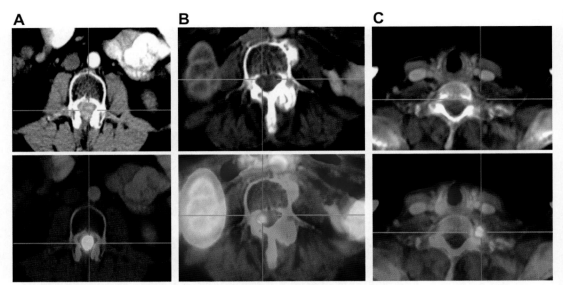

Fig. 3. Ga-68 DOTA-TATE PET/CT: Accuracy of disease localization. Intraspinal (*A, B*) and paravertebral (*C*) metastases of malignant pheochromocytoma.

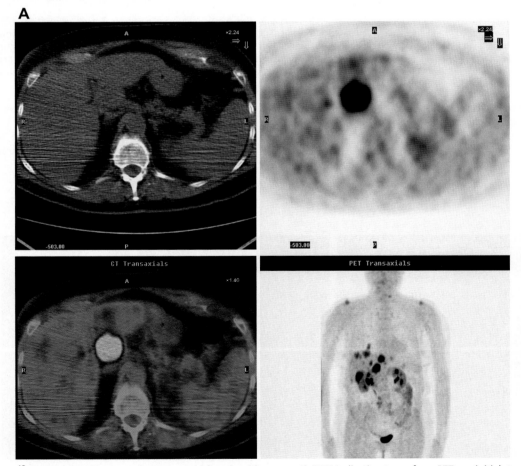

Fig. 4. ^{18}F-DOPA PET/CT images of a 63-year-old female with pancreatic NET. Indication to perform PET was initial staging. Conventional imaging showed peri-pancreatic nodes involvement, while SRS identified positive areas at liver level. ^{18}F-DOPA PET/CT images showed positive peri-pancreatic nodes (*A*), multiple liver metastasis (*B*) and sign of arthrosis.

B

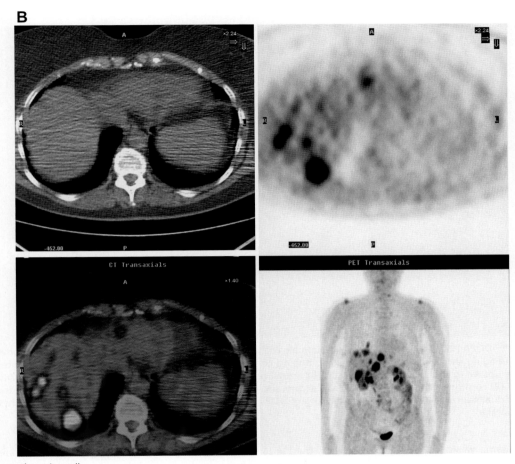

Fig. 4. (continued)

^{18}F-DOPA is an aromatic amino acid labeled with ^{18}fluorine that was first used for the assessment of patients who have Parkinson's disease.[31] More recently, ^{18}F-DOPA has been used to differentiate between focal and diffuse congenital hyperglycemia[32] and study NETs. Belonging to the APUD (amine precursor uptake and decarboxylation) cells system, many NET cells avidly take up ^{18}F-DOPA and can be visualized by ^{18}F-DOPA-PET scans.

At the central and the peripheral nervous system level, ^{18}F-DOPA is transformed by COMT enzyme (Catechol-O-Methyl-Transferase) into Catechol-O-Methyl-fuloro-L-DOPA and by aromatic amino acid decarboxylase into 6-fluorodopamine (FDA).[33,34] Both products are then stored in secretory granules. Recent studies have demonstrated increased L-DOPA decarboxylase activity in 80% of NETs, and it has been suggested that this could be used as a marker of tumor activity.[35] Physiologic ^{18}F-DOPA uptake has been seen because of its excretion in the bile ducts, gallbladder, and digestive and urinary tracts.[36] Physiologic uptake in the striatum and pancreas has been reported.

Pharmaceuticals that target catecholamine transport pathway

Pheochromocytoma, neuroblastoma, and other chromaffin tissues concentrate many synthetic amine precursors using catecholamine transporters. ^{11}C-epinephrine (^{11}C-E) and ^{11}C hydroxyepiphedrine (^{11}C-HED), both catecholamine analogs, and ^{18}F-fluorodopamine (^{18}F-FDA) are examples of such precursors (**Table 4**).[37]

Pharmaceuticals that target increased tumor glucose metabolism

One of the fundamental energy sources of many tumors is glucose. ^{18}F-2-fluoro-2-deoxyglucose (FDG) targets the glycolytic pathway, the main source of glucose consumption in tumors. FDG enters the glycolytic pathway like glucose in the

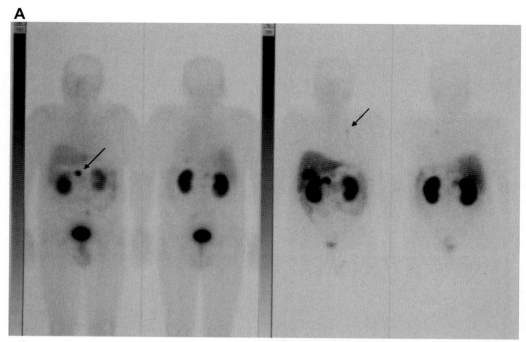

Fig. 5. ^{18}F-DOPA PET/CT images of a 60-year-old male with MEN1. Previous surgery: distal pancreatecomy. Conventional imaging showed a suspicious thoracic finding confirmed by SRS (*A*) that also detected the presence of intense uptake in the residual pancreas. (*Right arrow*) residual pancreas; (*Left arrow*) thoracic lesion. ^{18}F-DOPA PET/CT (*B*) confirmed the pathologic uptake at thoracic level (*C*) and also identified the presence of disease in the residual pancreas (*D*), although the reading of DOPA uptake at pancreas level is limited by the high physiologic uptake.

cytoplasm, where it is phosphorylated by the enzyme hexokinase to FDG-6-phosphate. It does not get metabolized further, however, and gets trapped inside the neoplastic cells.

Imaging Protocols

Receptor positron emission tomography/CT using ^{68}Ga-DOTA-NOC

Sandostatin long-acting release injections must be stopped 4 to 6 weeks before the scan, and subcutaneous treatment with octreotide should be stopped at least 2 days before. Care should be taken to ensure that the patient is properly hydrated. Just before the acquisition, 1.5 L of an oral contrast dispersion, such as gastrografin, is given. PET/CT acquisition starts 60 minutes after intravenous injection of approximately 100 MBq (75–250 MBq) of the radiolabeled peptide ^{68}Ga-DOTA-NOC. To increase renal elimination and reduce radiation exposure to the urinary bladder, furosemide is given at the time of injection of ^{68}Ga-DOTA-NOC. Before the ^{68}Ga-DOTA-NOC PET acquisition, a low-dose, contrast-enhanced CT scan is performed. Protocol for CT scan is outlined in the SNM

guidelines. Dynamic study gives more detailed and precise information about the kinetics of the radiopharmaceutical and allows absolute quantification.

Biodistribution and dosimetry

The excretion of DOTA-NOC is primarily through the kidneys, which makes them the critical organs. The urinary bladder, spleen, and liver—in that order—also receive a high radiation dose. Overall, however ^{68}Ga-DOTA-NOC delivers a radiation dose to the organs comparable to, and even lower than, other diagnostic analogs. Despite the fact that DOTA-NOC covers the wider range of somatostatin receptors, this fact makes it an interesting and important approach. Other organs having known physiologic SSTR expression, such as the pituitary glands, and adrenals show mild to moderate uptake of DOTA-NOC.

Metabolic imaging protocol (F-18 DOPA-PET)

^{18}F-DOPA-PET is performed in patients who have fasted for 6 hours (intravenous injected dose: 5–6 MBq/kg, uptake time 60–90 min). It has been reported that the oral premedication with carbidopa, a peripheral aromatic amino acid decarboxylase

B

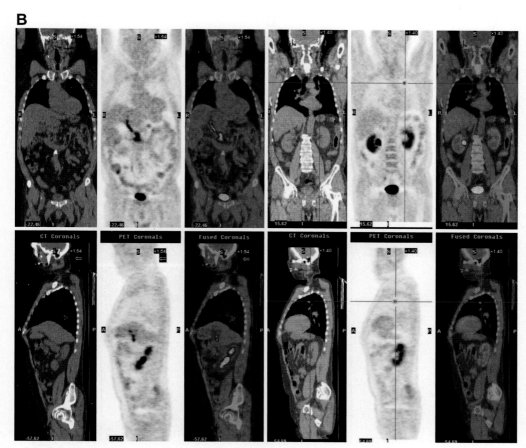

Fig. 5. (continued)

inhibitor, enhances sensitivity by increasing the tumor-to-background ratio of tracer uptake.[38] Carbidopa administration may be particularly useful for assessing lesions at sites with increased ^{18}F-DOPA physiologic uptake. Timmers and colleagues[39] recently described how premedication with carbidopa allowed visualization of three additional paraganglioma lesions that were undetected by ^{18}F-DOPA alone.

INDICATIONS FOR POSITRON EMISSION TOMOGRAPHY/CT
Diagnosis, Staging, and Restaging

Receptor positron emission tomography or positron emission tomography/CT

The variable nature, indolent course, and possibility of multiple and unpredictable primary anatomic sites make it difficult to evaluate patients with NETs. Until recently, ^{111}In-octreotide-SPECT has been considered to be the gold standard for NET diagnosis. Hofmann and colleagues[40] have shown that ^{68}Ga-DOTA-TOC is superior to ^{111}In-octreotide SPECT in detecting upper abdominal metastases when CT was taken as the reference for comparison. In a recent study by Buchmann and colleagues,[41] ^{68}Ga-DOTA-TOC PET/CT was proven to be superior to ^{111}In-DTPAOC in the detection of NET metastases to the lung and bone (Figs. 1–3).

In another study, Gabriel and colleagues[42] showed the feasibility and high accuracy of ^{68}Ga-DOTA-TOC PET as a promising tool for the detection of NET. The accuracy of PET (96%) was found to be significantly higher than that of CT (75%) and ^{111}In-DOTA-TOC SPECT (58%). In 32 patients, ^{68}Ga-DOTA-TOC PET was true positive, whereas SPECT results were false negative. PET also was able to detect more lesions than SPECT and CT. It was observed that for the staging of patients, PET was superior to CT or SPECT because it could pick up more lesions in lymph nodes, liver, and bone. Overall, PET provided additional clinically relevant information in 14% of patients when compared with SPECT and in 21% of patients when compared with CT. Other studies have

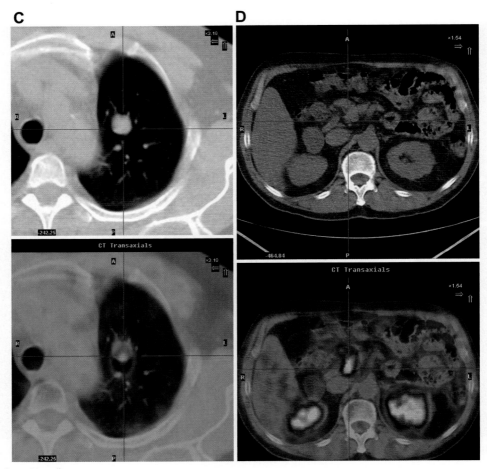

Fig. 5. (*continued*)

validated these observations. Kowalski and colleagues[43] reported that ^{68}Ga-DOTA-TOC PET was superior to ^{111}In-octreotide imaging, especially in detecting small tumors or tumors bearing only a low density of somatostatin receptors. Apart from GEP tumors, ^{68}Ga-DOTA-TOC PET also has been envisioned to have a potential role in small-cell lung cancer because this tumor is known to express somatostatin receptors.[44]

In a study that compared the diagnostic efficacy of ^{68}Ga-DOTA-NOC and ^{68}Ga-DOTA-TATE in the same subject, Antunes and colleagues[45] demonstrated that ^{68}Ga-DOTA-NOC might be superior to ^{68}Ga-DOTA-TATE. Our experience with more than 2500 receptor PET/CT studies performed at the Zentralklinik Bad Berka shows clearly that ^{68}Ga-DOTA-NOC PET is able to detect many more lesions than CT. The independence of the somatostatin receptor state of the tumor from their metabolic activity (functionality) makes it possible to detect nonfunctional NET using receptor PET/

CT. PET using ^{68}Ga-DOTA-TOC has been found to be superior to F-18 FDG-PET in the detection of NET by detecting 90% of the lesions in 15 patients when compared with only 68% on FDG-PET.[46]

Gluc-Lys [(^{18}F)FP]-TOCA is another radiopharmaceutical that targets somatostatin receptors. In a preliminary comparative study, Gluc-Lys [(^{18}F)FP]-TOCA PET was found to be superior to ^{111}In-DTPA-octreotide scan in the diagnosis of NETs. The results also suggested that the sensitivity and specificity of Gluc-Lys [(^{18}F)FP]-TOCA are comparable to the reported sensitivity and specificity of ^{68}Ga-DOTA-TOC PET findings in NET.[47]

Another interesting radiopharmaceutical is ^{64}Cu-TETA-octreotide. [64]Cu (half-life 12.7 hours) has been shown to have great potential as a positron emitting radionuclide for PET imaging and radiotherapy.[48–51] The possibility of performing dosimetry for peptide receptor radionuclide therapy (PRRT) based on ^{64}Cu is one other possible advantage. In a preliminary study,[64]

A

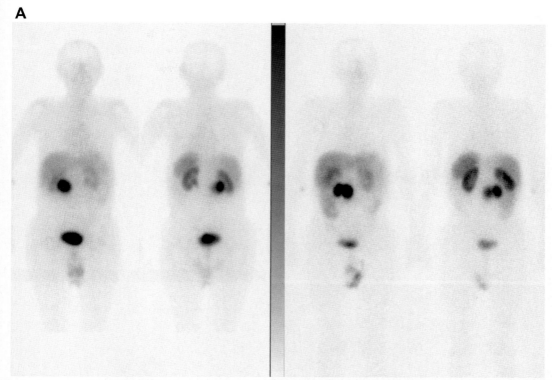

Fig. 6. ^{18}F-DOPA PET/CT images for staging of a 67-year old male with multiple duodenal gastrinomas with nodes metastasis (under therapy with sandostatin). Conventional imaging detected the presence of disease in the duodenum and at nodes level. SRS showed pathologic uptake only at nodes level (*A*) while PET/CT images identified the presence of both, pancreas (*B*) and positive nodes (*C*).

Cu-TETA-octreotide PET was found to have high sensitivity and favorable dosimetry and pharmacokinetics.[48]

Metabolic imaging
In recent years, studies have shown that ^{18}F-DOPA is useful for the assessment of NET and may be superior to conventional structural (US, CT, MR imaging) and somatostatin receptor scintigraphic (SRS) procedures, with sensitivities ranging from 65% to 100% (**Figs. 4–10**).[36,38,52–54]

In 2001, Hoegerle and colleagues[36] reported that ^{18}F-DOPA-PET detected a higher number of NET lesions in the gastrointestinal tract than SRS-based imaging or ^{18}F-FDG PET (true-positive findings at primary sites: 7 versus 4 versus 2; nodes metastasis: 41 versus 27 versus 14, respectively). In a prospective, single-center study, Koopmans and colleagues[38] compared ^{18}F-DOPA-PET results with SRS and CT in 53 patients with metastatic carcinoid tumor. ^{18}F-DOPA-PET was shown to have a higher sensitivity than SRS and CT alone (100% versus 92% and 87%, respectively) or

when the latter two modalities were combined (96%). ^{18}F-DOPA-PET detected more lesions, more regions with lesions, and more lesions per region than SRS and CT.

After imaging 23 advanced NET cases, Becherer and colleagues[52] reported that ^{18}F-DOPA-PET was more accurate than CT and SRS for the detection of NET, especially for bone lesions (^{18}F-DOPA sensitivity of 100% versus SRS sensitivity of 50%). The specificity of ^{18}F-DOPA-PET for the detection of liver involvement was 81% for skeletal disease 91%, and 100% for the abnormalities of the mediastinum, pancreas, and lymph nodes. Although wider availability, lower cost, and more specific mechanism of action render ^{68}Ga-DOTA peptides the tracers of choice for differentiated NET, ^{18}F-DOPA may offer advantages for the detection of tumors with a low or absent expression of SSR, such as medullary thyroid carcinoma[55] and undifferentiated NET. In 2001, Hoegerle and colleagues[56] reported good sensitivity for ^{18}F-DOPA-PET in medullary thyroid cancer (63%) with other imaging procedures (^{18}F-FDG-PET

B

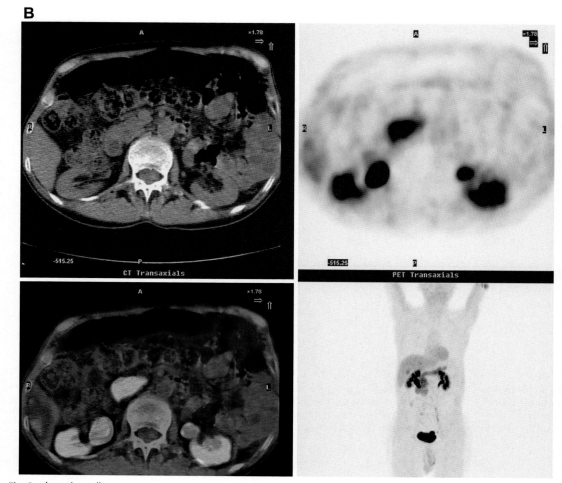

Fig. 6. (*continued*)

44%, SRS 52%, morphologic imaging 82%). The difficulty of interpreting the anatomic location of the primary tumor and the need to differentiate between scar tissue and local relapse of the primary tumor after surgery are major limitations of conventional imaging techniques in detecting thyroid carcinoma.

Currently, few studies have specifically investigated the role of ^{18}F-DOPA-PET in patients with medullary thyroid carcinoma, and the number of patients included in these studies is small. Findings on ^{18}F-DOPA scans were confirmed by either follow-up or pathology in only a few cases.[56–58]

Another condition in which ^{18}F-DOPA may offer advantages over ^{68}Ga-DOTA peptides is the assessment of adrenal neoplasms. Up to 50% of malignant pheochromocytomas and 15% of benign forms are undetected by CT, MR imaging, or ^{123}I-MIBG scans. Hoegerle and colleagues[53] and Mackenzie and colleagues[59] reported that

^{18}F-DOPA-PET can be particularly useful in these cases. ^{18}F-DOPA was also reported to be highly sensitive for the detection of glomus tumors.[60]

Regarding small-cell lung cancer, preliminary data in four patients suggested that ^{18}F-DOPA-PET is less accurate than FDG-PET and conventional imaging.[61] For this comparison, the agreement among FDG-PET, ^{18}F-DOPA-PET, and standard imaging procedures was made site by site. The results from ^{18}F-DOPA-PET and FDG-PET imaging were concordant in 4 out of 11 tumor sites, whereas FDG-PET and standard imaging procedures were in full agreement. ^{18}F-DOPA was negative in two of four cases in one study and in 7 of 11 sites in another study.

^{18}F-FDG positron emission tomography/CT

The use of FDG-PET in the diagnosis of NETs is limited to tumors that are undifferentiated and aggressive in nature.[29,62–66] It has been shown

C

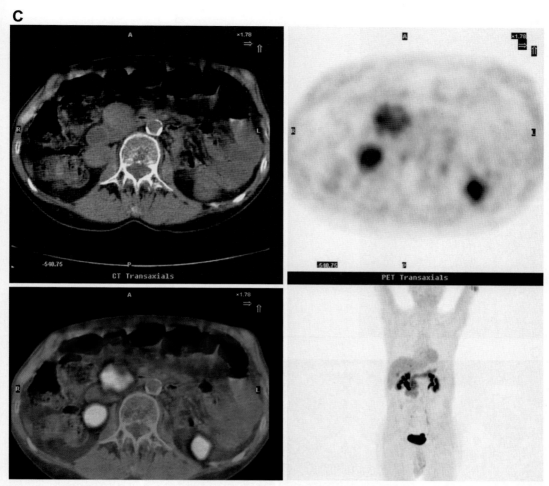

Fig. 6. *(continued)*

that FDG-PET is more sensitive than SSR (^{111}In-pentetreotide) in detecting poorly differentiated GEP tumors, but it was less sensitive in visualizing differentiated GEP tumors.[62] A multicenter study demonstrated that FDG-PET is a useful method for the staging and follow-up of patients with medullary thyroid cancer because it has the highest diagnostic accuracy compared with other imaging modalities, such as CT scan, SSR, and ^{99m}Tc(V) DMSA.[67]

^{11}C-epinephrine, ^{11}C-hydroxyepiphedrine positron emission tomography

In neuroblastoma, Shulkin and colleagues[68] compared the role of ^{123}I-MIBG and ^{11}C-hydroxyepiphedrine (^{11}C-HED) PET and demonstrated that ^{11}C-HED-PET has high sensitivity for detecting neuroblastoma. Most of the tumor lesions visible on the ^{11}C-HED-PET also could be seen on ^{123}I-MIBG. One of the limitations of ^{11}C-HED-PET was the high level of uptake in the liver, which

is a source of error for localization of tumors in this organ. In another study conducted by the same group,[69] similar results were observed in ten patients with pheochromocytoma, which suggested a potential role of ^{11}C-HED. High cost, short half-life, and limited availability of ^{11}C have made wider clinical use of ^{11}C-HED impractical. ^{11}C-epinephrine is also under evaluation and has the potential to be a potential agent for imaging neuroblastomas.

Detection of Unknown Primary Tumor

Receptor positron emission tomography/CT

Carcinoma of unknown primary origin is defined as a biopsy-proven secondary lesion with no detectable primary tumor after assessment by physical examination and conventional imaging tests (MR imaging, CT, and US). The site of the occult primary tumor may remain unidentified in a large number of patients after imaging with chest

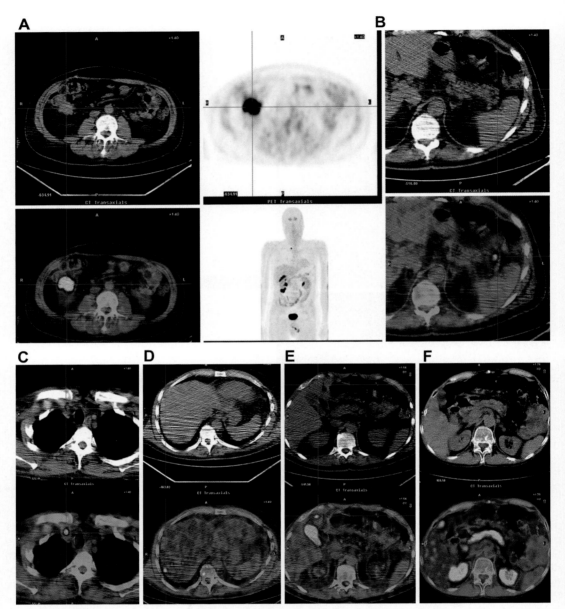

Fig. 7. ^{18}F-DOPA PET images of a 58-year old male with ileum NET investigated for re-staging. The normal physiologic distribution in the pancreas is often a hindrance in the detection of small pathologic lesion in the vicinity. Conventional imaging showed a solid mass at the ileo-cecal valve (A) while SRS was negative. PET/CT images confirmed the presence of a pathologic mass at the ileo-cecal valve level (SUV$_{max}$ 14) and showed uptake in a small area in the pancreatic tail (B), in paratracheal nodes (SUV$_{max}$ 9) (C) as well as multiple lesions in the liver (SUV$_{max}$ 13) (C, D). 18F-DOPA physiologic pancreatic uptake is shown in (E, F).

radiographs, abdominal and pelvic CT, and mammography in women or upon autopsy.[70–73] Overall, in approximately 3% of the patients, the site of origin of histologically documented carcinoma is not identified clinically. Lesion size smaller than the spatial resolution of the imaging modality being used, angiogenic incompetence leading to mass involution, and lesions in areas in which interpretation is difficult may account for the low detection rate.[74] The early identification of the primary tumor is a fundamental requisite for predicting the prognosis and improving survival.[75] This is also true for NETs.

Whole-body PET/CT using FDG has been used successfully for the detection of the most common cancers that present as carcinoma

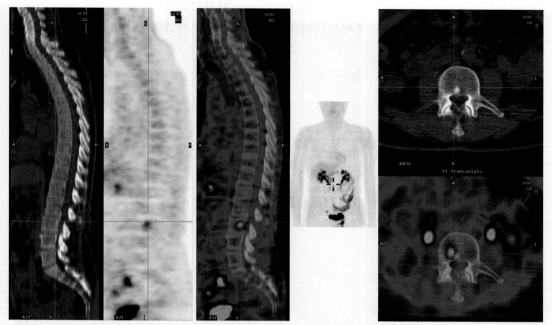

Fig. 8. ¹⁸F-DOPA PET/CT images of a 72-year-old male with pancreatic NET (re-staging after surgery). Conventional imaging was inconclusive (US was negative while CT identified a suspicious lesion at L3 level) and SRS showed poorly defined somatostatin receptor positive lesions in the thoracic and abdomen. ¹⁸F-DOPA PET/CT images confirmed the malignant nature of the L3 lesion and foci in the liver and pancreas.

of unknown primary origin, including adenocarcinomas, squamous cell carcinoma, and poorly differentiated carcinoma in which FDG-PET has identified the primary lesion in 24% to 40% of patients with negative conventional diagnostic investigations.[76–81] FDG-PET is of limited value in slow-growing, well-differentiated NETs, however.[62]

CT and MR imaging often fail to diagnose primary NET and endoscopic ultrasonography is

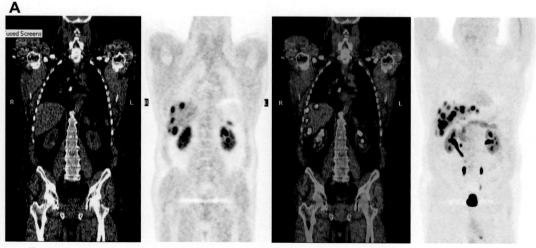

Fig. 9. ¹⁸F-DOPA PET/CT images of a 75-year-old male with ileum NET (re-staging after surgery). Conventional imaging and SRS showed the presence of multiple liver metastases while ¹⁸F-DOPA PET/CT confirmed the presence of liver metastasis (*A–C*) and also identified right mesenteric lymph node metastases (*D*).

B   **C**   **D**

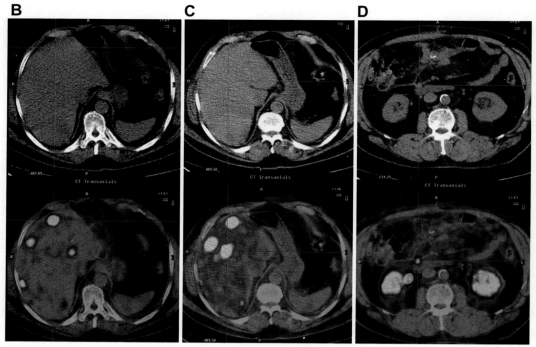

Fig. 9. (*continued*)

A

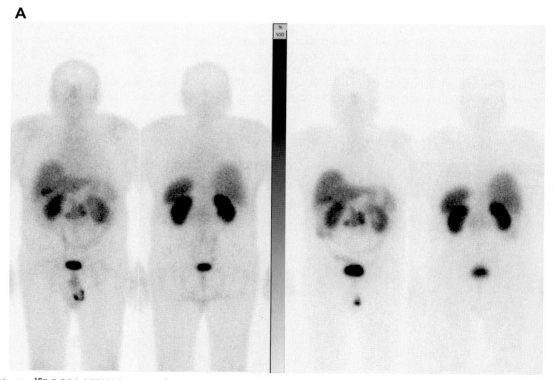

Fig. 10. ^{18}F-DOPA PET/CT images of a 64-year old male with ileum NET (re-staging after surgery) under sandostain therapy. Conventional imaging and SRS (*A*) showed the presence of abnormal peri-aortic nodes that were confirmed by ^{18}F-DOPA PET/CT (*B*) which, however, identified a larger number of lesions (multiple abdominal nodes and one supraclavicular node) (*C*).

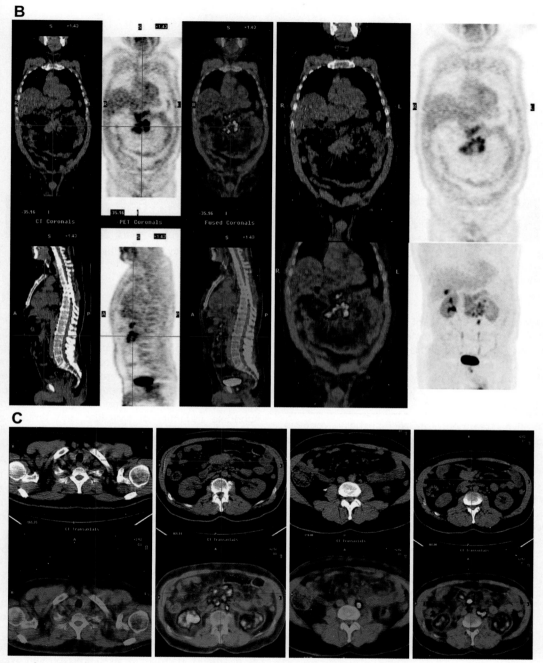

Fig. 10. (*continued*)

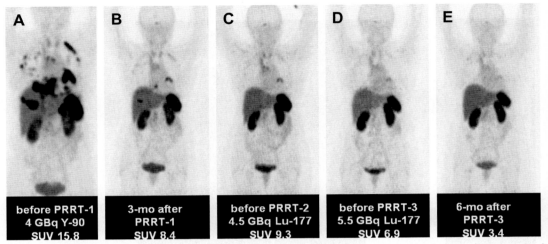

A	B	C	D	E
before PRRT-1 4 GBq Y-90 SUV 15.8	3-mo after PRRT-1 SUV 8.4	before PRRT-2 4.5 GBq Lu-177 SUV 9.3	before PRRT-3 5.5 GBq Lu-177 SUV 6.9	6-mo after PRRT-3 SUV 3.4

Fig. 11. Ga-68 DOTA-NOC PET/CT: MIP images (*A–E*) for evaluating therapy response by visual assessment in a patient with metastatic mediastinal NET (most probably arising from the thymus) under sequential PRRT using Y-90 and Lu-177 DOTA-TATE.

limited to the detection of gastroenteropancreatic NET. These factors make receptor PET/CT imaging an indispensable tool in the initial diagnosis of the primary site and staging of patients with carcinoma of unknown primary origin.

Therapy Stratification

Curative treatment of NET usually requires complete surgical resection of the primary tumor and perhaps regional lymph nodes with proven metastases. Effective palliative therapies are also available at all stages of the disease, however, and are indicated even at advanced stages of their tumors. Depending on tumor stage, size, and degree of differentiation, current treatment protocols for NET include the following options:

1. Surgery
2. Immunologic therapy (interferon)
3. Intra-arterial chemoembolization
4. Chemotherapy
5. Therapy with somatostatin analogs
6. PRRT
7. ISIRT and RFTA

Surgical resection and cold somatostatin analogs (intramuscular or subcutaneous octreotide) are most commonly used as the first line of treatment; chemotherapy is used as the last option. Recent years have seen the development of PRRT as a highly effective treatment option for metastasized progressive NET, and this approach is regarded as the third option for this purpose. For effective management of patients who have NET, receptor and metabolic PET/CT play an important role.

By directing surgeons to the site of primary tumor, ^{68}Ga-DOTA-NOC and ^{18}F-DOPA-PET/CT improve the prognosis and quality of life for these patients. For cold somatostatin therapy and somatostatin receptor-based radionuclide therapy, it is essential to document the expression of these sites on the tumor cells. The therapy schedule (quantity of radiation and timing) of PRRT using ^{177}Lu or ^{90}Y-DOTA-TATE/DOTA-TOC depends highly on the semiquantitative or visual interpretation of ^{68}Ga-DOTA-NOC/DOTA-TOC-PET/CT. Although conventional dosimetry is important to individualize PRRT, in our own experience, semiquantitative (SUV_{max}) evaluation seems to predict the degree of receptor concentration and response (**Figs. 11, 12**).

Intra-arterial PRRT is an option, partial hepatectomy, and SIRT are other possible options. The dose to be administered for such treatments also depends on receptor expression because size on CT and MR imaging is not a reliable parameter because of the possibility of cystic degeneration and other nonfunctional tissues in the tumor.

Ambrosini and colleagues[82] also reported that in a limited population of biopsy-proven NET, ^{18}F-DOPA-PET offered relevant information for the clinical management of patients with an unclear clinical presentation or with inconclusive findings on other imaging modalities (US, CT, SRS, MR imaging). In particular, ^{18}F-DOPA-PET changed patient management in 11 of 13 cases. Further surgery, other than that necessary to remove the primary tumor, was avoided in four cases. In three patients, a surgical extirpation of the metabolic lesion was guided by ^{18}F-DOPA-PET/CT findings,

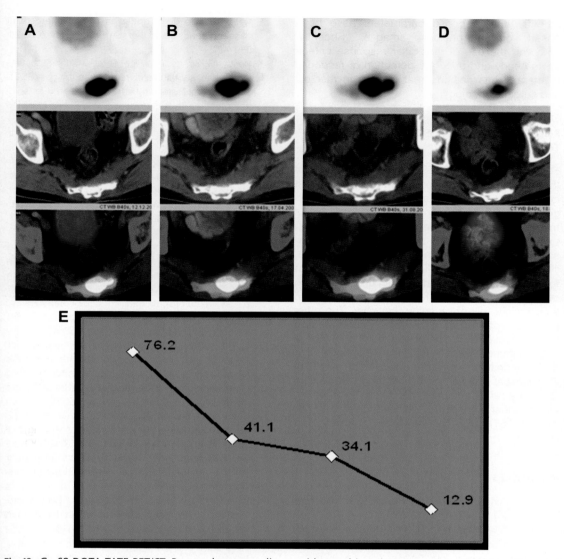

Fig. 12. Ga-68 DOTA-TATE PET/CT: Presacral paraganglioma with sacral invasion presenting with bone, liver and lymph node metastases, progressive at baseline (A) and responding well to peptide receptor radionuclide therapy (PRRT) administering three courses (B–D) of Y-90 and Lu-177 DOTA-TATE (total activity applied: 13,3 GBq). Time course of SUVmax of the presacral paraganglioma is also shown (E), dropping from 76.2 to 12.9 (partial response). Clinically dramatic pain reduction (the patient needed high doses of morphine before treatment and could give up completely on pain medication). Please mind that there is only little change on concurrent CT scan ("molecular response preceeds anatomical changes").

and in four nonoperable patients with bone marrow metastasis, chemotherapy was administered. One patient with a false-positive PET result had a lymph node removed and remained disease free during follow-up.

FDG-PET was noted to have the potential to change the treatment protocol in 17% of patients who had pancreatic-duodenal NETs. FDG-PET was best suited for patients suspected of having a malignant tumor or a pancreatic mass larger than

2 cm or a case of multiple neuroendocrine neoplasia I with at least one visible lesion. The authors also reported that FDG-PET is not useful in duodenal tumors, benign insulinomas, and small, single pancreatic neuroendocrine lesions.[83]

Evaluation of Therapy Response

PET/CT is increasingly being used for monitoring response to therapy for various tumors. Until recently, the response parameters have been based on morphologic images. Recently, however, the use of molecular response criteria for the early and accurate detection of response to therapy has gained great interest in medical and surgical oncology.

ROLE OF METABOLIC POSITRON EMISSION TOMOGRAPHY/CT

The role of metabolic PET/CT imaging techniques in the assessment of response to therapy is almost nonexistent, primarily because NETs are slow-growing tumors and no definitive therapy exists that influences cellular metabolism directly enough to be assessed by FDG or ^{18}F-DOPA-PET/CT. In a preliminary study at the Zentralklinik Bad Berka, ^{68}Ga-DOTA-NOC-PET/CT was found to be superior to FDG-PET/CT for the early and accurate prediction of response to PRRT.[84] More data are needed to substantiate this observation, however. The other potential application of receptor and metabolic PET/CT would be in the assessment of response to transarterial chemoembolization, chemotherapy, and sandostatin therapy (to predict relapse). Biochemical markers are not good indicators for early and accurate response to therapy, which further emphasizes the need to establish the role of PET/CT in the monitoring of treatment response.

REFERENCES

1. Oberndorfer S. Karzinoidtumore des Dünndarms. Frankf Z Pathol 1907;1:426–9.
2. Vinik AI, Woltering EA, O'Dorisio TM, et al. Neuroendocrine tumors: a comprehensive guide to diagnosis and management. Inter Science Institute; 2006.
3. Jensen RT. Endocrine tumors of the gastrointestinal tract and pancreas. In: Kasper DL, Fauci AS, Longo DL, et al, editors. Harrison's principles of internal medicine. 16th edition. McGraw-Hill; 2005. p. 2347–58.
4. Schmitt-Gräff A, Hezel B, Wiedenmann B. Pathologisch-diagnostische Aspekte neuroendokriner Tumoren des Gastrointestinaltrakts. Der Onkologe 2000;613–23.
5. Solcia E, Kloppel G, Sobin LH. Histological typing of tumors: international histological classification of tumors in collaboration with 9 pathologists from 4 countries. In: Organisation WHOPPWH. 2nd edition. Berlin (Germany): Springer; 2000.
6. Rindi G, Kloppel G, Alhman H, et al. TNM staging of foregut (neuro)endocrine tumors: a consensus proposal including a grading system. Virchows Arch 2006;449:395–401.
7. Reubi JC. Peptide receptors as molecular targets for cancer diagnosis and therapy. Endocr Rev 2003;24:389–427.
8. Reubi JC, Schar JC, Waser B, et al. Affinity profiles for human somatostatin receptor subtypes SST1-SST5 of somatostatin radiotracers selected for scintigraphic and radiotherapeutic use. Eur J Nucl Med 2000;27:273–82.
9. Reubi JC, Waser B, Schaer JC, et al. Somatostatin receptor sst1-sst5 expression in normal and neoplastic human tissues using receptor autoradiography with subtype-selective ligands. Eur J Nucl Med 2001;28:836–46.
10. Rufini V, Calcagni ML, Baum RP. Imaging of neuroendocrine tumors. Semin Nucl Med 2006;36:228–47.
11. Wild D, Macke HR, Waser B, et al. 68Ga-DOTANOC: a first compound for PET imaging with high affinity for somatostatin receptor subtypes 2 and 5. Eur J Nucl Med Mol Imaging 2005;32:724.
12. Wild D, Schmitt JS, Ginj M, et al. DOTA-NOC, a high-affinity ligand of somatostatin receptor subtypes 2, 3 and 5 for labelling with various radiometals. Eur J Nucl Med Mol Imaging 2003;30:1338–47.
13. Ginj M, Zhang H, Waser B, et al. Radiolabeled somatostatin receptor antagonists are preferable to agonists for in vivo peptide receptor targeting of tumors. Proc Natl Acad Sci USA 2006;103:16436–41.
14. Reubi JC, Schaer JC, Wenger S, et al. SST3-selective potent peptidic somatostatin receptor antagonists. Proc Natl Acad Sci USA 2000;97:13973–8.
15. Rösch F, Knapp WH. In: Radionuclide generators, vol. 4. Rotterdam (The Netherlands): Kluwer Academic Publishers; 2003.
16. Zhernosekov KP, Filosofov DV, Baum RP, et al. Processing of generator-produced 68Ga for medical application. J Nucl Med 2007;48:1741–8.
17. Meyer GJ, Macke H, Schuhmacher J, et al. 68Ga-labelled DOTA-derivatised peptide ligands. Eur J Nucl Med Mol Imaging 2004;31:1097–104.
18. Moody TW, Hill JM, Jensen RT. VIP as a trophic factor in the CNS and cancer cells. Peptides 2003;24:163–77.
19. Reubi JC, Waser B. Concomitant expression of several peptide receptors in neuroendocrine tumours: molecular basis for in vivo multireceptor tumour targeting. Eur J Nucl Med Mol Imaging 2003;30:781–93.
20. Thakur ML, Marcus CS, Saeed S, et al. 99mTc-labeled vasoactive intestinal peptide analog for rapid localization of tumors in humans. J Nucl Med 2000;41:107–10.
21. Virgolini I, Kurtaran A, Raderer M, et al. Vasoactive intestinal peptide receptor scintigraphy. J Nucl Med 1995;36:1732–9.
22. Virgolini I, Raderer M, Kurtaran A, et al. Vasoactive intestinal peptide-receptor imaging for the

localization of intestinal adenocarcinomas and endocrine tumors. N Engl J Med 1994;331:1116–21.

23. Behe M, Becker W, Gotthardt M, et al. Improved kinetic stability of DTPA- dGlu as compared with conventional monofunctional DTPA in chelating indium and yttrium: preclinical and initial clinical evaluation of radiometal labelled minigastrin derivatives. Eur J Nucl Med Mol Imaging 2003;30: 1140–6.

24. Behr TM, Behe M, Angerstein C, et al. Cholecystokinin-B/gastrin receptor binding peptides: preclinical development and evaluation of their diagnostic and therapeutic potential. Clin Cancer Res 1999;5: 3124s–38s.

25. Behr TM, Jenner N, Radetzky S, et al. Targeting of cholecystokinin-B/gastrin receptors in vivo: preclinical and initial clinical evaluation of the diagnostic and therapeutic potential of radiolabelled gastrin. Eur J Nucl Med 1998;25:424–30.

26. Breeman WA, De Jong M, Bernard BF, et al. Pre-clinical evaluation of [(111)In-DTPA-Pro(1), Tyr(4)]bombesin, a new radioligand for bombesin-receptor scintigraphy. Int J Cancer 1999;83:657–63.

27. Kwekkeboom DJ, Bakker WH, Kooij PP, et al. Cholecystokinin receptor imaging using an octapeptide DTPA-CCK analogue in patients with medullary thyroid carcinoma. Eur J Nucl Med 2000;27:1312–7.

28. Reubi JC, Waser B, Schaer JC, et al. Unsulfated DTPA- and DOTA-CCK analogs as specific high-affinity ligands for CCK-B receptor-expressing human and rat tissues in vitro and in vivo. Eur J Nucl Med 1998;25:481–90.

29. Eriksson B, Bergstrom M, Orlefors H, et al. Use of PET in neuroendocrine tumors: in vivo applications and in vitro studies. Q J Nucl Med 2000;44:68–76.

30. Orlefors H, Sundin A, Ahlstrom H, et al. Positron emission tomography with 5-hydroxytryprophan in neuroendocrine tumors. J Clin Oncol 1998;16:2534–41.

31. Eidelberg D, Moeller JR, Dhawan V, et al. The metabolic anatomy of Parkinson's disease: complementary [18F]fluorodeoxyglucose and [18F]fluorodopa positron emission tomographic studies. Mov Disord 1990;5:203–13.

32. Ribeiro MJ, Boddaert N, Bellanne-Chantelot C, et al. The added value of [(18)F]fluoro-L-DOPA PET in the diagnosis of hyperinsulinism of infancy: a retrospective study involving 49 children. Eur J Nucl Med Mol Imaging 2007;34:2120–8.

33. Creveling CR, Kirk KL. The effect of ring-fluorination on the rate of O-methylation of dihydroxyphenylalanine (DOPA) by catechol-O-methyltransferase: significance in the development of 18F-PET scanning agents. Biochem Biophys Res Commun 1985; 130:1123–31.

34. Melega WP, Luxen A, Perlmutter MM, et al. Comparative in vivo metabolism of 6-[18F]fluoro-L-dopa and [3H]L-dopa in rats. Biochem Pharmacol 1990;39:1853–60.

35. Eldrup E, Clausen N, Scherling B, et al. Evaluation of plasma 3,4-dihydroxyphenylacetic acid (DOPAC) and plasma 3,4-dihydroxyphenylalanine (DOPA) as tumor markers in children with neuroblastoma. Scand J Clin Lab Invest 2001;61:479–90.

36. Hoegerle S, Altehoefer C, Ghanem N, et al. Whole-body 18F DOPA PET for detection of gastrointestinal carcinoid tumors. Radiology 2001;220:373–80.

37. Kolby L, Bernhardt P, Levin-Jakobsen AM, et al. Uptake of meta-iodobenzylguanidine in neuroendocrine tumours is mediated by vesicular monoamine transporters. Br J Cancer 2003;89:1383–8.

38. Koopmans KP, de Vries EG, Kema IP, et al. Staging of carcinoid tumours with 18F-DOPA PET: a prospective, diagnostic accuracy study. Lancet Oncol 2006; 7:728–34.

39. Timmers HJ, Hadi M, Carrasquillo JA, et al. The effects of carbidopa on uptake of 6-18F-fluoro-L-DOPA in PET of pheochromocytoma and extraadrenal abdominal paraganglioma. J Nucl Med 2007;48: 1599–606.

40. Hofmann M, Maecke H, Borner R, et al. Biokinetics and imaging with the somatostatin receptor PET radioligand (68)Ga-DOTATOC: preliminary data. Eur J Nucl Med 2001;28:1751–7.

41. Buchmann I, Henze M, Engelbrecht S, et al. Comparison of 68Ga-DOTATOC PET and 111In-DTPAOC (Octreoscan) SPECT in patients with neuroendocrine tumours. Eur J Nucl Med Mol Imaging 2007;34:1617–26.

42. Gabriel M, Decristoforo C, Kendler D, et al. 68Ga-DOTA-Tyr3-octreotide PET in neuroendocrine tumors: comparison with somatostatin receptor scintigraphy and CT. J Nucl Med 2007;48:508–18.

43. Kowalski J, Henze M, Schuhmacher J, et al. Evaluation of positron emission tomography imaging using [68Ga]-DOTA-D Phe(1)-Tyr(3)-Octreotide in comparison to [111In]-DTPAOC SPECT: first results in patients with neuroendocrine tumors. Mol Imaging Biol 2003;5:42–8.

44. Maecke HR, Hofmann M, Haberkorn U. (68)Ga-labeled peptides in tumor imaging. J Nucl Med 2005;46(Suppl 1):172S–8S.

45. Antunes P, Ginj M, Zhang H, et al. Are radiogallium-labelled DOTA-conjugated somatostatin analogues superior to those labelled with other radiometals? Eur J Nucl Med Mol Imaging 2007;982–93.

46. Koukouraki S, Strauss LG, Georgoulias V, et al. Evaluation of the pharmacokinetics of 68Ga-DOTATOC in patients with metastatic neuroendocrine tumours scheduled for 90Y-DOTATOC therapy. Eur J Nucl Med Mol Imaging 2006;33:460–6.

47. Meisetschlager G, Poethko T, Stahl A, et al. Gluc-Lys ([18F]FP)-TOCA PET in patients with SSTR-positive tumors: biodistribution and diagnostic evaluation compared with [111In]DTPA-octreotide. J Nucl Med 2006;47:566–73.

48. Anderson CJ, Dehdashti F, Cutler PD, et al. 64Cu-TETA-octreotide as a PET imaging agent for patients with neuroendocrine tumors. J Nucl Med 2001;42:213–21.

49. Lewis JS, Lewis MR, Cutler PD, et al. Radiotherapy and dosimetry of 64Cu-TETA-Tyr3-octreotate in a somatostatin receptor-positive, tumor-bearing rat model. Clin Cancer Res 1999;5:3608–16.

50. Sprague JE, Peng Y, Sun X, et al. Preparation and biological evaluation of copper-64-labeled tyr3-octreotate using a cross-bridged macrocyclic chelator. Clin Cancer Res 2004;10:8674–82.

51. Wang M, Caruano AL, Lewis MR, et al. Subcellular localization of radiolabeled somatostatin analogues: implications for targeted radiotherapy of cancer. Cancer Res 2003;63:6864–9.

52. Becherer A, Szabo M, Karanikas G, et al. Imaging of advanced neuroendocrine tumors with (18)F-FDOPA PET. J Nucl Med 2004;45:1161–7.

53. Hoegerle S, Nitzsche E, Altehoefer C, et al. Pheochromocytomas: detection with 18F DOPA whole body PET: initial results. Radiology 2002;222:507–12.

54. Nanni C, Fanti S, Rubello D. 18F-DOPA PET and PET/CT. J Nucl Med 2007;48:1577–9.

55. Reubi JC, Chayvialle JA, Franc B, et al. Somatostatin receptors and somatostatin content in medullary thyroid carcinomas. Lab Invest 1991;64:567–73.

56. Hoegerle S, Altehoefer C, Ghanem N, et al. 18F-DOPA positron emission tomography for tumour detection in patients with medullary thyroid carcinoma and elevated calcitonin levels. Eur J Nucl Med 2001;28:64–71.

57. Beuthien-Baumann B, Strumpf A, Zessin J, et al. Diagnostic impact of PET with 18F-FDG, 18F-DOPA and 3-O-methyl-6-[18F]fluoro-DOPA in recurrent or metastatic medullary thyroid carcinoma. Eur J Nucl Med Mol Imaging 2007;34:1604–9.

58. Crippa F, Alessi A, Gerali A, et al. FDG-PET in thyroid cancer. Tumori 2003;89:540–3.

59. Mackenzie IS, Gurnell M, Balan KK, et al. The use of 18-fluoro-dihydroxyphenylalanine and 18-fluorodeoxyglucose positron emission tomography scanning in the assessment of metaiodobenzylguanidine-negative phaeochromocytoma. Eur J Endocrinol 2007;157:533–7.

60. Hoegerle S, Ghanem N, Altehoefer C, et al. 18F-DOPA positron emission tomography for the detection of glomus tumours. Eur J Nucl Med Mol Imaging 2003;30:689–94.

61. Jacob T, Grahek D, Younsi N, et al. Positron emission tomography with [(18)F]FDOPA and [(18)F]FDG in the imaging of small cell lung carcinoma: preliminary results. Eur J Nucl Med Mol Imaging 2003;30:1266–9.

62. Adams S, Baum R, Rink T, et al. Limited value of fluorine-18 fluorodeoxyglucose positron emission tomography for the imaging of neuroendocrine tumours. Eur J Nucl Med 1998;25:79–83.

63. Pasquali C, Rubello D, Sperti C, et al. Neuroendocrine tumor imaging: can 18F-fluorodeoxyglucose positron emission tomography detect tumors with poor prognosis and aggressive behavior? World J Surg 1998;22:588–92.

64. Scanga DR, Martin WH, Delbeke D. Value of FDG PET imaging in the management of patients with thyroid, neuroendocrine, and neural crest tumors. Clin Nucl Med 2004;29:86–90.

65. Sundin A, Eriksson B, Bergstrom M, et al. PET in the diagnosis of neuroendocrine tumors. Ann N Y Acad Sci 2004;1014:246–57.

66. Zhao DS, Valdivia AY, Li Y, et al. 18F-fluorodeoxyglucose positron emission tomography in small-cell lung cancer. Semin Nucl Med 2002;32:272–5.

67. Diehl M, Risse JH, Brandt-Mainz K, et al. Fluorine-18 fluorodeoxyglucose positron emission tomography in medullary thyroid cancer: results of a multicentre study. Eur J Nucl Med 2001;28:1671–6.

68. Shulkin BL, Wieland DM, Baro ME, et al. PET hydroxyephedrine imaging of neuroblastoma. J Nucl Med 1996;37:16–21.

69. Shulkin BL, Wieland DM, Schwaiger M, et al. PET scanning with hydroxyephedrine: an approach to the localization of pheochromocytoma. J Nucl Med 1992;33:1125–31.

70. Abbruzzese JL, Abbruzzese MC, Lenzi R, et al. Analysis of a diagnostic strategy for patients with suspected tumors of unknown origin. J Clin Oncol 1995;13:2094–103.

71. Didolkar MS, Fanous N, Elias EG, et al. Metastatic carcinomas from occult primary tumors: a study of 254 patients. Ann Surg 1977;186:625–30.

72. Le Chevalier T, Cvitkovic E, Caille P, et al. Early metastatic cancer of unknown primary origin at presentation: a clinical study of 302 consecutive autopsied patients. Arch Intern Med 1988;148:2035–9.

73. Steckel RJ, Kagan AR. Diagnostic persistence in working up metastatic cancer with an unknown primary site. Radiology 1980;134:367–9.

74. Naresh KN. Do metastatic tumours from an unknown primary reflect angiogenic incompetence of the tumour at the primary site? A hypothesis. Med Hypotheses 2002;59:357–60.

75. Raber MN, Faintuch J, Abbruzzese JL, et al. Continuous infusion 5-fluorouracil, etoposide and cis-diamminedichloroplatinum in patients with metastatic carcinoma of unknown primary origin. Ann Oncol 1991;2:519–20.

76. Alberini JL, Belhocine T, Hustinx R, et al. Whole-body positron emission tomography using fluorodeoxyglucose in patients with metastases of unknown primary tumours (CUP syndrome). Nucl Med Commun 2003;24:1081–6.

77. Bohuslavizki KH, Klutmann S, Kroger S, et al. FDG PET detection of unknown primary tumors. J Nucl Med 2000;41:816–22.

78. Freudenberg LS, Fischer M, Antoch G, et al. Dual modality of 18F-fluorodeoxyglucose-positron emission tomography/computed tomography in patients with cervical carcinoma of unknown primary. Med Princ Pract 2005;14:155–60.

79. Gutzeit A, Antoch G, Kuhl H, et al. Unknown primary tumors: detection with dual-modality PET/CT: initial experience. Radiology 2005;234:227–34.

80. Kole AC, Nieweg OE, Pruim J, et al. Detection of unknown occult primary tumors using positron emission tomography. Cancer 1998;82:1160–6.

81. Syed R, Bomanji JB, Nagabhushan N, et al. Impact of combined (18)F-FDG PET/CT in head and neck tumours. Br J Cancer 2005;92:1046–50.

82. Ambrosini V, Tomassetti P, Rubello D, et al. Role of 18F-dopa PET/CT imaging in the management of patients with 111In-pentetreotide negative GEP tumours. Nucl Med Commun 2007;28: 473–7.

83. Pasquali C, Sperti C, Scappin S, et al. Role and indications of fluorodeoxyglucose positron emission tomography (FDG-PET) in neuroendocrine pancreatico-duodenal tumors. J pancreas 2004;6(5 Suppl):528–9.

84. Oh SW, Prasad V, Lee DS, et al. Monitoring response to peptide receptor radionuclide therapy (PRRT) in patients with metastasised neuroendocrine tumours (NET): intraindividual comparison between Ga-68-DOTA-NOC, F-18-FDG-PET/CT, and CT alone [abstract EPOS]. European Society of Radiology Conference. Vienna, March 7-11, 2008.

PET, PET/CT, and PET/MR Imaging Assessment of Breast Cancer

Shamim Ahmed Shamim, MD[a], Drew A. Torigian, MD, MA[b], Rakesh Kumar, MD[a],*

KEYWORDS

- Breast cancer • Oncology
- Positron emission tomography (PET)
- Computed tomography (CT)
- Magnetic resonance imaging (MRI)
- PET/CT • PET/MRI • PET mammography

PET and CT are increasingly used in breast cancer for staging, restaging, treatment monitoring, and estimation of long-term prognosis. The radiotracer most widely used in clinical practice is the glucose analogue 2-[18F]-fluoro-2-deoxy-D-glucose (FDG). Combined PET/CT systems allow functional PET and anatomic CT images to be acquired in one session and coregistered. PET/CT has been reported to offer advantages over anatomically based imaging and PET alone modalities.[1–3] PET/CT has been shown to be particularly useful for restaging of breast cancer, for response evaluation to therapy, and for further analysis when the results of conventional imaging are equivocal. FDG PET often demonstrates locoregional or unsuspected distant metastatic disease that changes management. PET/CT is useful in the evaluation of chemotherapy response in patients with locally advanced breast carcinoma and in those with metastatic disease. This review focuses mainly on clinical applications of PET/CT in patients with breast cancer. It discusses the role of FDG PET/CT (and FDG PET) in the diagnosis and initial staging of breast cancer, in monitoring the response of disease to chemotherapy, and in identifying metastatic and recurrent disease. In addition, it discusses the role of MR imaging and potential future hybrid modalities such as PET/MR imaging.

DIAGNOSIS OF PRIMARY TUMOR

Early detection is the most effective strategy for reducing mortality from breast cancer. Currently, the diagnosis of primary breast cancer is principally based on mammography; however, this technique has a low specificity and sensitivity,[4–7] a limited value in distinguishing benign from malignant lesions, and is limited in detecting cancer in women with radiographically dense breasts.[8,9] Other diagnostic techniques such as ultrasonography and MR imaging are being used as well. The specificity of ultrasonography is reported to be superior to that of mammography, especially to distinguish solid and cystic lesions.[10,11] Ultrasonography has a higher detection rate than mammography for palpable breast masses but is not optimally sensitive to exclude breast cancer. Moreover, the diagnostic accuracy of ultrasonography is operator dependent. The sensitivity of MR imaging is greater than 90%, but its specificity is lower than that of mammography.[12,13] Various investigators have assessed the role of FDG PET to detect primary breast cancer and to differentiate benign from malignant disease. The sensitivity of FDG PET ranges from 80% to 96% and the specificity from 83% to 100%.[14–18] A meta-analysis was performed by Samson and

---

[a] Department of Nuclear Medicine, All India Institute of Medical Sciences, E-81, Ansari Nagar (East), AIIMS Campus, New Delhi 110029, India
[b] Department of Radiology, Hospital of the University of Pennsylvania, 3400 Spruce Street, Philadelphia, PA 19104, USA
* Corresponding author.
E-mail address: rkphulia@yahoo.com (R. Kumar).

PET Clin 3 (2008) 381–393
doi:10.1016/j.cpet.2009.01.001

colleagues[19] on 13 published studies evaluating the role of whole body FDG PET for breast cancer detection. From this analysis, FDG PET was reported to be 88% sensitive and 80% specific for breast cancer, with false-negative results occurring in 12% of cancer cases. The investigators concluded that whole body FDG PET should not be used to evaluate breast lesions. Currently, there is widespread agreement that whole body FDG PET does not have a clinical role in the detection of primary breast cancer. Because of its limited spatial resolution, PET is not recommended for lesions smaller than 1 cm in diameter. In addition, the accuracy of PET imaging is affected by the type of tumor histology. Slowly growing cancers such as tubular carcinoma or noninvasive cancers such as ductal or lobular carcinoma in situ can be missed on FDG PET.[20–25]

The truly functional nature of lesion detection by PET alone is not without limitations. Inaccurate anatomic localization of sites of radiotracer uptake along with difficulty in interpretation further compounds the problem. These limitations have led researchers to develop a hybrid imaging system in the form of PET/CT in which both anatomic and physiologic information can be

obtained. This system has led to a reduction in false-positive results with improved localization of lesions and accurate interpretation of the disease, leading to a drastic improvement in the specificity of the procedure.[26–28] Nevertheless, to date, few studies have been performed to assess the role of PET/CT in patients with breast cancer. Tatsumi and colleagues[2] compared the performance of FDG PET, CT, and FDG PET/CT and reported that PET/CT showed a higher rate of lesion detection when compared with PET or CT alone in more than 50% of the patient population. In a study by Yang and colleagues,[29] FDG PET/CT in 58 breast cancer patients was retrospectively compared with PET or CT scans alone. PET/CT was found to be better than PET or CT alone for detecting small tumors. Identification of the exact anatomic location of sites of increased tracer uptake was accurately performed through PET/CT (**Figs. 1** and **2**).

POSITRON EMISSION MAMMOGRAPHY

Positron emission mammography (PEM) is new technology that allows imaging specifically for the breast. When compared with conventional

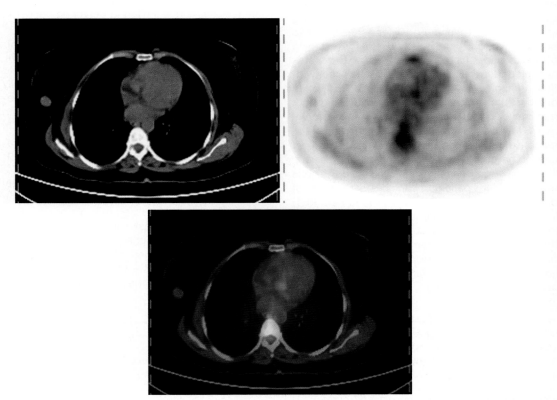

Fig. 1. Axial CT, PET, and PET/CT images of patient who presented with right breast nodule in upper outer quadrant. No FDG uptake was noted, suggestive of benign pathology. Final diagnosis was fibroadenoma.

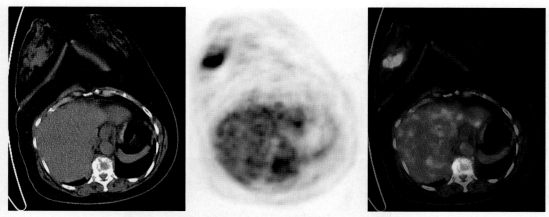

Fig. 2. Axial CT, PET, and PET/CT images of patient who presented with osseous metastasis with unknown primary. No breast mass was palpated due to pendulous configuration of breasts. Focal FDG uptake is noted in right breast lesion in keeping with primary breast cancer, which was confirmed via biopsy.

PET and PET/CT, PEM has better spatial resolution (~1.5 mm), requires a lower radiotracer dose (3–5 mCi), and has a shorter acquisition time (2–4 minutes) and lower cost. PEM has some advantages over MR imaging; it can be useful in patients who have posterior breast lesions and to distinguish fat necrosis from breast cancer. PEM is now being investigated in clinical trials at several sites to determine its sensitivity and specificity. Initial studies have reported a sensitivity of greater than 80% and a specificity of greater than 92% in the general population.[30] A recent study by Heusner and colleagues[31] demonstrated that FDG PET/CT mammography had similar accuracy to MR imaging for the detection of breast cancer lesions. Although MR imaging seems to be more accurate for assessment of the T stage of tumor, FDG PET/CT seems able to more accurately define lesion focality. The results of initial studies are encouraging. It appears that PEM may have an important role in the initial diagnosis of breast cancer.

FDG PET AND PET/CT IN LOCOREGIONAL STAGING OF BREAST CANCER

In breast cancer, lymph node involvement has important prognostic and therapeutic implications. There is no effective noninvasive modality for determining metastatic involvement of the axillary lymph nodes. Lymph node dissection fully evaluates the draining lymph nodes but can result in the long-term complication of upper extremity lymphedema. Identification of sentinel lymph nodes (SLN) for initial sampling and dissection is a well-established procedure for detecting axillary lymph node metastasis from primary breast

cancer.[32,33] CT is also used to assess axillary lymph node status based on nodal size but is limited, because a normal sized lymph node can harbor metastatic disease and an enlarged lymph node may be due to nonneoplastic etiologies.

FDG PET can demonstrate early axillary lymph node metastases by revealing increases in nodal metabolism before the occurrence of nodal enlargement; however, PET can miss small axillary lymph node metastases due to limitations in spatial resolution and difficulty in assessing the number of lymph nodes involved. In addition, FDG uptake may occur when nodal infection or noninfectious inflammation is present, resulting in a false-positive result. The sensitivity of FDG PET ranges from 79% to 100% and the specificity from 66% to 100%.[34] As such, the general opinion is that FDG PET is not sufficiently accurate for the purposes of axillary lymph node staging. In breast cancer, FDG PET can be helpful to assess the spread of tumor to regional nodal sites other than the axilla, such as the internal mammary chain and interpectoral nodes. These nodes are not routinely sampled due to their general inaccessibility. FDG PET has been shown to improve detection of metastatic disease in internal mammary nodes.[35–37]

The advantage of PET/CT in the detection of axillary lymph node involvement by metastatic disease is the improvement in the assessment of FDG uptake localization and of the number of lymph nodes involved. To the authors' knowledge, limited research has been performed to determine the role of PET/CT for assessing lymph node metastatic disease in breast cancer (**Figs. 3** and **4**). Wang and colleagues[38] performed a study on 15 breast cancer patients with lesion size ranging

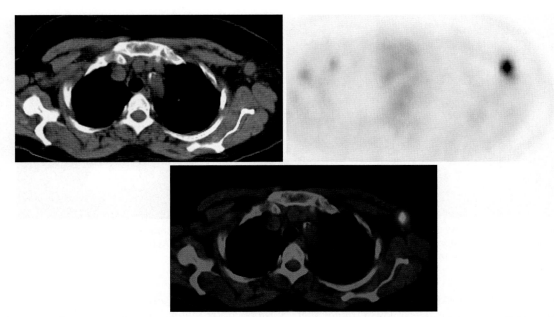

Fig. 3. Axial CT, PET, and PET/CT images of patient who was undergoing staging of left breast cancer. FDG uptake was noted in enlarged left axillary lymph node in keeping with metastatic lymphadenopathy.

from 3.1 to 8 mm. The sensitivity, specificity, and accuracy of FDG PET/CT for detection of lymph node metastases was 80%, 90%, and 86.7%, respectively, suggesting that PET/CT detection of axillary lymph node involvement was more accurate than other approaches using mammography, ultrasonography, or PET alone. Zhao and colleagues[39] reported a 60% sensitivity of FDG PET/CT for lymph node assessment. Another study by Groheux and colleagues[40] in patients with

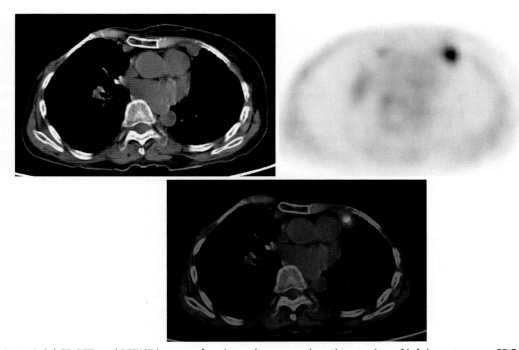

Fig. 4. Axial CT, PET, and PET/CT images of patient who was undergoing staging of left breast cancer. FDG uptake is noted in enlarged left internal mammary lymph node in keeping with metastatic lymphadenopathy.

clinical stage II or III breast cancer showed that FDG PET/CT could provide information regarding extra-axillary lymph node involvement.

PET AND PET/CT IN BREAST CANCER RECURRENCE

The detection of local recurrence is often difficult due to distortion of the local anatomy after surgery and radiotherapy. Recurrences can occur in about 30% of patients. The most common sites of recurrence are the breast and chest wall. With structural imaging modalities such as mammography, CT, and MR imaging, it is frequently difficult to differentiate posttreatment changes from tumor recurrence.[41,42] FDG PET is useful for discriminating between viable tumor and posttreatment changes such as necrosis or scarring in patients with equivocal structural imaging results.[43] Nevertheless, false-positive results can occur due to radiotherapy, muscle uptake, and inflammation. In these situations, a corresponding structural imaging technique will allow for the appropriate anatomic localization of sites of FDG uptake and will improve the specificity of diagnosis.

Combined FDG PET/CT is superior to PET alone for detecting recurrence of tumor in patients previously treated with surgery or radiotherapy (**Fig. 5**). Pelosi and colleagues[44] performed a study on 210 breast cancer patients, 40 of whom were previously treated, using PET/CT (n = 19) or PET combined with structural imaging (n = 21). Forty-five of 47 (96%) lesions were correctly localized by PET/CT in these patients. In the 21 patients studied by PET only, 58 of 63 (92%) lesions could be correctly localized with separate morphologic imaging. Radan and colleagues[45] performed FDG PET/CT in patients with suspected recurrent breast cancer who presented with elevated serum tumor markers, achieving an overall sensitivity, specificity, and accuracy of 90%, 71%, and 83%, respectively. When compared with contrast-enhanced CT, PET/CT had a higher sensitivity (85% versus 70%), specificity (76% versus 47%), and accuracy (81% versus 59%). In addition, PET/CT changed the management of 24 (51%) patients. Another study by Piperkova and colleagues[46] reported a sensitivity, specificity, accuracy, positive productive value, and negative productive value of PET/CT of 97.8%, 93.5%, 97.3%, 99.1%, and 85%, respectively, compared with 87.6%, 42%, 82.1%, 91.6%, and 31.7%, respectively, for contrast-enhanced CT. In that study, the investigators showed that PET/CT had a more important role than contrast-enhanced CT alone and could alter the management of breast cancer patients. Integrated PET/CT in

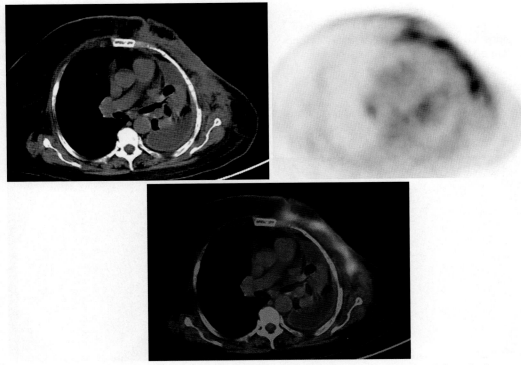

Fig. 5. Axial CT, PET, and PET/CT images of patient who was undergoing restaging after left radical mastectomy for breast cancer. FDG uptake is noted in left chest wall soft tissue in keeping with local recurrence.

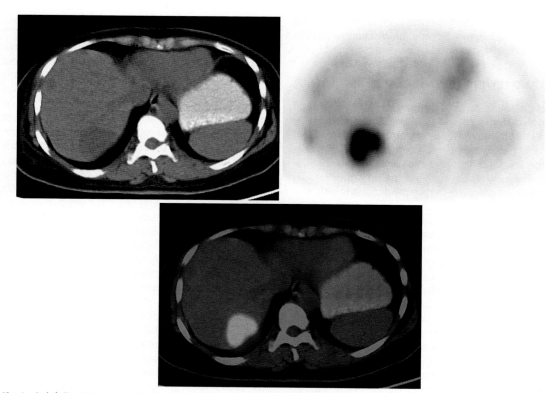

Fig. 6. Axial CT, PET, and PET/CT images of breast cancer patient undergoing restaging. Avid FDG uptake is noted in hypoattenuating lesion in posterior segment of liver in keeping with metastasis.

breast cancer patients has been shown to improve detection of recurrence when compared with PET or CT alone via the accurate localization of functional data on anatomic images.

DISTANT METASTATIC DISEASE

Common sites for distant metastasis from breast cancer include the lungs, liver, and bone marrow. Chest radiography, bone scintigraphy, and liver ultrasonography or abdominal CT are usually performed to assess for distant metastatic disease.[47–49] The advantage of whole body FDG PET imaging over conventional imaging modalities is that it can demonstrate the primary tumor and axillary lymph node metastases and also reveal distant metastatic disease involving different anatomic sites and organs (**Figs. 6–9**) during

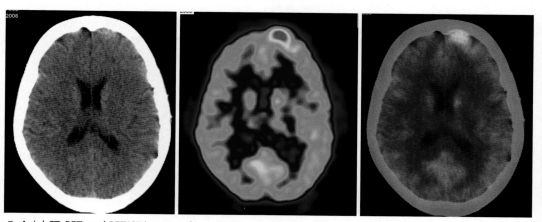

Fig. 7. Axial CT, PET, and PET/CT images of breast cancer patient undergoing restaging. FDG uptake is noted in left frontal lobe in keeping with brain metastasis.

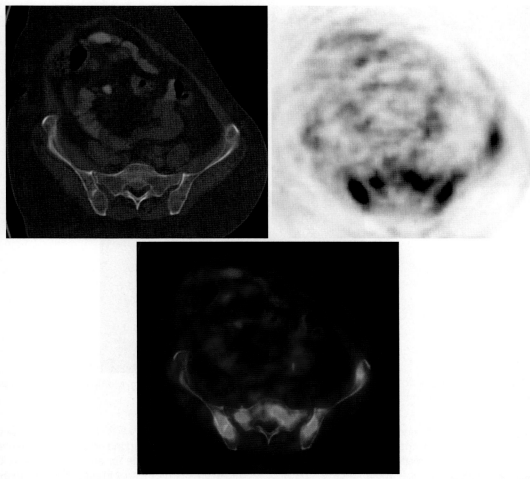

Fig. 8. Axial CT, PET, and PET/CT images of breast cancer patient undergoing restaging. Multiple areas of FDG uptake are noted in sacrum and iliac bones in keeping with bone marrow metastases.

a single examination.[50] Dose and colleagues[51] reported that the overall sensitivity and specificity of PET for the detection of distant metastatic disease were 86% and 90%, respectively. Moon and colleagues[43] reported that whole body PET had high diagnostic accuracy for patients with suspected recurrent or metastatic breast carcinoma. Based on an assessment of the number of lesions, the sensitivity for detecting distant metastasis was 85% and the specificity 79%. Overall, FDG PET has been shown to be superior to conventional diagnostic imaging for detecting distant metastases in breast cancer.[52,53] Bone marrow metastases from breast cancer may be osteolytic or osteoblastic, but most lesions are mixed with a combination of lytic and blastic components. Bone scintigraphy is a functional imaging procedure to survey the entire skeleton for metastatic disease, but purely osteolytic lesions may be missed. Several studies have shown that FDG PET is superior to bone

scintigraphy for detecting lytic and intramedullary metastases, although FDG PET may sometimes fail to demonstrate osteoblastic lesions.[2,43,54–58] Bone scintigraphy is limited in specificity because fractures and other nonneoplastic processes affecting the bones may lead to false-positive results and because images are not tomographic but are instead planar in configuration.

TREATMENT MONITORING

Neoadjuvant chemotherapy is used in patients with locally advanced breast cancer to reduce the size of the primary tumor and to eliminate metastatic disease. As such, it is effective in downstaging the primary tumor before surgery and is increasingly being used to manage patients with locally advanced breast cancer.[59,60] World Health Organization[61] and RECIST (response evaluation criteria in solid tumors) criteria[62] based on

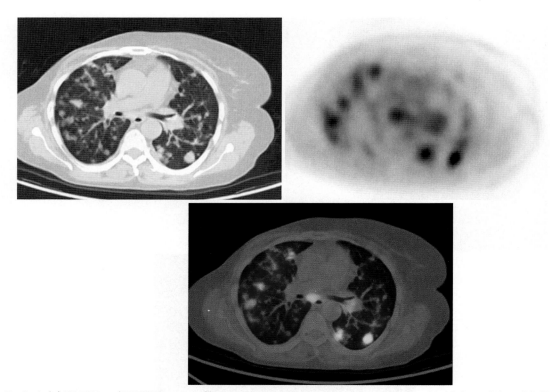

Fig. 9. Axial CT, PET, and PET/CT images of breast cancer patient undergoing restaging. Multiple nodules with FDG uptake are seen in lungs in keeping with metastases.

conventional imaging modalities (CT and MR imaging) have been described in the literature to define when a tumor response has or has not occurred. Despite the wide acceptance of these criteria in clinical practice, they have limitations. For example, the criteria assume that the chemotherapy agent being used is cytotoxic and will lead to cell death followed by a reduction in tumor size. This effect may not occur when cytostatic or immunomodulatory agents are used. Furthermore, several cycles of chemotherapy are generally required before the response can be assessed because changes in tumor size take time.

The most important step in the evaluation of treatment response is the identification of nonresponders as early as possible after the initiation of chemotherapy so that expensive, ineffective, and toxic drugs can be discontinued and alternative treatment methods instituted. Limitations of CT and MR imaging can be overcome by functional imaging techniques that can detect subclinical alterations in tumor metabolism resulting from therapy.[63] FDG PET has been used to assess the response of tumor during and after completion of treatment of breast cancer.[64–66] Integrated PET and CT using FDG have shown encouraging results in predicting breast cancer response to treatment,

helping to guide therapy.[67,68] Recently, Rousseau and colleagues[67] studied the efficacy of sequential FDG PET/CT to evaluate for an early response to neoadjuvant chemotherapy in stage II and III breast cancer patients. They demonstrated the ability of PET/CT to differentiate microscopic and macroscopic residual disease as early as after the first cycle of chemotherapy. Kumar and colleagues[68] had a similar experience in evaluating the response to treatment in 23 patients with locally advanced breast cancer after two cycles of neoadjuvant chemotherapy and reported a sensitivity, specificity, and accuracy of PET/CT for detecting responders of 93%, 75%, and 87%, respectively.

MR IMAGING IN BREAST CANCER

MR imaging is currently under investigation as another diagnostic tool in the field of oncology, especially in the setting of breast cancer.[69] Most of the published data on breast MR imaging have been accrued using 1.5 T magnets, with a few reports using 1.0 T scanners also noted in the literature. Pilot clinical studies involving exploration of the potential role of MR imaging in breast cancer have focused on further evaluation of a mammographically visible lesion or palpable lesion. MR

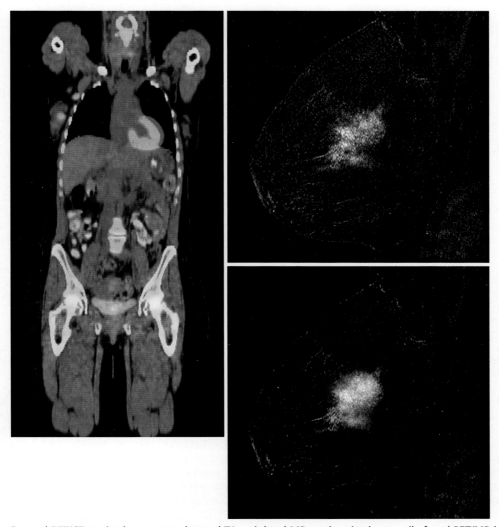

Fig. 10. Coronal PET/CT, sagittal contrast-enhanced T1-weighted MR, and sagittal manually fused PET/MR images of breast cancer patient undergoing staging. FDG avid irregular enhancing mass in right breast as well as FDG avid right axillary lymphadenopathy are seen.

imaging has been shown to have a high sensitivity but only moderate specificity when compared with mammography, ultrasonography, or clinical breast examination. The findings of a large multicenter study of 821 patients showed that MR imaging had a higher sensitivity than other imaging modalities for breast cancer. Nevertheless, although the positive predictive value of MR imaging is seen to be greater than that of mammography, MR imaging does not obviate the need for tissue sampling in the setting of a suspicious breast lesion.[70] Studies have also demonstrated that MR imaging provides the advantage of evaluating the contralateral breast for disease.[71] Patients presenting with axillary lymphadenopathy from an unknown primary also benefit from MR imaging

because it detects an occult cancer in 75% to 85% of patients, allowing many of them to undergo a lumpectomy rather than mastectomy.[72] MR imaging is also superior to mammography and clinical breast examination for evaluation of tumor response after neoadjuvant chemotherapy;[73] however, other studies have shown that the false-negative reporting rate of MR imaging increases with the use of neoadjuvant chemotherapy.[74,75]

MR imaging has a role in screening women at increased risk for developing early breast cancer when mammography is limited in sensitivity due to an increased mammographic density of normal breast tissue. Kuhl and colleagues[76] published the first study on screening MR imaging in high-risk women and reported that it detected six cancers

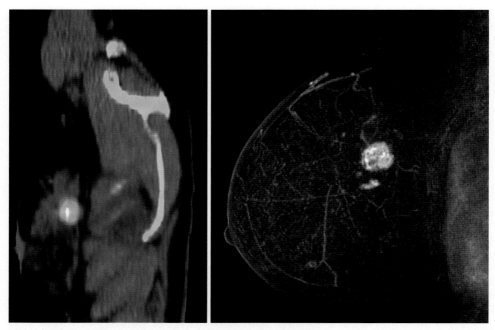

Fig. 11. Sagittal PET/CT and contrast-enhanced T1-weighted maximal intensity projection MR images of breast cancer patient undergoing staging. Focal avid FDG uptake is seen in right breast corresponding to several enhancing breast cancer lesions seen on MR image. FDG avid pulmonary mass due to metastasis (not shown) was also present.

in 192 women (3%) that were occult on mammography and ultrasonography. MR imaging also has a role in T staging of breast cancer in suspected multifocal or multicentric disease and in patients with suspected chest wall involvement as well. Currently, MR imaging is the best modality for the evaluation of breast implant integrity and the detection of cancer in the augmented breast. It is also highly accurate in the differentiation of axillary recurrence, chest wall recurrence, and brachial plexopathy following radiotherapy.

There are no data regarding the role of hybrid PET/MR imaging for the evaluation of patients with breast cancer; however, a few studies have explored the role of fused PET and MR imaging (**Figs. 10** and **11**). Semple and colleagues[77] investigated the relationship between vascular and metabolic characteristics of breast tumors using contrast-enhanced dynamic MR imaging and FDG PET imaging. They found a good correlation between tumor vascularity obtained by MR imaging and tumor metabolism obtained by PET. In another study comparing dynamic MR imaging and FDG PET, the results concerning the diagnosis of primary breast lesions were almost identical.[78]

SUMMARY

The application of FDG PET has shown significant improvement in the management of breast

cancer. Combined FDG PET/CT has shown further improvement in localizing and interpreting sites of abnormal FDG uptake, leading to improvements in sensitivity and specificity. Although only a few studies have been conducted to assess the potential role of PET/CT in the management of breast cancer patients, the advantages of this approach appear obvious. PET/CT has an important role in the staging of breast cancer, in the evaluation of therapeutic response, and in the monitoring of tumor recurrence and restaging. PET/CT may have limited diagnostic value for detecting small primary breast cancers and well-differentiated breast cancers but provides functional information relevant to tumor biology and patient outcome. In this era of rapidly changing technology, PET/MR imaging may be available in coming years for routine clinical use and research purposes. It will be interesting to see what role PET/MR imaging will ultimately have in this clinical realm.

REFERENCES

1. Mahner S, Schirrmacher S, Brenner W, et al. Comparison between positron emission tomography using 2-[fluorine-18]fluoro-2-deoxy-D-glucose, conventional imaging and computed tomography for staging of breast cancer. Ann Oncol 2008;19(7):1249–54.

2. Tatsumi M, Cohade C, Mourtzikos KA, et al. Initial experience with FDG-PET/CT in the evaluation of breast cancer. Eur J Nucl Med Mol Imaging 2006; 33(3):254–62.

3. Fueger BJ, Weber WA, Quon A, et al. Performance of 2-deoxy-2-[F-18]fluoro-D-glucose positron emission tomography and integrated PET/CT in restaged breast cancer patients. Mol Imaging Biol 2005;7(5): 369–76.

4. Fletcher SW, Black W, Harris R, et al. Report of the International Workshop on Screening for Breast Cancer. J Natl Cancer Inst 1993;85(20):1644–56.

5. Tabar L, Duffy SW, Krusemo UB. Detection method, tumour size and node metastases in breast cancers diagnosed during a trial of breast cancer screening. Eur J Cancer Clin Oncol 1987;23(7):959–62.

6. Kopans DB. The positive predictive value of mammography. AJR Am J Roentgenol 1992;158(3): 521–6.

7. Bird RE, Wallace TW, Yankaskas BC. Analysis of cancers missed at screening mammography. Radiology 1992;184(3):613–7.

8. Kerlikowske K, Grady D, Barclay J, et al. Positive predictive value of screening mammography by age and family history of breast cancer. JAMA 1993;270(20):2444–50.

9. Foxcroft LM, Evans EB, Joshua HK, et al. Breast cancers invisible on mammography. Aust N Z J Surg 2000;70(3):162–7.

10. Jackson VP. The current role of ultrasonography in breast imaging. Radiol Clin North Am 1995;33(6): 1161–70.

11. Stavros AT, Thickman D, Rapp CL, et al. Solid breast nodules: use of sonography to distinguish between benign and malignant lesions. Radiology 1995; 196(1):123–34.

12. Heywang SH, Wolf A, Pruss E, et al. MR imaging of the breast with Gd-DTPA: use and limitations. Radiology 1989;171(1):95–103.

13. Friedrich M. MRI of the breast: state of the art. Eur Radiol 1998;8(5):707–25.

14. Avril N, Dose J, Janicke F, et al. Metabolic characterization of breast tumors with positron emission tomography using F-18 fluorodeoxyglucose. J Clin Oncol 1996;14(6):1848–57.

15. Crowe JP Jr, Adler LP, Shenk RR, et al. Positron emission tomography and breast masses: comparison with clinical, mammographic, and pathological findings. Ann Surg Oncol 1994;1(2):132–40.

16. Scheidhauer K, Scharl A, Pietrzyk U, et al. Qualitative [18F]FDG positron emission tomography in primary breast cancer: clinical relevance and practicability. Eur J Nucl Med 1996;23(6):618–23.

17. Tse NY, Hoh CK, Hawkins RA, et al. The application of positron emission tomographic imaging with fluorodeoxyglucose to the evaluation of breast disease. Ann Surg 1992;216(1):27–34.

18. Buck A, Schirrmeister H, Kuhn T, et al. FDG uptake in breast cancer: correlation with biological and clinical prognostic parameters. Eur J Nucl Med Mol Imaging 2002;29(10):1317–23.

19. Samson DJ, Flamm CR, Pisano ED, et al. Should FDG PET be used to decide whether a patient with an abnormal mammogram or breast finding at physical examination should undergo biopsy? Acad Radiol 2002;9(7):773–83.

20. Avril N, Schelling M, Dose J, et al. Utility of PET in breast cancer. Clin Positron Imaging 1999;2(5): 261–71.

21. Crippa F, Agresti R, Seregni E, et al. Prospective evaluation of fluorine-18-FDG PET in presurgical staging of the axilla in breast cancer. J Nucl Med 1998;39(1):4–8.

22. Adler LP, Crowe JP, al-Kaisi NK, et al. Evaluation of breast masses and axillary lymph nodes with [F-18] 2-deoxy-2-fluoro-D-glucose PET. Radiology 1993;187(3):743–50.

23. Avril N, Dose J, Janicke F, et al. Assessment of axillary lymph node involvement in breast cancer patients with positron emission tomography using radiolabeled 2-(fluorine-18)-fluoro-2-deoxy-D-glucose. J Natl Cancer Inst 1996;88(17):1204–9.

24. Wahl RL, Siegel BA, Coleman RE, et al. Prospective multicenter study of axillary nodal staging by positron emission tomography in breast cancer: a report of the Staging Breast Cancer with PET Study Group. J Clin Oncol 2004;22(2):277–85.

25. Kumar R, Chauhan A, Zhuang H, et al. Clinicopathologic factors associated with false negative FDG-PET in primary breast cancer. Breast Cancer Res Treat 2006;98(3):267–74.

26. Buck A, Wahl A, Eicher U, et al. Combined morphological and functional imaging with FDG PET-CT for restaging breast cancer: impact on patient management. J Nucl Med 2003;44S:78P.

27. Tatsumi M, Cohade C, Mourtzikos KA, et al. Initial experience with FDG PET-CT in the evaluation of breast cancer. J Nucl Med 2003;44S:394P.

28. Czernin J. Summary of selected PET-CT abstracts from the 2003 Society of Nuclear Medicine Annual Meeting. J Nucl Med 2004;45:102S–3S.

29. Yang SK, Cho N, Moon WK. The role of PET/CT for evaluating breast cancer. Korean J Radiol 2007; 8(5):429–37.

30. Levine EA, Freimanis RI, Perrier ND, et al. Positron emission mammography: initial clinical results. Ann Surg Oncol 2003;10(1):86–91.

31. Heusner TA, Kuemmel S, Umutlu L, et al. Breast cancer staging in a single session: whole-body PET/CT mammography. J Nucl Med 2008;49(8): 1215–22.

32. Albertini JJ, Lyman GH, Cox C, et al. Lymphatic mapping and sentinel node biopsy in the patient with breast cancer. JAMA 1996;276(22):1818–22.

33. Kumar R, Jana S, Heiba SI, et al. Retrospective analysis of sentinel node localization in multifocal, multicentric, palpable, or nonpalpable breast cancer. J Nucl Med 2003;44(1):7–10.

34. Kumar R, Zhuang H, Schnall M, et al. FDG PET positive lymph nodes are highly predictive of metastasis in breast cancer. Nucl Med Commun 2006;27(3):231–6.

35. Gil-Rendo A, Zornoza G, Garcia-Velloso MJ, et al. Fluorodeoxyglucose positron emission tomography with sentinel lymph node biopsy for evaluation of axillary involvement in breast cancer. Br J Surg 2006;93(6):707–12.

36. Zornoza G, Garcia-Velloso MJ, Sola J, et al. 18F-FDG PET complemented with sentinel lymph node biopsy in the detection of axillary involvement in breast cancer. Eur J Surg Oncol 2004;30(1):15–9.

37. Bellon JR, Livingston RB, Eubank WB, et al. Evaluation of the internal mammary lymph nodes by FDG-PET in locally advanced breast cancer (LABC). Am J Clin Oncol 2004;27(4):407–10.

38. Wang Y, Yu J, Liu J, et al. PET-CT in the diagnosis of both primary breast cancer and axillary lymph node metastasis: initial experience. Int J Radiat Oncol Biol Phys 2003;57(2):S362–3.

39. Zhao TT, Li JG, Li YM. [Performance of 18F-FDG PET/CT in the detection of primary breast cancer and staging of the regional lymph nodes]. Zhonghua Zhong Liu Za Zhi 2007;29(3):206–9 [In Chinese].

40. Groheux D, Moretti JL, Baillet G, et al. Effect of (18)F-FDG PET/CT imaging in patients with clinical stage II and III breast cancer. Int J Radiat Oncol Biol Phys 2008;71(3):695–704.

41. Moore NR, Dixon AK, Wheeler TK, et al. Axillary fibrosis or recurrent tumour: an MRI study in breast cancer. Clin Radiol 1990;42(1):42–6.

42. Goerres GW, Michel SC, Fehr MK, et al. Follow-up of women with breast cancer: comparison between MRI and FDG PET. Eur Radiol 2003;13(7):1635–44.

43. Moon DH, Maddahi J, Silverman DH, et al. Accuracy of whole-body fluorine-18-FDG PET for the detection of recurrent or metastatic breast carcinoma. J Nucl Med 1998;39(3):431–5.

44. Pelosi E, Messa C, Sironi S, et al. Value of integrated PET/CT for lesion localisation in cancer patients: a comparative study. Eur J Nucl Med Mol Imaging 2004;31(7):932–9.

45. Radan L, Ben-Haim S, Bar-Shalom R, et al. The role of FDG-PET/CT in suspected recurrence of breast cancer. Cancer 2006;107(11):2545–51.

46. Piperkova E, Raphael B, Altinyay ME, et al. Impact of PET/CT in comparison with same day contrast enhanced CT in breast cancer management. Clin Nucl Med 2007;32(6):429–34.

47. Richie RC, Swanson JO. Breast cancer: a review of the literature. J Insur Med 2003;35(2):85–101.

48. Newman LA, Sabel M. Advances in breast cancer detection and management. Med Clin North Am 2003;87(5):997–1028.

49. Kubota M, Inoue K, Koh S, et al. Role of ultrasonography in treatment selection. Breast Cancer 2003;10(3):188–97.

50. Zimny M, Siggelkow W. Positron emission tomography scanning in gynecologic and breast cancers. Curr Opin Obstet Gynecol 2003;15(1):69–75.

51. Dose J, Bleckmann C, Bachmann S, et al. Comparison of fluorodeoxyglucose positron emission tomography and "conventional diagnostic procedures" for the detection of distant metastases in breast cancer patients. Nucl Med Commun 2002;23(9):857–64.

52. Kao CH, Hsieh JF, Tsai SC, et al. Comparison and discrepancy of 18F-2-deoxyglucose positron emission tomography and Tc-99m MDP bone scan to detect bone metastases. Anticancer Res 2000;20(3B):2189–92.

53. Eubank WB, Mankoff DA, Vesselle HJ, et al. Detection of locoregional and distant recurrences in breast cancer patients by using FDG PET. Radiographics 2002;22(1):5–17.

54. Cook GJ, Houston S, Rubens R, et al. Detection of bone metastases in breast cancer by 18FDG PET: differing metabolic activity in osteoblastic and osteolytic lesions. J Clin Oncol 1998;16(10):3375–9.

55. Even-Sapir E, Metser U, Flusser G, et al. Assessment of malignant skeletal disease: initial experience with 18F-fluoride PET/CT and comparison between 18F-fluoride PET and 18F-fluoride PET/CT. J Nucl Med 2004;45(2):272–8.

56. Isasi CR, Moadel RM, Blaufox MD. A meta-analysis of FDG-PET for the evaluation of breast cancer recurrence and metastases. Breast Cancer Res Treat 2005;90(2):105–12.

57. Kim TS, Moon WK, Lee DS, et al. Fluorodeoxyglucose positron emission tomography for detection of recurrent or metastatic breast cancer. World J Surg 2001;25(7):829–34.

58. Nakai T, Okuyama C, Kubota T, et al. Pitfalls of FDG-PET for the diagnosis of osteoblastic bone metastases in patients with breast cancer. Eur J Nucl Med Mol Imaging 2005;32(11):1253–8.

59. Bonadonna G, Valagussa P, Zucali R, et al. Primary chemotherapy in surgically resectable breast cancer. CA Cancer J Clin 1995;45(4):227–43.

60. Wang HC, Lo SS. Future prospects of neoadjuvant chemotherapy in treatment of primary breast cancer. Semin Surg Oncol 1996;12(1):59–66.

61. Miller AB, Hoogstraten B, Staquet M, et al. Reporting results of cancer treatment. Cancer 1981;47(1):207–14.

62. Therasse P, Arbuck SG, Eisenhauer EA, et al. New guidelines to evaluate the response to treatment in solid tumors: European Organization for Research

and Treatment of Cancer, National Cancer Institute of the United States, National Cancer Institute of Canada. J Natl Cancer Inst 2000;92(3):205–16.

63. Price P, Jones T. Can positron emission tomography (PET) be used to detect subclinical response to cancer therapy? The EC PET Oncology Concerted Action and the EORTC PET Study Group. Eur J Cancer 1995;31A(12):1924–7.

64. Wahl RL, Zasadny K, Helvie M, et al. Metabolic monitoring of breast cancer chemohormonotherapy using positron emission tomography: initial evaluation. J Clin Oncol 1993;11(11):2101–11.

65. Bassa P, Kim EE, Inoue T, et al. Evaluation of preoperative chemotherapy using PET with fluorine-18-fluorodeoxyglucose in breast cancer. J Nucl Med 1996;37(6):931–8.

66. Schelling M, Avril N, Nahrig J, et al. Positron emission tomography using [(18)F]fluorodeoxyglucose for monitoring primary chemotherapy in breast cancer. J Clin Oncol 2000;18(8):1689–95.

67. Rousseau C, Devillers A, Sagan C, et al. Monitoring of early response to neoadjuvant chemotherapy in stage II and III breast cancer by [18F]fluorodeoxyglucose positron emission tomography. J Clin Oncol 2006;24(34):5366–72.

68. Kumar A, Kumar R, Seenu V. Role of 18F-FDG PET-CT in evaluation of early response to neoadjuvant chemotherapy in patients with locally advanced breast cancer. Eur Radiol in press.

69. Heywang SH, Fenzl G, Hahn D, et al. MR imaging of the breast: comparison with mammography and ultrasound. J Comput Assist Tomogr 1986;10(4):615–20.

70. Bluemke DA, Gatsonis CA, Chen MH, et al. Magnetic resonance imaging of the breast prior to biopsy. JAMA 2004;292(22):2735–42.

71. Goldflam K, Hunt KK, Gershenwald JE, et al. Contralateral prophylactic mastectomy: predictors of significant histologic findings. Cancer 2004;101(9): 1977–86.

72. Orel SG, Weinstein SP, Schnall MD, et al. Breast MR imaging in patients with axillary node metastases and unknown primary malignancy. Radiology 1999; 212(2):543–9.

73. Gilles R, Guinebretiere JM, Toussaint C, et al. Locally advanced breast cancer: contrast-enhanced subtraction MR imaging of response to preoperative chemotherapy. Radiology 1994; 191(3):633–8.

74. Rosen EL, Blackwell KL, Baker JA, et al. Accuracy of MRI in the detection of residual breast cancer after neoadjuvant chemotherapy. AJR Am J Roentgenol 2003;181(5):1275–82.

75. Partridge SC, Gibbs JE, Lu Y, et al. Accuracy of MR imaging for revealing residual breast cancer in patients who have undergone neoadjuvant chemotherapy. AJR Am J Roentgenol 2002; 179(5):1193–9.

76. Kuhl CK, Schmutzler RK, Leutner CC, et al. Breast MR imaging screening in 192 women proved or suspected to be carriers of a breast cancer susceptibility gene: preliminary results. Radiology 2000; 215(1):267–79.

77. Semple SI, Gilbert FJ, Redpath TW, et al. The relationship between vascular and metabolic characteristics of primary breast tumours. Eur Radiol 2004; 14(11):2038–45.

78. Brix G, Henze M, Knopp MV, et al. Comparison of pharmacokinetic MRI and [18F] fluorodeoxyglucose PET in the diagnosis of breast cancer: initial experience. Eur Radiol 2001;11(10):2058–70.

PET, CT, and MR Imaging for Assessment of Thoracic Malignancy: Structure Meets Function

Sharyn Katz, MD*, Thomas Ferrara, BS,
Abass Alavi, MD, PhD (Hon), DSc (Hon),
Drew A. Torigian, MD, MA

KEYWORDS

- Thoracic • Malignancy
- Positron emission tomography (PET)
- Computed tomography (CT)
- Magnetic resonance imaging (MR imaging)
- PET/CT • PET/MR imaging

This article describes the use of positron emission tomography (PET), CT, and MR imaging in assessing thoracic malignancies, including pulmonary malignancies, such as lung cancer; pleural malignancies, such as malignant pleural mesothelioma (MPM); and esophageal cancer.

PULMONARY MALIGNANCY: LUNG CANCER

In the management of patients with known lung cancer, [18F]-2-fluoro-2-deoxy-D-glucose (FDG)–PET has an important role in staging. Contrast-enhanced CT is also typically acquired for detailed structural assessment of the lungs, thoracic lymph nodes, cardiovascular structures, pericardium, pleura, and chest wall, as well as for detailed evaluation of tumor morphology, with attention to local tumor extent and distant spread of disease to such structures as the liver, bone marrow, adrenal glands, and brain. MR imaging is also sometimes employed to detect or characterize potential lesions in these locations, as its major strength is its high soft-tissue contrast resolution in combination with high spatial resolution. A major strength of FDG-PET is its high sensitivity for the detection

of metastatic disease, particularly in thoracic lymph nodes, since CT and MR imaging have limited sensitivities and specificities for the detection of metastatic disease in normal-sized lymph nodes. In addition, FDG-PET is also useful in estimating patient prognosis, evaluating tumor response to therapy, and restaging of disease.[1]

Non–small Cell Lung Cancer

In the course of diagnosis and management of non–small cell lung cancer (NSCLC), a number of imaging techniques are central to clinical management. These techniques include CT and FDG-PET, frequently performed in combination using PET/CT. MR imaging may also play a role in lesion characterization and staging of disease. FDG-PET and CT are useful in defining tumor volume for planning radiation therapy.[2,3] Before therapeutic intervention, accurate staging of disease is required to maximize the chances of success while minimizing treatment-related morbidity or mortality. During therapy, accurate and precise measures of response assessment are needed, and are primarily performed using contrast-enhanced CT and FDG-PET,

Department of Radiology, Hospital of the University of Pennsylvania, School of Medicine, 3400 Spruce Street, Philadelphia, PA 19104, USA
* Corresponding author.
E-mail address: Sharyn.Katz@uphs.upenn.edu (S. Katz).

PET Clin 3 (2009) 395–410
doi:10.1016/j.cpet.2009.03.008

although several other novel PET radiotracers may also potentially be useful to obtain earlier functional measures of response compared with CT.

Staging

The TNM staging system is employed for the staging of NSCLC. The T-value describes the tumor size and extent, the N-value describes regional nodal involvement, and the M-value reflects the presence or absence of distant metastases. These three factors are then combined to generate the four stages of lung cancer. A critical staging threshold lies in the presence of T4, N3, or M1 disease, as the presence of any of these characteristics generally renders the patient unresectable and tends to predict a dismal prognosis.[4] To accurately stage disease, a variety of imaging techniques are available.

The T-value of staging non–small cell lung cancer Contrast-enhanced CT has superior spatial resolution and is most valuable for accurate determination of the T-value of staging. CT is able to resolve lesions that are 1 mm in size, is useful in establishing the size and extent of the primary tumor, and can detect the presence of satellite lesions or pulmonary metastases with high accuracy. In contrast, FDG-PET has been shown not to be reliable in the detection of primary lung malignancies under 1 cm.[5] With the potential of invasion of malignancy into the mediastinum, hila, pulmonary vasculature, or cardiac chambers, soft tissue contrast resolution on unenhanced CT is inadequate, which is the reason that intravenous

contrast administration is routinely administered for staging and restaging. However, even with contrast-enhanced CT, questions may still arise as to whether tumor invasion of mediastinal structures, such as pericardium, esophagus, and aorta, is present when no clear fat plane is identified between tumor and these structures.

In such cases, MR imaging may add value to separate invasion of mediastinal structures by tumor from those cases where tumor simply abuts the mediastinal structures. While MR imaging is not useful for staging disease extent in the lungs because of marked susceptibility artifacts created by gas in the lungs, it is very useful for assessing the heart, pericardium, aorta, great vessels, and esophagus. MR imaging can also be used to assess for invasion of structures challenging to assess on CT, including the superior sulcus, the brachial plexus, the subclavian vessels, the chest wall, the spine, and the diaphragm. Overall, the sensitivity and specificity of MR imaging for assessment of chest wall invasion are similar to those of CT, and are approximately 63% to 90% and 84% to 86%, respectively.[6,7]

Regarding determination of the T-value, FDG-PET can be useful for the characterization of pleural effusions as malignant, which, when present, would make a patient's T-value T4 (**Fig. 1**). FDG-PET can also sometimes be useful for assessment of potential chest wall or mediastinal invasion by tumor, and for delineation of the gross boundaries of tumor when it is surrounded by atelectatic lung, which is particularly important for planning radiation therapy. However, the main

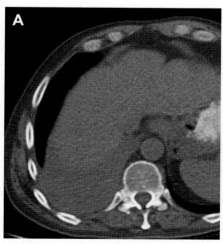
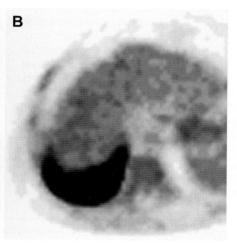

Fig. 1. Sixty-seven–year-old man with right lung NSCLC with suspected malignant pleural effusion undergoing staging evaluation. (*A*) Low-dose unenhanced axial CT image from PET/CT reveals nonspecific right pleural effusion measuring 20 to 30 Hounsfield units in attenuation. (*B*) Corresponding axial FDG-PET image reveals intense FDG uptake in right pleural effusion in keeping with pleural involvement by tumor.

strength of FDG-PET for lung cancer staging lies in the determination of the N-value and M-value staging parameters.

N-value of staging non–small cell lung cancer FDG-PET is highly sensitive in the detection of mediastinal nodal involvement with a lower limit of detection reported at 4 mm.[8] FDG-PET has been estimated to have a sensitivity as high as 91% to 96% and specificity as high as 86% to 93%, as compared with a sensitivity as high as 68% to 75% and specificity as high as 65% to 66% for CT in staging the mediastinal lymph nodes.[9,10] Thus, FDG-PET is very useful for detecting metastatic disease in normal-sized lymph nodes as detected on CT or MR imaging. It has been suggested that with a negative FDG-PET scan for mediastinal nodes and absence of N1 disease, mediastinoscopy can be omitted,[11] although there is still disagreement on the matter.[12] Recent studies suggest that FDG-PET/CT is more accurate than CT, MR imaging, or FDG-PET alone for staging of the mediastinum.[13–15] For example, Plathow and colleagues[14] compared the performances of whole-body MR imaging and FDG-PET/CT in 52 patients with stage III NSCLC, and reported a sensitivity of 88.5% and specificity of 96.1% for N staging by MR imaging, compared with a sensitivity of 96.1% and specificity of 100% for FDG-PET/CT.

The M-value of staging non–small cell lung cancer The most common sites of metastasis from NSCLC are the liver, brain, adrenal glands, and bone marrow. CT remains central to the evaluation for metastatic disease, but has been greatly complemented by the addition of FDG-PET. FDG-PET is highly sensitive for the detection of metastases and, in one reported study, FDG-PET resulted in upstaging of lung cancer stage in 15% of patients with M0 disease status by CT.[11] In solid organs, subcentimeter metastases are frequently not accurately characterized by CT, but are often detectable by FDG-PET. It should be noted that gross standardized uptake value (SUV) measurements of lesions less than 1 to 2 cm cannot be relied upon to discriminate between benign and malignant tissue by simple comparison to a threshold SUV cutoff level of 2.5 because of partial volume averaging effects that erroneously result in misleadingly low apparent SUVs. However, partial volume corrected SUV measurements, as well as dual time-point FDG-PET imaging technique, where two sets of PET images are acquired at two time points following FDG administration, can improve the sensitivity, specificity, and accuracy of FDG-PET to characterize lesions as truly malignant.[16–18]

Because of its excellent soft tissue contrast resolution, MR imaging is often helpful in providing a definitive diagnosis of metastasis for small lesions, even without contrast material. MR imaging is particularly valuable in characterizing potential metastatic disease in the brain, liver, bone marrow, adrenal glands, and other solid organs. Heavily T2-weighted and fat-suppressed T2-weighted images of the liver are used to differentiate between solid tumors, hemangiomas, and simple cysts with an accuracy of up to 100%, as cysts and hemangiomas generally remain very high in signal intensity on heavily T2-weighted images, whereas metastases, with a signal intensity similar to that of the spleen, tend to be lower in signal intensity.[19] A recent prospective study by Ohno and colleagues[20] reported that whole-body MR imaging with diffusion-weighted imaging can be used for M-stage assessment in patients with NSCLC with accuracy as good as that of FDG-PET/CT. MR imaging is very sensitive and specific in characterizing brain lesions, whereas CT is limited by suboptimal soft tissue contrast resolution, and FDG-PET is limited by the normal increased background FDG uptake in the cerebral gray matter, deep nuclei, and cerebellum.

MR imaging is very useful in characterizing adrenal lesions indeterminate on CT or on FDG-PET (as benign adrenal lesions, such as adenomas, may have attenuation values greater than 10–12 Hounsfield units on unenhanced CT or may sometimes demonstrate FDG uptake on FDG-PET). A definitive diagnosis of adrenal adenoma can be made on MR imaging when the signal intensity of the lesion drops from in-phase to out-of-phase in the T1-weighted gradient-recalled echo chemical shift images. This drop results from the cancellation of signal of water and lipid molecules present in the same voxels.[21–23] MR imaging evaluation of the adrenal glands with chemical shift imaging has a sensitivity of 91% to 100%, specificity of 94% to 100%, and accuracy of 93% to 100% in the diagnosis of an adrenal adenoma, the most common cause of an adrenal mass.[21,22] FDG-PET has been reported to have a sensitivity of 100% and a specificity of 80% to 90% for the identification of adrenal metastases in patients with lung cancer (**Fig. 2**).[24,25]

FDG-PET is useful in the detection of osseous metastatic disease, and has a much higher sensitivity than CT for detecting metastases of the bone marrow. However, confirmatory characterization of suspicious osseous lesions can be performed

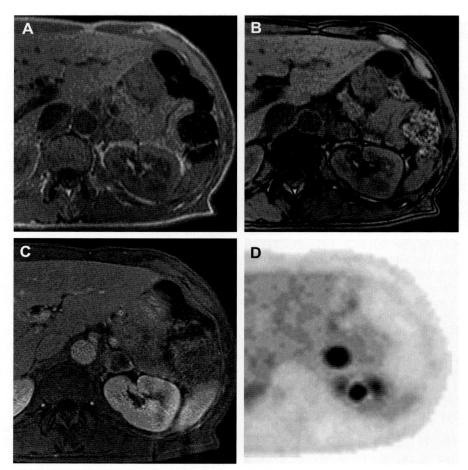

Fig. 2. Seventy-three–year-old man with NSCLC and indeterminate adrenal nodule. (*A*) Axial in-phase T1-weighted MR image reveals mass in left adrenal gland. (*B*) Axial out-of-phase T1-weighted MR image shows no loss of signal intensity within mass, indicating absence of microscopic lipid. (*C*) Axial fat-suppressed T1-weighted contrast-enhanced MR image demonstrates rim of enhancement in mass. (*D*) Axial FDG-PET image reveals avid FDG uptake in mass with maximum SUV of 10.9. Findings are diagnostic of adrenal metastasis.

with MR imaging, particularly for isolated bone marrow lesions detected on FDG-PET. MR imaging is also particularly useful in evaluating the relationships of spinal osseous metastatic disease to the spinal cord, thecal sac, nerve roots, and leptomeninges (**Fig. 3**). A recent study revealed that MR imaging had an average sensitivity of 96% when a combination of T1-weighted, T2-weighted short tau inversion recovery, and diffusion-weighted imaging sequences were employed.[26]

Restaging and response assessment

Restaging of non–small cell lung cancer Months after the initiation of chemotherapy or surgery, patients typically undergo restaging FDG-PET and CT to assess for disease progression or regression (**Fig. 4**). Once the new state of the disease is

characterized, patients are upstaged or downstaged accordingly to direct future treatment plans. FDG-PET is generally superior for the detection of subtle malignant disease in the solid organs, usually the adrenal glands, brain, liver, bone marrow, and lymph nodes, whereas CT generally remains superior for characterization of changes in the size and local extent of primary and metastatic tumor in the lungs, although evaluation of portions of the lung affected by postradiation changes is more limited.

FDG uptake may be seen in the thorax following radiation therapy, talc pleurodesis, or surgery, which may sometimes be difficult to differentiate from residual or recurrent tumor.[27,28] Morphologic changes detected on CT may have features characteristic of posttherapeutic changes (eg, linear margins in the setting of radiation pneumonitis,

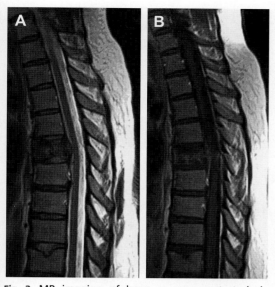

Fig. 3. MR imaging of bone marrow metastasis in thoracic spine in patient with NSCLC. Sagittal T2-weighted MT image (*A*) and sagittal contrast-enhanced T1-weighted MR image (*B*) reveal abnormal signal intensity in T5 vertebral body with pathologic compression fracture and extension of enhancing soft tissue into epidural space, resulting in mild central canal stenosis.

and high attenuation foci within the pleural space due to talc pleurodesis), although sometimes the detected findings may be indistinguishable from residual or recurrent tumor (**Fig. 5**). Dual time-point FDG-PET may be especially useful in this setting to distinguish areas of tumor from areas of posttreatment change.[29]

Early response assessment of non–small cell lung cancer FDG-PET has shown much promise for functionally assessing early response to therapy as early as 1 week after initiation of chemotherapy.[30–32] This is important because most patients are diagnosed at an advanced stage of disease with limited time for optimization of therapy. The ability to determine efficacy or failure of a treatment regimen early on provides more opportunities to tailor the therapeutic approach for the most benefit. In a study by Hellwig and colleagues,[33] patients with a lung cancer with a maximum SUV less than four measured 1 month after therapy had a survival benefit of 56 months compared with 19 months when the maximum SUV was greater than four. Also currently under study are other PET radiotracers to measure intratumoral cellular proliferation, angiogenesis, and hypoxia, which may also prove useful for monitoring early response to therapy.

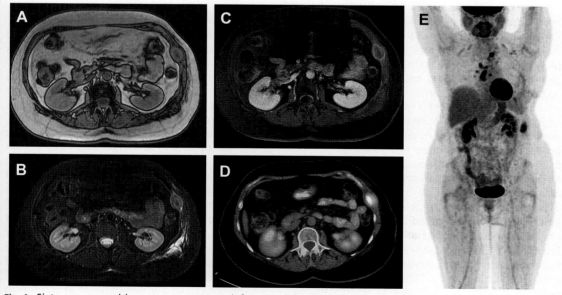

Fig. 4. Sixty-one–year-old woman status post–left upper lobectomy for NSCLC now presents with left chest wall palpable abnormality. (*A*) Axial out-of-phase T1-weighted MR image shows ovoid mass of left lower anterior rib with intermediate signal intensity relative to skeletal muscle. (*B*) Axial fat-suppressed T2-weighted MR image reveals intermediate-high signal intensity of mass. (*C*) Axial contrast-enhanced fat-suppressed T1-weighted MR image demonstrates enhancement of mass. (*D*) Axial FDG-PET/CT image shows avid FDG uptake in mass. (*E*) Coronal PET maximal intensity projection image reveals additional FDG uptake in mediastinal and hilar lymph nodes. Findings are in keeping with chest wall, hilar, and mediastinal lymph node metastases.

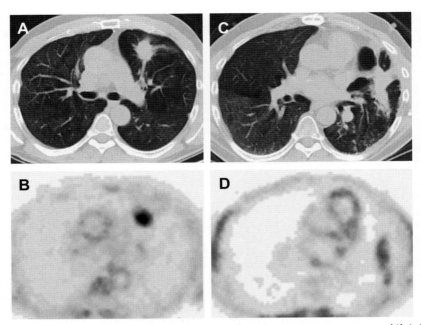

Fig. 5. Fifty-two–year-old man with left upper lobe NSCLC undergoing response assessment. (*A*) Axial baseline CT image shows 3-cm spiculated mass in left upper lobe. (*B*) Axial baseline FDG-PET image demonstrates avid FDG uptake in mass with maximum SUV of 5.4. No lymphadenopathy or distant metastases were detected. As patient could not undergo surgical treatment, chemoradiotherapy was administered. (*C*) Axial posttherapy CT image reveals new irregular opacity in left lung, much of which is due to postradiation change, although it is difficult to determine whether residual tumor is present. (*D*) Axial FDG-PET image shows minimal FDG uptake in left lung opacity due to postradiation change but more focal nodular area of increased FDG uptake suspicious for residual tumor.

Prognosis

The estimated 5-year survival rate for T1 NSCLC is 70%,[34] with 30% mortality due to recurrent progressive disease. Since this mortality is thought to be due to undetected micrometastases, additional methods of assessing tumor aggressiveness are needed to signal when a more intense treatment regimen is needed to eliminate such undetected sites of disease. A recent study by Ohtsuka and colleagues[35] demonstrated that tumor avidity for FDG was predictive of disease-free survival for stage I lung adenocarcinoma, where a tumor maximum SUV of 3.3 or more correlated with a worse prognosis compared with tumors with less FDG uptake. In another study, by Watanabe and colleagues,[36] maximum SUV of tumor on baseline FDG-PET was positively correlated with histologic measures of proliferation and frequency of lymph node metastasis. Other reports have also noted the utility of FDG-PET to prognosticate patient outcome in the setting of NSCLC.[37–39]

Small Cell Lung Cancer

Staging

Small cell lung cancer (SCLC), representing approximately 20% of all lung cancers, is usually locally advanced at presentation such that surgery is no longer a therapeutic option. Patients are categorized into one of two staging categories: limited disease, when disease is limited to one hemithorax; and extensive disease, when disease extends beyond one hemithorax.[40] Patients with limited disease are candidates for chemotherapy and radiation therapy whereas those with extensive disease are generally treated for palliation due to the generally dismal prognosis and limited usefulness of chemotherapy.

Conventional staging is typically performed with contrast-enhanced CT. Recently, the addition of FDG-PET to CT has demonstrated value for therapy planning.[41] FDG-PET is more sensitive to lymph node involvement and for detection of disease beyond one hemithorax.[42,43] FDG-PET has a sensitivity of 100% and specificity of 98% (compared with a sensitivity of 70% and specificity of 94% for CT) in the detection of extrathoracic lymph node involvement. FDG-PET also has a sensitivity of 98% and specificity of 92% (compared with a sensitivity of 83% and specificity of 72% for CT) for the detection of distant metastasis with exclusion of the brain.[42] These data suggest that FDG-PET contributes significantly to treatment planning in patients with SCLC, particularly when used in conjunction with CT (**Fig. 6**). MR imaging may also be used as a problem-solving tool when needed to improve the assessment of tumor invasion into adjacent structures and to characterize lesions in organs (such as the liver, adrenal glands, brain, and axial skeletal bone marrow) that are indeterminate by CT or FDG-PET.

Response assessment

Unfortunately, despite a reported tumor response rate of 60% to 85% with initial therapy, SCLC characteristically recurs rapidly, resulting in a 5-year survival rate of 10% to 13%. An accurate and timely means to measure response to therapy and to identify residual tumor, often obscured by posttreatment changes, would likely improve survival. There are limited data available related to the potential role of FDG-PET to assess response to therapy. One recent report by Onitilo and colleagues[44] demonstrated that those patients with a negative FDG-PET scan at 4 months after treatment had a mean survival of 29.2 months (compared with 10.3 months for other patients).

SCLC has also been noted to have neuroendocrine receptor expression with accumulation of dihydroxyphenylalanine. As such, [18F]-fluoro-di-hydroxyphenylalanine (FDOPA) has been used as a novel PET radiotracer in clinical trials to assess SCLC. Initial studies have demonstrated tumor uptake of FDOPA, although the sensitivity was reported to be limited.[45]

Prognosis

There are limited data demonstrating that baseline FDG-PET has prognostic value in patients with SCLC. A study by Pandit and colleagues[46] revealed a strong negative correlation between pretherapy tumor maximum SUV and survival. Similarly, a negative correlation between tumor maximum SUV and survival in patients with neuroendocrine tumors was also observed by Chong and colleagues.[47] Future investigations are still needed to explore the prognostic role of FDG-PET in patients with SCLC.

PLEURAL MALIGNANCY
Pleural Metastasis

Pleural metastasis is the most common malignancy of the pleura, and is commonly encountered with lung, breast, esophageal, and ovarian cancers. Pleural malignancy is often suspected in the setting of unexplained pleural effusions in patients with a known primary malignancy. Contrast-enhanced CT or MR imaging can detect nodular pleural thickening and pleural effusions. FDG-PET has a reported accuracy of 82% in the diagnosis of malignant pleural effusions when a threshold maximum SUV of 2.2 is used.[48] However, care should be taken to correlate FDG-PET findings with those of CT as talc

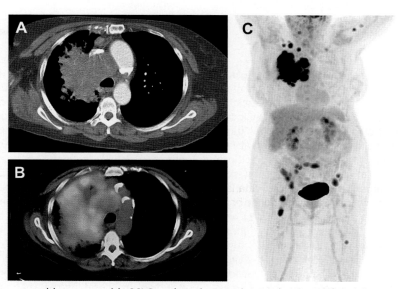

Fig. 6. Sixty-three–year-old woman with SCLC undergoing staging evaluation. (*A*) Axial contrast-enhanced CT image shows large right lung mass with local invasion of right hilum and mediastinum. (*B*) Axial FDG-PET/CT image reveals avid FDG uptake in mass with maximum SUV of 12.1, as well as intratumoral heterogeneity of glucose metabolism. (*C*) Coronal PET maximal intensity projection image demonstrates FDG avid foci within right supraclavicular lymph nodes, pelvic bones, and bilateral femora, in keeping with metastatic disease.

pleurodesis can cause a long-standing increase in SUV within the pleural space, potentially mimicking pleural malignancy.[28,49] In general, suspected pleural effusions are further assessed by fluid aspiration and cytologic analysis. As contrast-enhanced CT generally has high specificity, MR imaging is not often used in the diagnosis of metastatic pleural thickening, unless there are contraindications against the intravenous administration of iodinated contrast material for CT or if there is suspected chest wall or diaphragmatic invasion.[50,51]

Malignant Pleural Mesothelioma

MPM is an uncommon but extremely aggressive and invasive malignancy that is nearly uniformly fatal within 12 months of diagnosis. This malignancy is a long-term consequence of asbestos exposure and is currently on the rise in Europe. The diagnosis is suggested on CT and MR imaging by nodular rindlike pleural thickening that is frequently unilateral, associated with decreased volume of the ipsilateral hemithorax, and often accompanied by a malignant pleural effusion.[52] In fact, the presence of a persistent pleural effusion in the setting of calcified asbestos-related pleural plaques should raise suspicion for MPM. However, MPM often cannot be reliably differentiated from metastatic pleural disease on imaging features alone. FDG-PET is useful in patients with MPM for staging purposes, as staging follows the TNM system. However, FDG-PET also plays a role in the assessment of patient prognosis and for early response assessment.

Staging

The T-value in staging malignant pleural mesothelioma The critical distinction to be made in assessment of T stage is the differentiation between T3 and T4. T3 is characterized by locally advanced but potentially resectable tumor involving all ipsilateral pleural surfaces with at least one of the following: involvement of the endothoracic fascia, extension into the mediastinal fat, nontransmural involvement of the pericardium, or a solitary completely resectable focus of tumor extending into the soft tissues of the chest wall. Meanwhile, T4 is characterized by locally advanced but technically unresectable tumor involving all ipsilateral pleural surfaces with at least one of the following: diffuse extension or multifocal masses of tumor in the chest wall, direct transdiaphragmatic extension of tumor to the peritoneum, direct extension of tumor to the contralateral pleura, direct extension of tumor to one or more mediastinal organs, direct extension

of tumor into the spine, tumor extending through to the internal surface of pericardium, or tumor involving the myocardium. Those tumors that are resectable may be considered for extrapleural pneumonectomy or radial pleurectomy-decortication followed by adjuvant chemotherapy and radiation therapy, and are associated with improved survival.[53,54] Thus accurate T staging is critical to proper management of these patients.

CT is useful in the determination of T-value but can be limited when assessing for possible mediastinal, chest wall, or diaphragmatic transgression. In this situation, MR imaging can be employed to provide improved soft tissue contrast and multiplanar images to make a determination of the presence of tissue invasion (**Fig. 7**). Heelan and colleagues[50] reported that MR imaging was superior to CT for demonstration of diaphragmatic invasion (with MR imaging accuracy of 82% versus and CT accuracy of 55%) and endothoracic fascia or solitary resectable foci of chest wall invasion (with MR imaging accuracy of 69% versus CT accuracy of 46%). Stewart and colleagues[55] showed that contrast-enhanced MR imaging reclassified about 30% of surgical candidates with MPM to a nonoperable stage of disease. MR imaging has also been reported to be superior to CT in the differentiation of malignant pleural disease from benign pleural disease.[56] FDG-PET also plays a role in revealing the extent of tumor into these locations, and is useful in differentiating benign from malignant pleural disease.[57,58]

The N-value in staging malignant pleural mesothelioma Nodal involvement usually occurs in the hilum or mediastinum, areas that can be challenging for accurate staging by CT or MR imaging. The addition of FDG-PET to the staging algorithm has resulted in increased sensitivity for nodal disease, improving the accuracy of overall staging and improving the selection of patients for extrapleural pneumonectomy.[57,59] Furthermore, FDG-PET is useful in helping to select the most metabolically active site for tissue sampling of nodes, thereby increasing the yield of positive biopsy results.[60] In the TNM staging system for MPM, N0 is defined by the lack of evidence of nodal disease; N1 is defined by presence of ipsilateral bronchopulmonary or hilar lymphadenopathy; N2 is defined by subcarinal or ipsilateral mediastinal lymphadenopathy, including ipsilateral internal mammary lymph nodes; and N3 is defined by contralateral mediastinal, contralateral internal mammary, or ipsilateral or contralateral supraclavicular lymphadenopathy.[53,54]

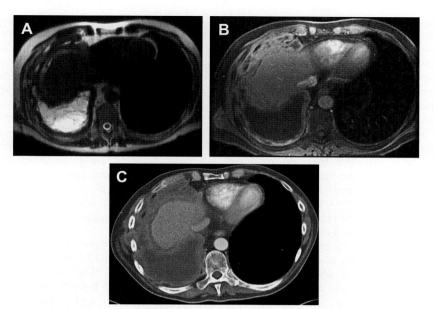

Fig. 7. Sixty-four–year-old man undergoing staging evaluation for known MPM. Axial T2-weighted MR image (*A*), axial contrast-enhanced fat-suppressed T1-weighted MR image (*B*), and axial contrast-enhanced CT image (*C*) through inferior chest demonstrate thickening, nodularity, and enhancement of right visceral and parietal pleura with complex pleural effusion containing multiple low signal intensity septations seen on T2-weighted image in keeping with mesothelioma. Note irregularity of hepatic contour and small perihepatic fluid on contrast-enhanced images, indicative of tumor invasion through diaphragm to perihepatic peritoneal space.

The M-value in staging malignant pleural mesothelioma Metastasis is a late and uncommon occurrence in MPM, and is usually in association with extensive local invasion by tumor. FDG-PET has been shown to improve the accuracy of staging compared with CT or MR imaging alone, as it increases the sensitivity of detection of distant metastatic disease, particularly when performed as part of a FDG-PET/CT examination (**Fig. 8**).[57,59,61] In the TNM staging system, M0 indicates the absence of distant metastatic disease, whereas M1 indicates the presence of distant metastatic disease.[53,54]

Response assessment

MPM often has a rapid pace of progression with resistance to chemotherapy. Timely and accurate assessment of response to therapy is therefore important to provide maximal opportunity for optimization of the therapeutic regimen and improvement in patient outcome. In recent years, the response evaluation criteria in solid tumors (RECIST) have been modified to address the challenges for accurate measurement on CT or MR imaging posed by this insinuating malignancy. The revised criteria, called the modified RECIST, assign response using a value generated as

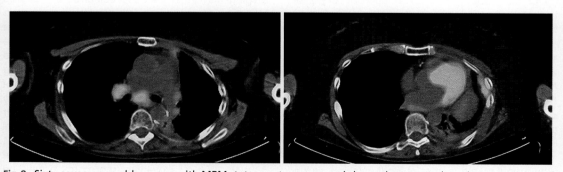

Fig. 8. Sixty-seven–year-old woman with MPM status post–surgery and chemotherapy, undergoing restaging evaluation. Axial FDG-PET/CT images through midchest (*top*) and lower chest (*bottom*) demonstrate FDG avid right hilar and subcarinal lymphadenopathy as well as thickening and nodularity of the left pleura with focal areas of FDG uptake, in keeping with recurrent disease.

follows: Three transverse slices are selected (each 1 cm or more from the other), two radial tumor diameters are measured per slice, and the six radial diameters are summed. Temporal differences in these summed diameters indicate a complete response when there is complete resolution of disease, a partial response when there is a greater than 30% decrease, progressive disease when there is a greater than 20% increase, and stable disease otherwise.[62] Plathow and colleagues[63] have reported that the modified RECIST, particularly in combination with MR imaging, is accurate and reproducible for response assessment in MPM. However, CT and MR imaging do not reveal the changes that occur in tumors at the molecular level but only at the macroscopic tissue level, and therefore suffer from limitations in sensitivity of early detection of response assessment and from limitations in specificity to distinguish viable tumor from nonviable tumor or non-neoplastic tissue.

Recently, FDG-PET tumor uptake has been proposed as a measure of functional tumor response to therapy to be used alongside CT or MR imaging assessments of disease response.[64–66] Ceresoli and colleagues[66] demonstrated stratification of patient response to therapy and survival through use of maximum SUV of tumor measured after two cycles of chemotherapy. Metabolic responders, defined as having a 25% or more decrease in maximum SUV, demonstrated a survival of 14 months compared with 7 months in nonresponders. Francis and colleagues[65] demonstrated the superiority of changes in volumetric uptake of FDG, termed *total glycolytic volume*, to maximum SUV and modified RECIST for assessment of MPM response to therapy and for prediction of time-to-progression and survival.

This preliminary evidence suggests that FDG-PET will be useful and likely more accurate than CT or MR imaging in the evaluation of response to therapy as early as after one cycle of chemotherapy. Measurements of tumor FDG volume of uptake may be more useful than maximum SUV in assessing tumor response.

Prognosis

Prognostic stratification has implications for clinical management and appropriate enrollment in clinical trials. Recent literature suggests that FDG-PET tumor maximum SUV may serve as a prognostic marker in MPM along with histologic type, nodal status, extent of local invasion, extrathoracic metastasis, and elevated vascular endothelial growth factor expression.[65,67] Flores and colleagues[68] concluded that FDG-PET tumor

uptake with a high maximum SUV was associated with a median survival of 14 months compared with 24 months in patients with low maximum SUV of the tumor, and that high-SUV tumors were associated with 3.3 times greater risk of death than low-SUV tumors. A maximum SUV of four or more and mixed histology were noted to be poor risk factors in patients with MPM.[68] Furthermore, Gerbaudo and colleagues[69] reported that the pattern, intensity, and kinetics of FDG uptake in MPM are good indicators of tumor aggressiveness and are superior to histologic grade in this regard.

ESOPHAGEAL CANCER

Esophageal cancer is an aggressive malignancy generally associated with a poor prognosis, largely due to advanced stage at diagnosis. The best chance of a good patient outcome depends on accurate staging and assessment of tumor response so that the best clinical management is employed.

Staging

The staging system for esophageal cancer follows the TNM system, providing an accurate common language for surgeons and oncologists to manage the course of this aggressive malignancy. FDG-PET, CT, MR imaging, and endoscopic ultrasound (EUS) have complementary roles in the staging of esophageal malignancy.

The T-value of staging esophageal cancer

The T-value for esophageal cancer, one of the most important prognostic factors of outcome, characterizes the extent of local tumor and, in particular, the depth of tumor invasion in the esophageal wall and invasion of adjacent structures.[70] Assessment of T-value is primarily conducted with EUS and biopsy, as EUS can directly reveal all layers of the esophageal wall.[71] CT and MR imaging are comparable in their diagnostic performance in defining the extent of tumor invasion beyond the esophagus to involve the mediastinal fat and other surrounding structures, but are not reliable for evaluation of the depth of tumor invasion when confined to the layers of the esophageal wall or for demonstration of microscopic invasion of periesophageal fat by tumor.[72,73] In one study, the overall accuracy of CT or MR imaging for the detection of periesophageal fat invasion by tumor was reported to range from 88% to 100%.[71] However, in a meta-analysis by Rosch and colleagues,[74] the accuracy of EUS for overall T-staging was 85% compared with 45% for CT.

For evaluation of potential involvement of medi-astinal structures, MR imaging is useful to differen-tiate tumor from uninvolved surrounding tissues, and is most effectively employed when there is no clear fat plane between tumor and adjacent soft tissue structures on CT or EUS (**Fig. 9**). However, the usefulness of MR imaging is limited in the evaluation of the airways and lungs because of susceptibility artifacts. If airway involvement is suspected based on imaging findings or location of the primary tumor in the upper esophagus, then bronchoscopy with biopsy is typically performed.[75] Assessment of extension of tumor into the stomach is also important for surgical planning, and is primarily achieved with EUS and sometimes with a fluoroscopic upper gastrointes-tinal examination.[75] CT and MR imaging can also be used to assess for gastric involvement by tumor, with overall accuracy ranging from 79% to 97%, but may be limited when the stomach is incompletely distended.[71,76]

The N-value of staging esophageal cancer

The N-value of staging esophageal cancer relates to the presence (N1) or absence (N0) of regional nodal involvement, and is defined relative to the site of primary malignancy. Involvement of nodes regional to the primary malignancy is considered as N1 disease whereas involvement of more remote lymph nodes is considered as M1 disease.[70]

The characterization of nodal disease is primarily performed with a combination of EUS and biopsy, which, with an accuracy of 77% to 94%, is regarded as the most reliable method to assess for regional nodal metastases, but is often complemented by FDG-PET, CT, or MR imaging.[70,77–79] FDG-PET can detect nodal metastases even when the lymph nodes are normal in size, but has been reported to have poor sensitivity for regional nodal metastases, probably because of limitations in spatial resolu-tion, making it difficult to evaluate lymph nodes adjacent to the primary tumor.[80,81] A meta-anal-ysis by van Vliet and colleagues[81] evaluated the relative sensitivity and specificity of EUS, CT, and FDG-PET for the various components of the staging system for esophageal cancer, and deter-mined that, for regional nodal staging, EUS was more sensitive (80% sensitivity for EUS compared

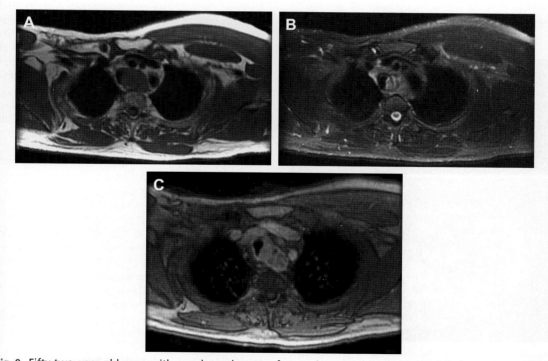

Fig. 9. Fifty-two–year-old man with esophageal cancer for staging. Axial T1-weighted (*A*), fat-suppressed T2-weighted (*B*), and contrast-enhanced T1-weighted (*C*) MR images through upper chest demonstrate large upper thoracic esophageal mass with intermediate T1-weighted and high T2-weighted signal intensity relative to skel-etal muscle with heterogeneous enhancement in keeping with esophageal carcinoma. Note mass effect upon low signal intensity gas-filled trachea to right of mass with extension of tumor through left tracheal wall into tracheal lumen, indicating tracheal invasion.

with 50% for CT and 57% for FDG-PET), while CT and FDG-PET were more specific (70% specificity for EUS compared with 83% for CT and 85% for FDG-PET). Conventional MR imaging has been reported to have similar accuracy to that of CT for the detection of malignant mediastinal lymph nodes.[82] However, Nishimura and colleagues[83] reported that MR imaging performed after the intravenous administration of ferumoxtran-10, an ultrasmall superparamagnetic iron oxide contrast agent, had a sensitivity of 100%, specificity of 95%, and accuracy of 96% for detection of nodal metastases in 16 patients with esophageal cancer.

The M-value of staging esophageal cancer

For the detection of distant metastatic disease, a combination of FDG-PET and CT or MR imaging is generally used (**Fig. 10**). In a meta-analysis by van Vliet and colleagues[81] involving staging of patients with esophageal cancer, FDG-PET had a sensitivity of 71% and a specificity of 93% for the detection of distant metastatic disease, whereas CT had a sensitivity of 52% and a specificity of 91%. In another report, FDG-PET was shown to detect metastatic disease in approximately 20% of patients considered as having only locoregional disease on CT.[84] MR imaging is useful for improved characterization of indeterminate lesions detected on CT or FDG-PET, particularly when there is involvement of the liver, bone marrow, or adrenal glands, whereas CT is superior for the detection of pulmonary metastases, particularly when those are small.

Response Assessment

Given the high morbidity and mortality in patients with esophageal cancer, there has been interest in metabolic imaging to measure response to therapy. Many studies have shown that FDG-PET is useful for the assessment of the therapeutic response of esophageal cancer, and is superior to the assessment provided by CT or EUS, particularly when neoadjuvant therapy is employed, as the latter imaging modalities are unable to distinguish inflammation and fibrosis from residual cancer.[85–88] A significant drop in FDG uptake in tumor sites has been shown to be predictive of ultimate response to therapy as measured by conventional measures, such as CT, as well as of survival rate and tumor recurrence rate.[89–92] For example, data from the Municon (Metabolic Response Evaluation for Individualisation of Neoadjuvant Chemotherapy in Oesophageal and Oesophogastric Adeneocarcinoma) trial in 119 patients with locally advanced esophageal adenocarcinoma demonstrated the feasibility and utility of FDG-PET performed 2 weeks after the start of chemotherapy for early metabolic response evaluation and individualized adjustment of the therapeutic regimen for patients. In this study, metabolic responders (defined as those who had a decrease in tumor SUV by 35% or more after therapy) had a median event-free survival of about 30 months compared with about 14 months in nonresponders.[93] In a study by Swisher and colleagues[92] of 103 patients with locoregionally advanced esophageal cancer, a tumor SUV of four or more on FDG-PET performed after chemoradiation therapy had the highest accuracy (76%) of pathologic response compared with CT and EUS, and was an independent predictor of long-term survival. However, FDG-PET after chemoradiation therapy cannot exclude the presence of microscopic residual disease, even if no FDG uptake is seen in the tumor, and so esophagectomy should still be considered even in the presence of a normal posttherapy FDG-PET scan.

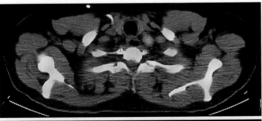
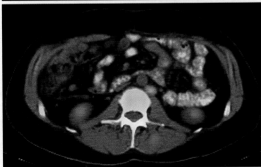

Fig. 10. Fifty-four–year-old man status post–esophagectomy and gastric pull-through for esophageal cancer undergoing restaging evaluation. Axial FDG-PET/CT images through upper chest (*top*) and midabdomen (*bottom*) demonstrate avid FDG uptake in enlarged left supraclavicular and left para-aortic lymph nodes, in keeping with metastatic disease.

POSITRON EMISSION TOMOGRAPHY/MR IMAGING

The fusion of PET and MR imaging into a hybrid PET/MRI scanner is attractive for many of the same reasons that PET/CT is preferred over either

PET or CT alone. This approach to evaluate patients with thoracic malignancies will likely result in a synergism of the strengths of a highly sensitive functional imaging modality with those of a structural imaging modality with excellent soft tissue contrast and high spatial resolution. Specificity and accuracy of diagnosis will also likely improve compared with those of either imaging modality alone. With MR imaging, additional benefits compared with CT include the lack of additional radiation exposure and superior soft tissue contrast, even when intravenous contrast material is not administered. However, the major limitation of PET/MR imaging for the evaluation of patients with thoracic malignancy would most likely be related to the limitations of MR imaging to assess the lung parenchyma, likely necessitating the continued need for CT to evaluate the lungs in the majority of patients. Furthermore, PET/MR imaging equipment will be expensive, technologists will require extra training in both PET and MR imaging for safe and proper operation, and certain patients with implantable metallic or electronic devices, such as automatic defibrillators or pacemakers, may not undergo MR imaging.

SUMMARY

Imaging of patients with thoracic malignancy usually requires a multimodality approach. Each of these modalities has its own strengths and weaknesses. CT remains central to the staging and restaging of thoracic malignancies, but has recently been complemented with FDG-PET imaging to maximize its potential. Furthermore, FDG-PET/CT has taken hold in the clinical realm for evaluation of patients with thoracic malignancy, as it is useful at all stages of the workup and treatment of these patients, and is rapidly replacing PET-only imaging. MR imaging is also occasionally used in some patients with thoracic malignancies to improve disease staging or lesion characterization. Lastly, PET/MR imaging may one day be used to evaluate patients with thoracic malignancies as well.

REFERENCES

1. Torigian DA, Huang SS, Houseni M, et al. Functional imaging of cancer with emphasis on molecular techniques. CA Cancer J Clin 2007;57(4):206–24.
2. Gregoire V, De Neve W, Eisbruch A, et al. Intensity-modulated radiation therapy for head and neck carcinoma. Oncologist 2007;12(5):555–64.
3. Greco C, Rosenzweig K, Cascini GL, et al. Current status of PET/CT for tumour volume definition in radiotherapy treatment planning for non-small cell lung cancer (NSCLC). Lung Cancer 2007;57(2):125–34.
4. Wynants J, Stroobants S, Dooms C, et al. Staging of lung cancer. Radiol Clin North Am 2007;45(4):609–25, v.
5. Watanabe K, Nomori H, Ohtsuka T, et al. [False negative cases of F-18 fluorodeoxyglucose-positron emission tomography (FDG-PET) imaging in small lung cancer less than 3 cm in size]. Nihon Kokyuki Gakkai Zasshi 2004;42(9):787–93 [in Japanese].
6. Webb WR, Gatsonis C, Zerhouni EA, et al. CT and MR imaging in staging non-small cell bronchogenic carcinoma: report of the Radiologic Diagnostic Oncology Group. Radiology 1991;178(3):705–13.
7. Padovani B, Mouroux J, Seksik L, et al. Chest wall invasion by bronchogenic carcinoma: evaluation with MR imaging. Radiology 1993;187(1):33–8.
8. Nomori H, Watanabe K, Ohtsuka T, et al. The size of metastatic foci and lymph nodes yielding false-negative and false-positive lymph node staging with positron emission tomography in patients with lung cancer. J Thorac Cardiovasc Surg 2004;127(4):1087–92.
9. Gupta NC, Graeber GM, Bishop HA. Comparative efficacy of positron emission tomography with fluorodeoxyglucose in evaluation of small (3 cm) lymph node lesions. Chest 2000;117(3):773–8.
10. Pieterman RM, van Putten JW, Meuzelaar JJ, et al. Preoperative staging of non-small-cell lung cancer with positron-emission tomography. N Engl J Med 2000;343(4):254–61.
11. Verhagen AF, Bootsma GP, Tjan-Heijnen VC, et al. FDG-PET in staging lung cancer: How does it change the algorithm? Lung Cancer 2004;44(2):175–81.
12. Gonzalez-Stawinski GV, Lemaire A, Merchant F, et al. A comparative analysis of positron emission tomography and mediastinoscopy in staging non-small cell lung cancer. J Thorac Cardiovasc Surg 2003;126(6):1900–5.
13. Lardinois D, Weder W, Hany TF, et al. Staging of non-small-cell lung cancer with integrated positron-emission tomography and computed tomography. N Engl J Med 2003;348(25):2500–7.
14. Plathow C, Aschoff P, Lichy MP, et al. Positron emission tomography/computed tomography and whole-body magnetic resonance imaging in staging of advanced nonsmall cell lung cancer—initial results. Invest Radiol 2008;43(5):290–7.
15. Aquino SL, Asmuth JC, Alpert NM, et al. Improved radiologic staging of lung cancer with 2-[18F]-fluoro-2-deoxy-D-glucose-positron emission tomography and computed tomography registration. J Comput Assist Tomogr 2003;27(4):479–84.
16. Basu S, Zaidi H, Houseni M, et al. Novel quantitative techniques for assessing regional and global function and structure based on modern imaging modalities:

implications for normal variation, aging and diseased states. Semin Nucl Med 2007;37(3):223–39.

17. Basu S, Kung J, Houseni M, et al. Temporal profile of fluorodeoxyglucose uptake in malignant lesions and normal organs over extended time periods in patients with lung carcinoma: implications for its utilization in assessing malignant lesions. Q J Nucl Med Mol Imaging 2009;53(1):9–19.

18. Matthies A, Hickeson M, Cuchiara A, et al. Dual time point 18F-FDG PET for the evaluation of pulmonary nodules. J Nucl Med 2002;43(7):871–5.

19. Ito K, Mitchell DG, Outwater EK, et al. Hepatic lesions: discrimination of nonsolid, benign lesions from solid, malignant lesions with heavily T2-weighted fast spin-echo MR imaging. Radiology 1997;204(3):729–37.

20. Ohno Y, Koyama H, Onishi Y, et al. Non-small cell lung cancer: whole-body MR examination for M-stage assessment—utility for whole-body diffusion-weighted imaging compared with integrated FDG PET/CT. Radiology 2008;248(2):643–54.

21. Savci G, Yazici Z, Sahin N, et al. Value of chemical shift subtraction MRI in characterization of adrenal masses. AJR Am J Roentgenol 2006; 186(1):130–5.

22. Heinz-Peer G, Honigschnabl S, Schneider B, et al. Characterization of adrenal masses using MR imaging with histopathologic correlation. AJR Am J Roentgenol 1999;173(1):15–22.

23. Remer EM, Obuchowski N, Ellis JD, et al. Adrenal mass evaluation in patients with lung carcinoma: a cost-effectiveness analysis. AJR Am J Roentgenol 2000;174(4):1033–9.

24. Erasmus JJ, Patz EF Jr, McAdams HP, et al. Evaluation of adrenal masses in patients with bronchogenic carcinoma using 18F-fluorodeoxyglucose positron emission tomography. AJR Am J Roentgenol 1997; 168(5):1357–60.

25. Yun M, Kim W, Alnafisi N, et al. 18F-FDG PET in characterizing adrenal lesions detected on CT or MRI. J Nucl Med 2001;42(12):1795–9.

26. Nakanishi K, Kobayashi M, Nakaguchi K, et al. Whole-body MRI for detecting metastatic bone tumor: diagnostic value of diffusion-weighted images. Magn Reson Med Sci 2007;6(3):147–55.

27. Ahmadzadehfar H, Palmedo H, Strunk H, et al. False positive 18F-FDG-PET/CT in a patient after talc pleurodesis. Lung Cancer 2007;58(3):418–21.

28. Kwek BH, Aquino SL, Fischman AJ. Fluorodeoxyglucose positron emission tomography and CT after talc pleurodesis. Chest 2004;125(6):2356–60.

29. Alavi A, Gupta N, Alberini JL, et al. Positron emission tomography imaging in nonmalignant thoracic disorders. Semin Nucl Med 2002;32(4):293–321.

30. Weber WA, Wieder H. Monitoring chemotherapy and radiotherapy of solid tumors. Eur J Nucl Med Mol Imaging 2006;33(Suppl 1):27–37.

31. Su H, Bodenstein C, Dumont RA, et al. Monitoring tumor glucose utilization by positron emission tomography for the prediction of treatment response to epidermal growth factor receptor kinase inhibitors. Clin Cancer Res 2006;12(19):5659–67.

32. Nahmias C, Hanna WT, Wahl LM, et al. Time course of early response to chemotherapy in non-small cell lung cancer patients with 18F-FDG PET/CT. J Nucl Med 2007;48(5):744–51.

33. Hellwig D, Graeter TP, Ukena D, et al. Value of F-18-fluorodeoxyglucose positron emission tomography after induction therapy of locally advanced bronchogenic carcinoma. J Thorac Cardiovasc Surg 2004; 128(6):892–9.

34. Pairolero PC, Williams DE, Bergstralh EJ, et al. Postsurgical stage I bronchogenic carcinoma: morbid implications of recurrent disease. Ann Thorac Surg 1984;38(4):331–8.

35. Ohtsuka T, Nomori H, Watanabe K, et al. Prognostic significance of [(18)F]fluorodeoxyglucose uptake on positron emission tomography in patients with pathologic stage I lung adenocarcinoma. Cancer 2006; 107(10):2468–73.

36. Watanabe K, Nomori H, Ohtsuka T, et al. [F-18]Fluorodeoxyglucose positron emission tomography can predict pathological tumor stage and proliferative activity determined by Ki-67 in clinical stage IA lung adenocarcinomas. Jpn J Clin Oncol 2006; 36(7):403–9.

37. Nguyen XC, Lee WW, Chung JH, et al. FDG uptake, glucose transporter type 1, and Ki-67 expressions in non-small-cell lung cancer: correlations and prognostic values. Eur J Radiol 2007;62(2):214–9.

38. Hicks RJ, Kalff V, MacManus MP, et al. (18)F-FDG PET provides high-impact and powerful prognostic stratification in staging newly diagnosed non-small cell lung cancer. J Nucl Med 2001;42(11): 1596–604.

39. Kramer H, Post WJ, Pruim J, et al. The prognostic value of positron emission tomography in non-small cell lung cancer: analysis of 266 cases. Lung Cancer 2006;52(2):213–7.

40. Simon GR, Wagner H. Small cell lung cancer. Chest 2003;123(Suppl 1):259S–71S.

41. Zhao DS, Valdivia AY, Li Y, et al. 18F-fluorodeoxyglucose positron emission tomography in small-cell lung cancer. Semin Nucl Med 2002;32(4):272–5.

42. Brink I, Schumacher T, Mix M, et al. Impact of [18F]FDG-PET on the primary staging of small-cell lung cancer. Eur J Nucl Med Mol Imaging 2004; 31(12):1614–20.

43. Bradley JD, Dehdashti F, Mintun MA, et al. Positron emission tomography in limited-stage small-cell lung cancer: a prospective study. J Clin Oncol 2004;22(16):3248–54.

44. Onitilo AA, Engel JM, Demos JM, et al. Prognostic significance of 18 F-fluorodeoxyglucose–positron

emission tomography after treatment in patients with limited stage small cell lung cancer. Clin Med Res 2008;6(2):72–7.

45. Jacob T, Grahek D, Younsi N, et al. Positron emission tomography with [(18)F]FDOPA and [(18)F]FDG in the imaging of small cell lung carcinoma: preliminary results. Eur J Nucl Med Mol Imaging 2003;30(9):1266–9.

46. Pandit N, Gonen M, Krug L, et al. Prognostic value of [18F]FDG-PET imaging in small cell lung cancer. Eur J Nucl Med Mol Imaging 2003;30(1):78–84.

47. Chong S, Lee KS, Kim BT, et al. Integrated PET/CT of pulmonary neuroendocrine tumors: diagnostic and prognostic implications. AJR Am J Roentgenol 2007;188(5):1223–31.

48. Duysinx BC, Larock MP, Nguyen D, et al. 18F-FDG PET imaging in assessing exudative pleural effusions. Nucl Med Commun 2006;27(12):971–6.

49. Weiss N, Solomon SB. Talc pleurodesis mimics pleural metastases: differentiation with positron emission tomography/computed tomography. Clin Nucl Med 2003;28(10):811–4.

50. Heelan RT, Rusch VW, Begg CB, et al. Staging of malignant pleural mesothelioma: comparison of CT and MR imaging. AJR Am J Roentgenol 1999; 172(4):1039–47.

51. Lorigan JG, Libshitz HI. MR imaging of malignant pleural mesothelioma. J Comput Assist Tomogr 1989;13(4):617–20.

52. Yamamuro M, Gerbaudo VH, Gill RR, et al. Morphologic and functional imaging of malignant pleural mesothelioma. Eur J Radiol 2007.

53. Rusch VW. A proposed new international TNM staging system for malignant pleural mesothelioma from the International Mesothelioma Interest Group. Lung Cancer 1996;14(1):1–12.

54. Patz EF Jr, Rusch VW, Heelan R. The proposed new international TNM staging system for malignant pleural mesothelioma: application to imaging. AJR Am J Roentgenol 1996;166(2):323–7.

55. Stewart D, Waller D, Edwards J, et al. Is there a role for pre-operative contrast-enhanced magnetic resonance imaging for radical surgery in malignant pleural mesothelioma? Eur J Cardiothorac Surg 2003;24(6):1019–24.

56. Hierholzer J, Luo L, Bittner RC, et al. MRI and CT in the differential diagnosis of pleural disease. Chest 2000;118(3):604–9.

57. Benard F, Sterman D, Smith RJ, et al. Metabolic imaging of malignant pleural mesothelioma with fluorodeoxyglucose positron emission tomography. Chest 1998;114(3):713–22.

58. Gerbaudo VH, Sugarbaker DJ, Britz-Cunningham S, et al. Assessment of malignant pleural mesothelioma with (18)F-FDG dual-head gamma-camera coincidence imaging: comparison with histopathology. J Nucl Med 2002;43(9):1144–9.

59. Erasmus JJ, Truong MT, Smythe WR, et al. Integrated computed tomography–positron emission tomography in patients with potentially resectable malignant pleural mesothelioma: staging implications. J Thorac Cardiovasc Surg 2005;129(6): 1364–70.

60. Gerbaudo VH, Mamede M, Trotman-Dickenson B, et al. PET/CT patterns of treatment failure of malignant pleural mesothelioma. J Nucl Med 2007;48: 360.

61. von Schulthess GK, Steinert HC, Hany TF. Integrated PET/CT: current applications and future directions. Radiology 2006;238(2):405–22.

62. Byrne MJ, Nowak AK. Modified RECIST criteria for assessment of response in malignant pleural mesothelioma. Ann Oncol 2004;15(2):257–60.

63. Plathow C, Klopp M, Thieke C, et al. Therapy response in malignant pleural mesothelioma—role of MRI using RECIST, modified RECIST and volumetric approaches in comparison with CT. Eur Radiol 2008;18(8):1635–43.

64. Steinert HC, Santos Dellea MM, Burger C, et al. Therapy response evaluation in malignant pleural mesothelioma with integrated PET-CT imaging. Lung Cancer 2005;49(Suppl 1):S33–5.

65. Francis RJ, Byrne MJ, van der Schaaf AA, et al. Early prediction of response to chemotherapy and survival in malignant pleural mesothelioma using a novel semiautomated 3-dimensional volume-based analysis of serial 18F-FDG PET scans. J Nucl Med 2007;48(9):1449–58.

66. Ceresoli GL, Chiti A, Zucali PA, et al. Early response evaluation in malignant pleural mesothelioma by positron emission tomography with [18F]fluorodeoxyglucose. J Clin Oncol 2006; 24(28):4587–93.

67. Benard F, Sterman D, Smith RJ, et al. Prognostic value of FDG PET imaging in malignant pleural mesothelioma. J Nucl Med 1999;40(8):1241–5.

68. Flores RM. The role of PET in the surgical management of malignant pleural mesothelioma. Lung Cancer 2005;49(Suppl 1):S27–32.

69. Gerbaudo VH, Britz-Cunningham S, Sugarbaker DJ, et al. Metabolic significance of the pattern, intensity and kinetics of 18F-FDG uptake in malignant pleural mesothelioma. Thorax 2003;58(12):1077–82.

70. Diederich S. Staging of oesophageal cancer. Cancer Imaging 2007;7(Spec No A):S63–6.

71. Holscher AH, Dittler HJ, Siewert JR. Staging of squamous esophageal cancer: accuracy and value. World J Surg 1994;18(3):312–20.

72. Petrillo R, Balzarini L, Bidoli P, et al. Esophageal squamous cell carcinoma: MRI evaluation of mediastinum. Gastrointest Radiol 1990;15(4):275–8.

73. Iyer RB, Silverman PM, Tamm EP, et al. Diagnosis, staging, and follow-up of esophageal cancer. AJR Am J Roentgenol 2003;181(3):785–93.

74. Rosch T. Endosonographic staging of esophageal cancer: a review of literature results. Gastrointest Endosc Clin N Am 1995;5(3):537–47.

75. Quint LE, Bogot NR. Staging esophageal cancer. Cancer Imaging 2008;8(Suppl A):S33–42.

76. Takashima S, Takeuchi N, Shiozaki H, et al. Carcinoma of the esophagus: CT vs MR imaging in determining resectability. AJR Am J Roentgenol 1991; 156(2):297–302.

77. Marsman WA, Fockens P. State of the art lecture: EUS for esophageal tumors. Endoscopy 2006; 38(Suppl 1):S17–21.

78. Vazquez-Sequeiros E. Nodal staging: number or site of nodes? How to improve accuracy? Is FNA always necessary? Junctional tumors—What's N and what's M? Endoscopy 2006;38(Suppl 1):S4–8.

79. Bataille L, Lonneux M, Weynand B, et al. EUS-FNA and FDG-PET are complementary procedures in the diagnosis of enlarged mediastinal lymph nodes. Acta Gastroenterol Belg 2008;71(2):219–29.

80. Fletcher JW, Djulbegovic B, Soares HP, et al. Recommendations on the use of 18F-FDG PET in oncology. J Nucl Med 2008;49(3):480–508.

81. van Vliet EP, Heijenbrok-Kal MH, Hunink MG, et al. Staging investigations for oesophageal cancer: a meta-analysis. Br J Cancer 2008;98(3):547–57.

82. Lehr L, Rupp N, Siewert JR. Assessment of resectability of esophageal cancer by computed tomography and magnetic resonance imaging. Surgery 1988;103(3):344–50.

83. Nishimura H, Tanigawa N, Hiramatsu M, et al. Preoperative esophageal cancer staging: magnetic resonance imaging of lymph node with ferumoxtran-10, an ultrasmall superparamagnetic iron oxide. J Am Coll Surg 2006;202(4):604–11.

84. Ott K, Weber W, Siewert JR. The importance of PET in the diagnosis and response evaluation of esophageal cancer. Dis Esophagus 2006;19(6):433–42.

85. Jones DR, Parker LA Jr, Detterbeck FC, et al. Inadequacy of computed tomography in assessing patients with esophageal carcinoma after induction chemoradiotherapy. Cancer 1999;85(5):1026–32.

86. Westerterp M, van Westreenen HL, Reitsma JB, et al. Esophageal cancer: CT, endoscopic US, and FDG PET for assessment of response to neoadjuvant therapy—systematic review. Radiology 2005; 236(3):841–51.

87. Cerfolio RJ, Bryant AS, Ohja B, et al. The accuracy of endoscopic ultrasonography with fine-needle aspiration, integrated positron emission tomography with computed tomography, and computed tomography in restaging patients with esophageal cancer after neoadjuvant chemoradiotherapy. J Thorac Cardiovasc Surg 2005;129(6):1232–41.

88. Jamil LH, Gill KR, Wallace MB. Staging and restaging of advanced esophageal cancer. Curr Opin Gastroenterol 2008;24(4):530–4.

89. Wieder HA, Ott K, Lordick F, et al. Prediction of tumor response by FDG-PET: comparison of the accuracy of single and sequential studies in patients with adenocarcinomas of the esophagogastric junction. Eur J Nucl Med Mol Imaging 2007;34(12):1925–32.

90. Mamede M, Abreu ELP, Oliva MR, et al. FDG-PET/CT tumor segmentation-derived indices of metabolic activity to assess response to neoadjuvant therapy and progression-free survival in esophageal cancer: correlation with histopathology results. Am J Clin Oncol 2007;30(4):377–88.

91. Ott K, Weber WA, Lordick F, et al. Metabolic imaging predicts response, survival, and recurrence in adenocarcinomas of the esophagogastric junction. J Clin Oncol 2006;24(29):4692–8.

92. Swisher SG, Maish M, Erasmus JJ, et al. Utility of PET, CT, and EUS to identify pathologic responders in esophageal cancer. Ann Thorac Surg 2004;78(4):1152–60 [discussion: 60].

93. Lordick F, Ott K, Krause BJ, et al. PET to assess early metabolic response and to guide treatment of adenocarcinoma of the oesophagogastric junction: the MUNICON phase II trial. Lancet Oncol 2007; 8(9):797–805.

Cardiovascular Imaging with PET, CT, and MR Imaging

Amol Takalkar, MD[a,b,*], Wengen Chen, MD, PhD[c],
Benoit Desjardins, MD, PhD[c], Abass Alavi, MD, PhD (Hon), DSc (Hon)[c],
Drew A. Torigian, MD, MA[c]

KEYWORDS
- Cardiac PET • Cardiac CT • Cardiac MR
- Myocardial viability • FDG

Positron emission tomography (PET) is a functional nuclear medicine imaging technique that provides high-resolution tomographic images of the administered radiopharmaceutical biodistribution in vivo. The radiopharmaceuticals used in PET imaging are typically compounds of interest (such as glucose) tagged with a positron emitter (such as fluorine-18 [F18]). F18-labeled fluorodeoxyglucose (FDG) is by far the most commonly used radiopharmaceutical and is used mostly for oncologic imaging. There are a few other PET radiopharmaceuticals that are Food and Drug Administration (FDA) approved for additional indications (such as rubidium [Rb]-82 and N-13 ammonia [NH_3] for myocardial perfusion imaging [MPI]) and many radiopharmaceuticals are under preclinical and development stages of development. The concept and technique of FDG-PET imaging primarily was developed in the 1970s and initially used mainly for functional brain imaging. Subsequently, in the early 1980s, FDG-PET imaging was used to assess cardiac metabolism. Throughout the 1980s and most of the 1990s, however, PET was restricted mostly to research and large academic centers and failed to become a routine clinical tool. Hence, its cardiac and brain applications did not get widespread attention. Since the late 1990s there has been an explosion of PET use

due to its impact on oncologic management. This has contributed to increased availability of PET imaging throughout the United States and made it cost effective. Today, FDG-PET is an established entity in the work-up of several oncologic disorders and is making forays in the diagnosis of inflammatory diseases. This has led to increased use of PET for cardiac and neurologic applications.

Traditionally, nuclear cardiology techniques have evolved from planar cardiac scintigraphy to single photon emission CT (SPECT)–MPI to gated SPECT imaging with attenuation correction. PET has further improved the usefulness of nuclear cardiology in evaluating cardiovascular diseases. PET offers several advantages over traditional SPECT imaging, including better spatial and temporal resolution and absolute quantification of regional radiotracer uptake. In addition to its use in assessing myocardial perfusion, PET has been successful in evaluating myocardial viability. Combination of MPI (using PET or SPECT techniques) and metabolism imaging using FDG-PET is considered the gold standard for noninvasive assessment of myocardial viability.[1]

Recent advancements in imaging instrumentation (including CT and MR imaging technology) facilitate noninvasive assessment of an array of

[a] PET Imaging Center, Biomedical Research Foundation of Northwest Louisiana, 1505 Kings Highway, Shreveport, LA 71103, USA
[b] Department of Radiology, LSUHSC-S, 1501 Kings Highway, Shreveport, LA 71103, USA
[c] Department of Radiology, University of Pennsylvania School of Medicine, Philadelphia, PA, USA
* Corresponding author. PET Imaging Center, Research Foundation of Northwest Louisiana, 1505 Kings Highway, Shreveport, LA 71103, USA.
E-mail address: amoltakalkar@yahoo.com (A. Takalkar).

PET Clin 3 (2009) 411–434
doi:10.1016/j.cpet.2009.03.004

cardiovascular pathologies. Coronary CT angiography (CCTA) has become another major disruptive imaging modality and may revolutionize cardiac imaging. Previously, the role of CT in coronary evaluation was restricted to electron beam CT for calcium scoring. However, with the advances in CT instrumentation and availability of the 64-slice CT (or even higher slice CT), however, CCTA is set to become the default imaging technique for nontherapeutic coronary angiography for structural assessment of the coronary arterial system. CCTA in combination with MPI studies, such as PET with Rb-82 or N-13 NH$_3$ can provide a thorough cardiac evaluation of the coronary arterial tree, myocardial perfusion derived from the coronary vasculature, and left ventricular function in a single imaging session.

Cardiac MR imaging can be used to assess a wide array of heart conditions, such as congenital heart disease, ventricular dysplasias, cardiac masses, coronary arterial abnormalities, ventricular dysfunction, valvular disorders, and others. Although there are other competing and sometimes better imaging modalities, such as SPECT, PET, CT, or echocardiography (ECHO), for individual clinical indications of cardiac MR imaging, MR imaging is best placed to become the single imaging modality that can provide the most comprehensive cardiac evaluation. Moreover, it lacks ionizing radiation, has superior temporal and contrast resolution, and has excellent spatial resolution, which has improved with recent advances in instrumentation. Thus cardiac MR imaging also has the potential to provide a complete cardiac evaluation in a single imaging session. The potential for hybrid PET/MR imaging in a single setting further increases the possibilities for cardiovascular imaging. This article addresses evaluation of the cardiovascular system by PET, CT, and MR imaging.

POSITRON EMISSION TOMOGRAPHY MYOCARDIAL PERFUSION IMAGING

Traditionally, SPECT with technetium (Tc)-or thallium (Tl)-based agents are used to assess myocardial perfusion. However, myocardial perfusion can be more accurately assessed with PET MPI using Rb-82 or N-13 NH$_3$. PET offers several advantages over SPECT: better spatial and temporal resolution, superior attenuation correction, feasibility of absolute quantification of regional radiotracer uptake, and less radiation exposure with more efficient protocols (due to faster protocols and shorter-lived radionuclides). Thus, PET myocardial perfusion is better suited to patients prone to attenuation artifacts (for

instance, women who have large breasts or men who have a thick chest wall), allowing detection of less apparent perfusion abnormalities, facilitating detection of endothelial dysfunction, and providing more precise measurement of heart volumes and function.

Several PET radiopharmaceuticals can be used to assess myocardial perfusion. These include the cyclotron-produced N-13 NH$_3$ and O-15 water and the generator-produced Rb-82 chloride (Cl) and copper-64–pyruvaldehyde–bis(N^4-methyl-thiosemicarbazone) (64Cu-PTSM). N-13 NH$_3$ and Rb-82 Cl are FDA approved for assessing myocardial perfusion with PET whereas O-15 water and 64Cu-PTSM are used mostly in the research realm.

N-13 is a cyclotron-produced radioisotope with a physical half-life of approximately 9.9 minutes, positron energy of 1.19 MeV, and an average positron range of approximately 0.4 mm. It shows a high extraction rate and remains metabolically trapped because of the glutamine synthetase pathway, resulting in prolonged myocardial retention. By virtue of its favorable physical characteristics and biologic properties, it generates excellent PET images. **Fig. 1** shows a typical rest-stress myocardial perfusion study protocol using N-13 NH$_3$. It starts with a transmission scan followed by intravenous administration of approximately 10 to 15 mCi (370–555 MBq) of N-13 NH$_3$. Dedicated PET images of the chest that include the entire heart are then obtained approximately 5 minutes later. The tracer is allowed to completely decay over 50 to 60 minutes and the patient then is stressed pharmacologically (preferred) or with exercise (slightly cumbersome technically but

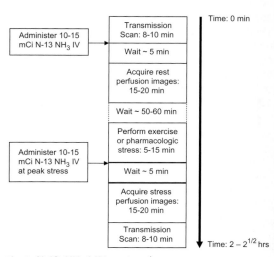

Fig. 1. N-13–NH$_3$ MPI protocol.

feasible). Another 10 to 15 mCi (370–555 MBq) of N-13 NH_3 are administered intravenously at peak stress and another set of dedicated PET images of the chest that include the entire heart is obtained. A second transmission scan is obtained after this stress imaging to use for attenuation correction for this data set. Images can be processed and displayed in the conventional three-axes format (short axis, vertical long axis, and horizontal long axis) (**Fig. 2**). The 9.9-minute half-life facilitates gated acquisition. In addition, the stress images obtained after the rest images are more pure stress images with almost no contamination of residual radiotracer from the prior rest injection. The protocol also is shorter than the traditional SPECT study. The procedure to acquire quantitative myocardial perfusion data using dynamic imaging with N-13–NH_3 PET has been well validated.[2–9] An advantage of N-13–NH_3 PET MPI over Rb-82–Cl PET MPI is the ability to obtain exercise-induced stress images as opposed to pharmaceutical stress images alone with Rb-82–Cl PET myocardial perfusion.

Rb-82 is a generator-produced radioisotope with a physical half-life of approximately 75 seconds, positron energy of 3.15 MeV, and an average positron range of approximately 2.8 mm. These physical characteristics (high positron energy and average positron range) are not optimal for imaging and result in slightly impaired spatial resolution. The extremely short half-life enables the study to be completed quickly (within 1 hour) but also necessitates administration of higher doses of the radiopharmaceutical. However, the major advantage of Rb-82 over N-13 NH_3 is that it does not require an in-house cyclotron to produce the radioisotope. The parent isotope for Rb-82 generator is Sr-82, and one generator can be used for up to a month (the physical half-life of Sr-82 is 25 days). Rb-82 Cl is transported into the cells by active Na/K-ATPase pumps similar to potassium and T1-201. **Fig. 3** shows a typical rest-stress myocardial perfusion study protocol using Rb-82 Cl. It also starts with a transmission scan followed by intravenous administration of approximately 60 mCi (2220 MBq) of Rb-82 Cl. Dedicated PET images of the chest that include the entire heart then are obtained approximately 1 to 3 minutes later. By virtue of its extremely short half-life, a patient can be immediately stressed pharmacologically (exercise stress not feasible). Another 60 mCi (2220 MBq) of Rb-82 Cl are administered intravenously at peak stress and another set of dedicated PET images of the chest that also includes the entire heart is obtained 1 to 3 minutes later. A second transmission scan is obtained after this stress imaging to use for attenuation correction for this data set. Images can be processed and displayed in the conventional three-axes format (short axis, vertical

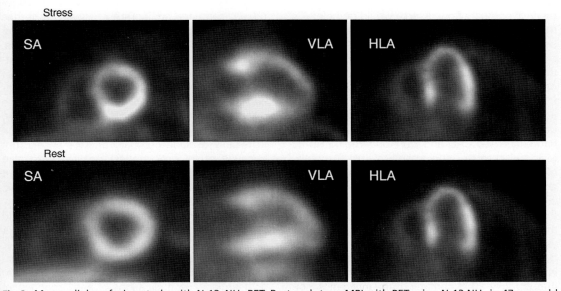

Fig. 2. Myocardial perfusion study with N-13–NH_3 PET. Rest and stress MPI with PET using N-13 NH_3 in 47-year-old man who had history of essential hypertension complaining of exertional chest pain. Selected images of stress and rest myocardial perfusion in short axis (SA), vertical long axis (VLA), and horizontal long axis (HLA) demonstrate large area of moderate reduction in tracer uptake in mid and distal anterior wall and apex at peak exercise stress with normal myocardial perfusion at rest. (*Reproduced from* Takalkar A, Mavi A, Alavi A, et al. PET in cardiology. Radiol Clin North Am 2005;43(1):107–19; with permission.)

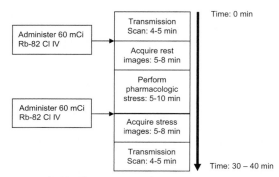

Fig. 3. Rb-82–Cl MPI protocol.

long axis, and horizontal long axis). The rapid study enables imaging during pharmacologic stressing permitting acquisition of pure stress images (not poststress images) that also are not contaminated by residual radiotracer from the rest injection and have minimal background activity.

The current indications for PET MPI include: (i) patients needing MPI who have a body habitus that is prone to cause a suboptimal SPECT scan (female patients, obese patients, or muscular patients), (ii) patients needing MPI who have had a prior suboptimal/equivocal SPECT scan, (iii) patients needing MPI in whom prior SPECT scan results did not correlate with other findings (such as results of a subsequent angiogram) or with clinical impression, (iv) patients in whom measurement of coronary flow reserve would be helpful in management decisions, and (v) patients requiring serial studies for assessment of disease progression/regression. Several studies have validated the high accuracy of PET MPI. Sampson and colleagues[10] in 2006 showed a sensitivity of 93%, specificity of 91%, and an overall diagnostic accuracy of 87% for diagnosis of coronary artery disease (CAD) in 64 consecutive patients who had suspected CAD and were undergoing Rb-82 MPI and coronary angiography within 6 months of each other. Moreover, the results remained accurate in different subgroups based on gender or obesity, confirming the overall robustness of this modality. PET has been confirmed to be better than SPECT in several studies.[11–13] A meta-analysis of the diagnostic performance of PET in detection of CAD by Nandalur and colleagues[14] in 2008 that reviewed studies from January 1977 through July 2008 confirmed an excellent sensitivity (92%) and specificity (85%) for detecting luminal stenoses greater than or equal to 50% with exceptional positive and negative likelihood ratios. They concluded that PET MPI seems superior to perfusion imaging with Tl-201 and sestamibi

or anatomic imaging with CCTA or magnetic resonance angiography (MRA).

The cost-effectiveness of PET MPI is important to consider, given the current total health care expenditure. Although SPECT MPI has been in practice for decades and has been proven to be cost effective, there has been significant data accumulation for PET perfusion imaging over the past 10 to 15 years. As early as 1995, Patterson and colleagues[15] reported PET to be cost effective in the work-up of CAD relative to exercise testing, SPECT, and immediate angiography. The cost of PET imaging has decreased substantially since 1995 as PET/CT scanners have become more prevalent in the United States, potentially making it even more cost-effective now.

CORONARY CT ANGIOGRAPHY AND CALCIUM SCORING

Almost synchronous with advancement in PET imaging, cardiac evaluation with multidetector row CT (MDCT) also has evolved significantly. Today, CCTA with a 64-slice CT system has become a major disruptive technology. It is believed to be well suited to assess CAD because it provides detailed anatomic information of the coronary arterial tree and any existing atherosclerotic plaque by virtue of its exquisite spatial resolution in the submillimeter range (0.4–0.6 mm).[16–18] It is significantly faster to perform and less invasive than the traditional catheter and fluoroscopy-based coronary angiography. However, it has certain limitations, especially in patients who have an irregular or rapid heart rate, small vessels, coronary artery calcification, and stents or extensive calcification.[19] CCTA may miss detection of arterial occlusions in patients who have total coronary occlusions but good collateral flow, as the distal vessel may fill from the collateral flow. CCTA has an excellent negative predictive value to reliably exclude coronary artery stenosis, but because of its only modest positive predictive value to detect hemodynamically significant stenosis, its application for routine diagnostic testing needs more validation.[18,20]

In addition to the use of MDCT for imaging of the coronary arteries (calcium scoring and CCTA) it also can be used to evaluate coronary plaque, cardiac function, myocardial perfusion, myocardial infarcts, cardiac tumors, pericardial disease, postsurgical complications, and congenital malformations.[21]

The presence of calcium in the coronary arteries indicates that there may be coronary atherosclerosis, whereas its absence suggests that there probably is no atherosclerosis. However, some coronary artery lesions do not contain any calcifications. Therefore, coronary calcium is of limited use for the detection of coronary artery stenosis. The load of calcium in the coronary arteries increases with age by approximately 15% to 25% per year without treatment and slows down or stops under statin therapy.[22] A large amount of calcium in coronary arteries is a sensitive but not a specific marker for CAD[23] and the value of coronary calcium as an independent or superior risk factor to predict cardiac events has not been fully established yet.[24] The distribution of calcium in the coronary arteries can be assessed by CT imaging (**Fig. 4**A), and its total amount can be quantified by a numeric score. The American College of Cardiology and American Heart Association guidelines[23] describe two indications for calcium scoring: to detect coronary calcium in patients who have atypical chest pain, and to quantify and follow-up calcified coronary plaque in asymptomatic patients who have other positive cardiovascular risk factors. Although electron beam CT initially was the modality used to evaluate calcified coronary plaque, it has now been almost completely replaced by MDCT.

A typical MDCT protocol used for calcium scoring utilizes prospective gating at 70% of the R-R interval, 0.4-second gantry rotation, 40-mm table motion between each acquisition, 2.5-mm slice reconstruction, 0.5-mm in plane resolution, scan from carina to cardiac apex, kilovolt (peak) 120, mAs 300 to 320, 15-second single breath-hold acquisition with 3-second exposure time, and a total radiation dose of 1 to 2 mSv without administration of intravenous contrast. Determination of the total coronary calcium load is performed semiautomatically. A threshold of 130 Hounsfield units (HU) is used to identify and quantify all clusters of calcifications in the coronary arteries by a region growth algorithm. Clusters less than two pixels in size are considered to be noise and are not included in the final assessment. The Agatston calcium score is the most widely used.[25] The total Agatston score is the sum of all scores of clusters of coronary calcium on all images of the scan. The score of each single lesion on each image is the product of its area multiplied by a cofactor reflecting calcium density in each lesion. The cofactor indicates maximal attenuation in the lesion (1: 130–199 HU, 2: 200–299 HU, 3: 300–399 HU, 4: $\geq$400 HU). The Agatston score is highly dependent on the imaging parameters, and shows variable reproducibility, especially for small amounts of calcium, with variations in the scores by 20% or more from scan to scan.[26] Volumetric quantification algorithms also are available for calcium scoring. They have a higher reproducibility (7%–25% variability)[27] and could replace the Agatston score in the future.

By far the most exciting new development of MDCT is noninvasive motion-free imaging of the lumen of the coronary arteries after administration of an iodine-based intravenous contrast agent (**Fig. 4**B). The latest 64- to 320-slice technologies[28] enable submillimeter isotropic resolution in all three axes and, therefore, excellent reformatting in any imaging plane. This makes possible evaluation of many small structures, such as distal submillimeter coronary artery branches. It also makes feasible reliable visualization and assessment of grafts for stent patency and in-stent stenosis. Clinical indications for CTA include evaluation of chest pain with intermediate pretest probability of CAD, lack of electrocardiogram (ECG) changes or negative serial cardiac enzymes, uninterpretable or equivocal stress test results, or suspected coronary anomalies. CCTA also can assess the patency of coronary vessels after

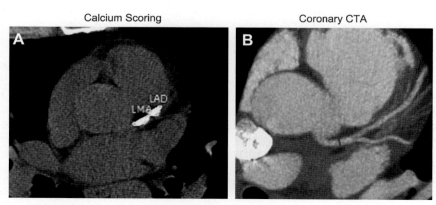

Calcium Scoring   Coronary CTA

Fig. 4. Coronary CT. (*A*) Calcium scoring. (*B*) Coronary CTA.

balloon angioplasty, stenting, or grafting. It may be useful for follow-up in patients undergoing statin therapy.[29]

A typical acquisition protocol for MDCT is retrospective gating, 0.4-second gantry rotation, continuous table motion with pitch of 0.3:1, 0.6-mm slice reconstruction, 0.5-mm in plane resolution, scan from carina to cardiac apex, kilovolt (peak) 120, mAs 340 to 400, and 7-second single breath-hold, with a total radiation dose of 10 to 15 mSv. One hundred to 150 mL of nonionic iodinated contrast material is administered via an antecubital vein using a power injector at 4 mL per second. The images are retrospectively reconstructed at different phases of the cardiac cycle, typically with at least one sequence at full resolution in diastole and another in systole and lower resolution images sampling the entire cardiac cycle for functional analysis. The images then are transferred to a postprocessing workstation for further analysis with specialized software. Examination of the coronary arteries then is performed, using 2-D multiplanar reformations (MPRs), 2-D maximum intensity projections, 2-D curved coronary artery MPRs, and 3-D surface shaded reconstructions.[30] The American College of Cardiology and American Heart Association guidelines for segmental anatomy[31] and lesion morphology[32] are used for lesion characterization. Each stenosis is graded by percentage diameter, with reference to the coronary artery diameter size proximal and distal to the stenosis. Bypass grafts are included in the scan and are evaluated from their proximal to distal anastomosis.

A recent meta-analysis of CCTA versus coronary angiography for 64-slice MDCT[33] reveals a sensitivity of 98%, a specificity of 93%, and a negative predictive value of 97%. Grafts are larger and less calcified than the native coronary arteries and easier to analyze, with 95% to 100% sensitivity and specificity for the detection of stenosis or occlusion. Evaluation of stents[34] revealed a sensitivity of 92%, a specificity of 81%, and a negative predictive value of 98%. At least three elements have an impact on the quality of the images produced by CTA. First, the presence of heavy calcification creates streak artifacts and markedly limits assessment of coronary lumen. The development of calcium subtraction techniques may minimize or eliminate this artifact. Second, excessive motion can markedly degrade image quality. The duration of the period of low motion decreases at high heart rates, rendering imaging more difficult. A heart rate above 75 beats per minute or an arrhythmia, therefore, are limiting factors for single source scanners. Dual-source CT scanners have twice the temporal resolution than single-source scanners and tolerate higher heart rates with minimal degradation of image quality. The motion of the left main, left anterior descending, and circumflex coronary arteries mainly follows the motion of the left ventricle. The motion of the right coronary artery is related to the contraction of the right atrium and ventricle, and is non-negligible at end diastole. Third, CCTA becomes less reliable for smaller vessels with lumen diameter in the 0.5- to 1.5-mm range.

From the same acquisition dataset as the CCTA, lower-resolution images sampling the entire cardiac cycle (typically 20 different phases) are reconstructed for functional analysis. Cardiac chamber volumes, ejection fraction, wall thickness, and global and segmental wall motion can be assessed. The end-systolic sequence is centered on the T wave, whereas the end-diastolic sequence is centered between the R wave and following P wave. Wall motion is qualitatively assessed from cine loops in the long and short axis planes. Automated left ventricular endocardial and epicardial contour detection is performed using specialized software for each reconstructed phase of the cardiac cycle. Following conventions used for ECHO, the papillary muscles are included inside the endocardial borders.[35] From the generated contours, the software computes two sets of measurements. First, the volumes bounded by the endocardium and epicardium are computed using Simpson's rule,[35–37] and their variation throughout the cardiac cycle is determined.[38] From these basic measurements, the end-systolic and end-diastolic volumes, ejection fraction, stroke volume, cardiac output, and cyclic variations in the myocardial wall thickness are derived. The results are displayed graphically. Second, the radial excursion of each point of the endocardium throughout the cardiac cycle is computed and displayed graphically for three levels (base, mid-left ventricle, and apex), to determine regional left ventricular regional wall motion.

INTEGRATED CARDIAC POSITRON EMISSION TOMOGRAPHY–CORONARY CT ANGIOGRAPHY

CCTA is suboptimal for detecting CAD in distal smaller vessels, and although only stenosis in larger vessels (>2 mm) is amenable to percutaneous revascularization, accurately detecting disease in smaller coronary arteries is equally important for optimal medical management. Moreover, it is equally crucial to determine the functional significance of a stenosis/plaque detected on a CCTA study as to whether or not it actually is causing ischemia. In this regard, PET (or SPECT) MPI and CCTA are highly complementary. PET

MPI can detect clinically relevant ischemia in patients who have factors limiting the accuracy of CCTA and can confirm the functional significance of a lesion detected on CCTA by assessing ischemia downstream to it. Thus, the combined and complementary functional and anatomic information from an integrated stress perfusion PET and CCTA can help identify the culprit stenosis in patients presenting with chest pain.

At the same time, PET MPI has a slightly limited ability to delineate the presence of multivessel CAD. In a study by Sampson and colleagues[10] only 55% of patients who had multivessel CAD showed evidence of multivessel perfusion defects on PET/CT imaging. This is because although stress MPI (with SPECT or PET) is highly sensitive in detecting obstructive CAD, it relies strongly on relative perfusion abnormalities to detect ischemia in various coronary territories. Hence, it usually discovers ischemia only in the territory downstream to the most severe stenosis. In patients who have CAD, however, coronary vasodilator reserve frequently is diminished even in territories supplied by hemodynamically noncritical stenosis. This reduces the relative flow differences between normal, noncritical, and critical stenosis territories and leads to underestimation of the extent of actual CAD.[39–41] This can be avoided by using the high-resolution anatomic information supplied by the CCTA study in an integrated PET/CT–CCTA study. Thus, an integrated PET/CT–CCTA cardiac evaluation overcomes limitations of each individual modality and provides a more comprehensive evaluation.

Fig. 5 shows a usual integrated cardiac PET/CT–CCTA protocol. Essentially, it is the same as PET myocardial perfusion study (with a CT attenuation scan instead of a transmission scan using an external radioactive source in traditional PET imaging) with an added CCTA component. The CCTA can be performed at the beginning or at the end of the PET perfusion study. Just before the CCTA portion of the study, the heart rate is controlled with oral or intravenous β-blockers, and once the heart rate is in the optimal range, rapid CCTA images are obtained after the intravenous injection of iodinated contrast material. Some protocols also include sublingual nitroglycerin before administration of contrast material.

The traditional work-up of patients who have chest pain suspected to be of cardiac origin and of patients who have high risk for CAD includes stress MPI to detect potential ischemic regions. If positive, further work-up includes catheter-based angiography, which also can be used as therapeutic procedure in case a critical stenosis is detected. The majority of invasive

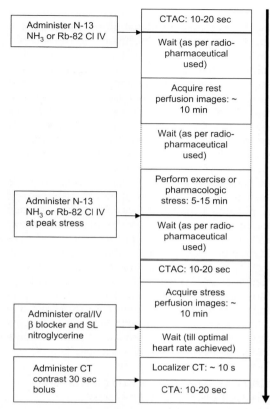

Fig. 5. Integrated cardiac PET/CT–CCTA protocol.

catheter-based coronary angiograms, however, are only diagnostic (as opposed to therapeutic) because patients may have diffuse disease not amenable to surgical or percutaneous revascularization or due to normal vessels (related to a false-positive MPI study). Furthermore, on several occasions, there may be incongruence between coronary angiography and MPI findings. This is because anatomic assessment of the luminal stenosis provided by coronary angiography may not be a reliable indicator of its downstream hemodynamic effects. In spite of having significant stenosis, the territory supplied by that coronary artery may still have adequate perfusion from collateral blood supply and may not be at risk for ischemia.

An integrated PET/CT–CCTA study evaluates the presence and severity of coronary artery luminal stenosis (by CCTA) along with its downstream hemodynamic consequences, including stress-induced ischemia or microvascular dysfunction (by MPI) in a single imaging session. This combined approach provides structural and functional information and offers several benefits in the management of patients who have CAD. It accurately identifies the culprit lesion (in the setting of single and multivessel disease) and helps to direct optimal management toward the offending stenosis. In patients who have endothelial/microvascular dysfunction without critical coronary artery stenosis, it helps avoid unnecessary further invasive coronary angiography and steers patients to appropriate medical management. In addition, because the positive predictive value of CTA for identifying hemodynamically significant coronary stenoses (those that produce stress-induced ischemia) is suboptimal, the integrated PET/CT–CCTA study provides the necessary additional functional information to aid in the decision-making process of further management of patients (whether or not with percutaneous angioplasty, bypass surgery, or medical therapy). Without the combined approach of a PET/CT–CCTA study, the use of CCTA as the sole imaging tool for assessing CAD (instead of the traditional noninvasive MPI followed by catheter-based coronary angiography if needed) could result in an enormous increase in health care expenses due to unnecessary therapeutic invasive coronary catheterizations and revascularization procedures on the basis of CCTA findings alone.

INTEGRATED CARDIAC POSITRON EMISSION TOMOGRAPHY/CORONARY ARTERY CALCIUM SCORING

For PET/CT scanners with a slightly lower-end CT component (less than 16-slice CT), a dedicated CCTA study may not be feasible. However, even with a 4-slice CT as a part of the PET/CT scanner, it is easily possible to combine coronary artery calcium scoring along with PET MPI. Again, the protocol for such an integrated cardiac PET/CT–coronary artery calcium scoring study is essentially the same as a PET myocardial perfusion study with an added noncontrast gated cardiac CT study for calcium scoring. Coronary calcium scoring increasingly is used to assess preclinical CAD.[42] It is estimated that a significant number of patients who have normal myocardial perfusion study but have other cardiac risk factors may have widespread underlying coronary artery atherosclerotic calcification.[43] Because these are noncritical lesions, they may not cause detectable ischemia on MPI. Although a normal myocardial perfusion study justifies no further invasive testing in most cases, patients who have a normal perfusion study but have a high coronary calcium score need further management in the form of aggressive risk factor modification to halt progression of the hemodynamically stable CAD. Hence, an integrated cardiac PET/CT–coronary artery calcium scoring approach may provide a better approach toward risk stratification and management of this cohort of patients.

POSITRON EMISSION TOMOGRAPHY MYOCARDIAL VIABILITY EVALUATION

Patients who have severe left ventricular dysfunction and ischemic heart disease continue to pose a significant management dilemma in spite of tremendous progress in understanding the pathophysiology of CAD and great strides in treatment approaches and preventive strategies addressing CAD. Therapeutic options remain limited to medical management, revascularization (surgical or percutaneous), and cardiac transplantation.[44] Cardiac transplantation almost always is the last resort due to the associated morbidity and mortality and the lack of availability of donor hearts.[44,45] In the setting of confirmed myocardial ischemia, revascularization offers superior long-term survival rates compared with medical management, despite considerable advances in medical therapeutic options.[46–54] Revascularization procedures, however, are associated with significant periprocedural risks. Hence, it is critical to select appropriately only those patients who will benefit the most from revascularization treatment to optimize the risk-benefit ratio.

The myocardium responds in several ways to an ischemic insult (acute or chronic) and may adopt any of the several immediate or sustained mechanisms of adjustment to withstand the trauma of ischemic injury. These responses include stunning, hibernation, and ischemic preconditioning, and, depending on the severity and duration of the underlying cause for ischemia, it may become permanently damaged and necrosed/scarred, revert to fully functional myocardium without residual damage, or show an array of findings ranging between these two extremes. Scarred necrosed myocardium is nonviable and thus revascularization is of no benefit in this situation. Myocardium that is stunned or hibernating, however, is dysfunctional but viable and has the potential to become normal or show significant improvement in contractile function with proper revascularization therapy. This reversibility of contractile dysfunction is the most crucial determinant of postrevascularization functional improvement and overall benefit to patients. Viable myocardium denotes a dysfunctional myocardium that is reversible to functional myocardium with restoration of blood supply. Hence, accurate identification of viable myocardium from necrosed/scarred (ie, nonviable) myocardium is the single most decisive factor to determine revascularization as the optimal therapy for particular patients.

Several techniques, including rest-redistribution TI-201 studies, low-dose dobutamine stress ECHO, cardiac MR imaging,[55] and others, can evaluate myocardial viability. In 1986, Tillisch and colleagues,[56] however, were the first to successfully predict functional reversibility of myocardium on the basis on FDG-PET imaging. Since then, the value of FDG-PET imaging to assess myocardial viability in multiple clinical scenarios has been extensively validated in the literature,[57–65] and MPI combined with FDG-PET myocardial metabolic imaging is considered the gold standard for assessing myocardial viability.[1]

Dysfunctional myocardium with drastically reduced blood flow probably is scarred nonviable myocardium whereas that with relatively normal blood flow most likely is stunned but viable myocardium. These situations lie at the extreme ends of the spectrum of dysfunctional myocardial imaging findings and usually pose no dilemma with regard to their assessment. More commonly, however, dysfunctional myocardium with an intermediate decline in blood flow is encountered and in such cases the presence of myocardial viability cannot be adequately assessed with regional myocardial blood flow alone. Hence, myocardial viability typically is determined by evaluating myocardial metabolism (using FDG-PET imaging) in combination with myocardial blood flow (using PET or SPECT-MPI).

There are several PET radiopharmaceuticals (such as C-11 palmitate, C-11 acetate, and FDG) that can assess myocardial metabolism depending on the energy substrate being used by the myocardium, which is highly variable and dependent on the hormonal milieu and the available substrate concentration. Fasting conditions with low plasma glucose and insulin levels and high plasma free fatty acid (FFA) levels all promote FFA as the primary myocardial substrate. In postprandial conditions with increased plasma glucose and, consequently, increased insulin levels, however, and under ischemic and hypoxic conditions, the substrate switches from FFA to glucose as the substrate of choice for its metabolic needs.[44,60,66–74] Hence, FDG is the radiopharmaceutical of choice for PET myocardial metabolic imaging.

Because ischemic myocardium prefers glucose as its energy substrate, when ischemic myocardium has at least some blood supply to keep it viable, it shows increased FDG uptake on FDG-PET myocardial metabolic imaging. Conversely, when there is no blood supply to the myocardium, there is no FDG uptake in that myocardial segment on FDG-PET myocardial imaging. This is the underlying principle for assessing myocardial

viability with FDG-PET metabolic imaging combined with MPI. The protocol for myocardial viability assessment consists of an integrated PET myocardial perfusion and metabolism study or a SPECT myocardial perfusion study and an FDG-PET myocardial metabolism study performed on separate days but within a short time interval. The PET-MPI requires glucose loading before FDG administration to overcome the variability in myocardial FDG uptake under normal testing conditions. Glucose loading ensures good myocardial FDG uptake by increasing plasma glucose and insulin levels during the FDG uptake period promoting increased intramyocardial FDG transport.

There are several methods for performing glucose loading. The most practical and commonly used technique, consists of oral glucose administration with or without insulin supplementation depending on diabetic status and plasma glucose levels. However, in approximately 10% of patients, this causes suboptimal myocardial FDG uptake and uninterpretable images (more often in diabetics). Because diabetes frequently is associated with cardiac disease, it remains a challenging and sometimes limiting issue. Alternative approaches to promoting myocardial glucose uptake include administration of intravenous glucose (in patients who have altered gastrointestinal glucose absorption and in those unable to tolerate oral glucose), administration of acipimox, and the hyperinsulinemic/euglycemic clamp technique. The drug, acipimox, a nicotinic acid derivative, indirectly promotes myocardial glucose uptake and has been used successfully by a few investigators.[8,75,76] It is not available in the United States and is used mostly in Europe. The hyperinsulinemic/euglycemic clamp technique provides controlled metabolic conditions for the study and consistently provides good images, although it is cumbersome and technically challenging to implement in routine clinical practice.[77] A simplified technique using glucose-insulin-potassium solution infusion protocol also has been implemented successfully by Martin and colleagues.[78]

The typical PET myocardial metabolism imaging protocol with FDG consists of having a patient fast for at least 4 to 6 hours before the study. Blood sugar level (BSL) is obtained on arrival at the imaging center. In nondiabetic patients who have BSL less than 110 mg/dL, 50 to 75 g glucose (usually in solution form) is administered orally approximately 30 to 60 minutes before intravenous administration of 185 to 555 MBq (5–15 mCi) of FDG. Dedicated PET images of the chest to include the complete heart (consisting of transmission and emission scans) then typically are obtained approximately 60 minutes after the administration of FDG. In diabetic patients or for BSL greater than 110 mg/dL, insulin supplementation also is given along with the oral glucose dose to maintain a BSL between 100 and 140 mg/dL at the time of FDG administration. **Fig. 6** depicts a myocardial viability assessment protocol using PET-MPI with N-13 NH_3 combined with PET myocardial metabolism imaging with FDG and oral glucose loading.

Myocardial blood flow combined with myocardial glucose metabolism can have three distinct patterns (depicted schematically in **Fig. 7**): (1) normal blood flow and normal glucose metabolism, (2) decreased blood flow and decreased glucose metabolism, and (3) decreased blood flow but retained/normal glucose metabolism. Pattern 1 represents normal viable myocardium but generally under circumstances of normal blood flow, viability assessment usually is not warranted. Pattern 2 represents necrosed/scarred myocardium, which is nonviable. Pattern 3 is the classic flow-metabolism mismatch that is the hallmark of dysfunctional but viable myocardium.[44,45]

Myocardial viability assessment has several important implications on clinical management of patients who have left ventricular failure due to CAD. Pretreatment myocardial viability assessment can accurately predict functional recovery after revascularization treatment. This has been well documented by several investigators.[56,79–82] Moreover, the size and number of viable segments

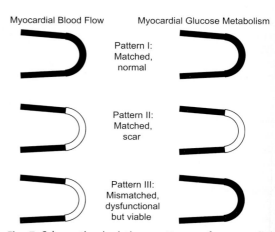

Fig. 7. Schematic depicting patterns of myocardial blood flow and myocardial metabolism for myocardial viability studies.

also positively affect functional outcome post revascularization.[83–85] Thus, pretreatment assessment of myocardial viability aids in predicting the amount of expected improvement from congestive heart failure symptoms after revascularization, playing a crucial role in determining the risk-benefit ratio for revascularization. Myocardial viability assessment also predicts perioperative complications for revascularization. Documentation of viable myocardium by flow-metabolic imaging using FDG-PET and incorporating this information along with the clinical and angiographic data in the decision-making process for revascularization results in less perioperative complications, less need for inotropic drugs, low early mortality, and better short-term survival.[86,87] Identification of viable myocardium in patients who have left ventricular dysfunction due to CAD is an indication for prompt revascularization therapy, as in the presence of sustained myocardial ischemia, the adaptive responses ultimately fail, leading to irreversible myocardial damage. Delaying revascularization in the presence of documented viable myocardium usually leads to suboptimal outcome and can have other serious consequences, including death.[88] Furthermore, presence of viable myocardium on PET imaging appears to be a risk factor for future ischemic events, and medical management of such patients without revascularization does not decrease this risk. Hence, the presence of viable myocardium and lack of revascularization are independent predictors of ischemic events.[89,90] Consequently, patients who have viable myocardium treated with revascularization also tend to have improved long-term survival compared with those treated with medical therapy alone.[91,92]

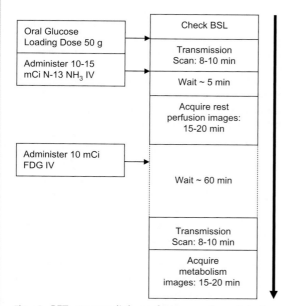

Fig. 6. PET myocardial perfusion and metabolism imaging protocol for myocardial viability.

At the same time, failure to definitely identify significant viable myocardium strengthens the decision to treat these patients medically or by cardiac transplantation, if warranted.

CARDIAC MR IMAGING/MAGNETIC RESONANCE ANGIOGRAPHY

MR imaging has become the gold standard in morphologic and functional imaging of the heart. The noninvasive techniques of CTA and MRA have almost completely replaced diagnostic catheter angiography of the thoracic vessels at major institutions. MRA still faces competition from CTA but avoids the large volumes of intravenous contrast material and ionizing radiation and is the preferred approach for patients who have allergies to iodine-based contrast agents. MPRs from MR imaging provide a unique insight to the complex anatomy of the heart; surrounding structures, such as pericardium; coronary arteries; and great vessels and eliminates the problem of overlapping structures as seen with catheter angiography.[93]

Accurate measurements of cardiac chambers, wall thickness, and vessel diameters can be obtained.[94] Dynamic imaging of wall motion by MR imaging is now the gold standard. MRA can measure flow information in chambers and vessels, providing quantitative measures of increased flow through stenoses and of shunt vascularity.[95] MR imaging also can image vessel walls and surrounding tissues.[96] Cardiac MR imaging is increasingly becoming the one-stop-shop examination for cardiac imaging, as it enables acquisition of most clinically relevant information on cardiovascular disease within the course of a single examination.[97] This is possible because of an ever-increasing set of pulse sequences that offer different approaches to acquire MR imaging data. Some of these are discussed briefly later, with image examples shown in **Fig. 8**.[98,99]

Spin-echo (Black Blood) Sequences

These sequences include T1-weighted images with and without intravenous contrast, T2-weighted

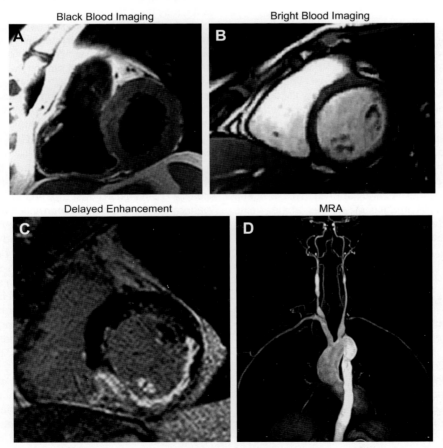

Fig. 8. Cardiac MR imaging. (A) Black blood imaging. (B) Bright blood imaging. (C) Delayed enhancement. (D) MRA.

spin-echo images with fat saturation, and double inversion recovery and triple inversion recovery sequences. These are used for imaging general cardiac morphology with or without fat nulling, imaging edema, and imaging the vessel walls and the mediastinal and perivascular tissues.

Gradient-echo (Bright Blood) Sequences

These sequences include rapid imaging techniques with and without intravenous contrast, such as steady-state free precession or spoiled gradient-echo images for dynamic imaging, and fast gradient echoplanar images for perfusion imaging. Of special interest is inversion recovery gradient-echo imaging, which nulls the signal of normal myocardium for viability imaging. After a 10- to 15-minute delay, intravenously administered gadolinium-based contrast agents are retained in scar tissue longer than in normal myocardium and show the scar as an area of bright signal in an otherwise dark normal myocardium.

Time-of-flight Imaging

Radiofrequency pulses are used to saturate all protons in an imaging slice or volume and suppress the signal from all stationary tissue within that volume. Blood flowing into the imaging volume brings "unsaturated" protons that have not experienced the prior excitation pulses of the other protons and produce higher signal. Additional saturation pulses immediately above or below the plane of imaging selectively suppress signal from either veins or arteries. This is useful to obtain MRA images of arteries alone, veins alone, or arteries and veins simultaneously without the administration of intravenous contrast material.

Phase-contrast Imaging

Bipolar magnetic gradient fields perpendicular to the plane of imaging can be used to quantify the speed of spatially moving protons. Protons acquire different precession phases depending on their position. Two opposite and equal gradients separated by a time delay give protons varying precession phases depending on their speed. The intensity of the bipolar gradient fields is adjusted to avoid aliasing. This allows precise quantification of blood flow through valves of vessels.

3-D Contrast-enhanced Magnetic Resonance Angiography

This technique uses a 3-D spoiled gradient-echo pulse sequence to optimize imaging of the first pass of a T1 shortening gadolinium-based contrast agent in blood vessels. The dose of gadolinium may range from 0.1 to 0.3 mmol/kg injected at a rate of at least 2.0 mL per second. Timing of the contrast bolus with respect to image acquisition is important. 3-D contrast-enhanced MRA (CE-MRA) has become the most commonly used approach to MRA for all vessels in the body.

Time-resolved Sequences

With repetitive rapid acquisition of the low-frequency spectral information (center of k-space) as a contrast bolus is injected, followed by later filling of the remaining of k-space, it is possible to obtain a sequence of CE-MRA images showing the time course of the contrast bolus as it progressively fills the vessels.

Although intravenous gadolinium-based contrast agents were previously perceived as safe, they have recently been reported to be associated with nephrogenic systemic fibrosis and nephrogenic fibrosing dermatopathy in patients who have renal failure, which can produce debilitating and sometimes fatal outcomes.[100,101] Intravenous gadolinium-based contrast agent administration thus is avoided in subjects who have a glomerular filtration rate (GFR) below 30 mL/min, and administered volumes of contrast typically are decreased when the GFR is between 30 and 60 mL per minute.

A typical cardiac MR imaging study takes 30 to 45 minutes and starts with multiplanar localizer heavily T2-weighted fast spin-echo images for general patient orientation information and an axial black blood double inversion recovery sequence to image morphology. A T2-weighted sequence then can be performed to detect the presence of fluid or edema, followed by dynamic short- and long-axis steady-state free precession sequences to image morphology and wall motion. ECG gating is used as part of this sequence to track cardiac motion and produce stop-frame images of the heart. Intravenous contrast material then is administered while first-pass perfusion imaging is performed. After a delay of 10 to 15 minutes, delayed enhancement imaging is performed, which concludes the study. All sequences are performed during breath holding to eliminate respiratory motion artifacts. Alternatively, free breathing with navigator pulse tracking of the diaphragm excursion can be used to eliminate respiratory motion artifacts.[102] Perfusion imaging also can be performed after administration of adenosine as a pharmacologic stress agent.[103] Common clinical applications for cardiac MR imaging are discussed.

Ischemic Cardiomyopathy

Reversible ischemia due to flow-limiting CAD can be visualized by dynamic perfusion imaging.[104] First-pass perfusion imaging at rest after administration of an intravenous gadolinium-based contrast agent is compared with another first-pass perfusion sequence under pharmacologic stress, such as with adenosine or dipyridamole. Flow-limiting stenoses present as areas of slow myocardial uptake (hypoperfusion) under stress not present at rest. Acute myocardial infarction can present with increased signal on T2-weighted images, a nonspecific finding, and with wall motion abnormalities. Chronic myocardial infarction may be seen as myocardial wall thinning, lack of myocardial thickening during systole on dynamic bright blood sequences, and sometimes decreased signal intensity in areas of scar on spin-echo sequences. Myocardial scar, which retains gadolinium-based contrast material longer than normal myocardium because of increased extracellular space (in the chronic setting) and disruption of cell membrane integrity (in the acute setting), appears with high signal intensity on delayed enhanced images. The area of increased signal intensity stabilizes after 1 to 2 weeks after myocardial infarction.[105] By virtue of its excellent spatial resolution, MR imaging can readily distinguish transmural infarcts from subendocardial infarcts. They also present with characteristic patterns of myocardial wall enhancement different from those found in nonischemic cardiomyopathy, hypertrophic cardiomyopathy, arrhythmogenic cardiomyopathy, and myocarditis.[106,107]

Hypertrophic Cardiomyopathy

Both black blood and bright blood sequences reveal myocardial wall thickening (>12 mm), which can be concentric or asymmetric, basal, mid, or apical in location. If the basal septum is hypertrophied, dynamic bright blood imaging, which also shows blood flow pattern disruption can reveal abnormal septal displacement of the anterior leaflet of the mitral valve during systole, causing functional subaortic valvular stenosis and functional mitral regurgitation. Delayed enhancement imaging often shows abnormal intramural signal intensity within the hypertrophied myocardium due to fibrotic changes.[108]

Pericardial Disease

Cardiac MR imaging often is used to help distinguish constrictive pericarditis from restrictive cardiomyopathy.[109,110] Multiplanar black blood and bright blood sequences can readily evaluate diffuse abnormal pericardial thickening (>2–3 mm) with an accuracy of 93%. Unlike CT, MR imaging is poor at assessing pericardial calcifications, which if seen appear as low signal intensity areas on most sequences. MR imaging can assess the size and composition of pericardial effusions. T1-weighted black blood sequences show low signal intensity for transudative effusions and higher signal intensity for proteinaceous, hemorrhagic, or exudative effusions. Areas of loculation and adhesions also may be seen due to an inflammatory process. Dynamic bright blood imaging can show septal wall straightening and abnormal septal wall motion, narrowing of the ventricles, or atrial dilation. During normal cardiac contraction, there is a twist motion in the myocardium, with the base rotating clockwise and the apex rotating counterclockwise. The reverse rotations are present during isovolumetric relaxation. This twist motion can decrease or disappear if there are pericardial adhesions. In the presence of cardiac tamponade, diastolic collapse of the chambers is demonstrated.

Cardiac Tumors

Black blood and bright blood sequences show precise anatomic extent of cardiac tumors and help to determine whether or not a tumor is extracardiac, intramural, or intraluminal in location and to distinguish tumors from prominent normal cardiac structures. MR imaging also can characterize the gross composition of tumors.[111] A pericardial cyst shows low signal intensity fluid on T1-weighted sequences and high signal intensity on T2-weighted sequences, with a location adjacent to the pericardium. A lipoma or lipomatous hypertrophy of the interatrial septum shows high signal intensity on T1-weighted sequences and loss of signal intensity on fat-suppressed T1-weighted images. Although tumors and thrombus can show low or intermediate signal intensity on black blood sequences, a thrombus typically shows low signal intensity on bright blood sequences and, unlike tumor, does not enhance after the administration of intravenous contrast material. Frequently, cardiac tumors, such as myxoma, show high signal intensity on T2-weighted images or location at the interatrial septum, with possible prolapse through an atrioventricular valve during cardiac contraction.

424   Takalkar et al

INTEGRATED CARDIAC POSITRON EMISSION TOMOGRAPHY/MR IMAGING

The hardware integration of PET and MR imaging is more difficult than for PET and CT. Current PET detector modules do not operate in high magnetic fields. Once a positron is emitted by a radiopharmaceutical, it annihilates with an electron and produces a pair of 511-keV high-energy photons, which are absorbed by detector crystals surrounding the patient.[112] These produce lower-energy photons detected by photomultiplier tubes, which in turn produce electrons that are amplified. These electrons are displaced by even smaller magnetic fields as low as 10 mT, which render detection by photomultiplier tubes useless. Experimental systems have been produced[113] using long light guides to transfer the postannihilation photons to detectors outside the main magnetic field but so far show limited PET performance and small fields of view.[114] The few initial clinical PET/MR imaging systems are expected to be in place at a few beta sites in the United States as of mid 2009.

Although the technical hurdles are slowly being worked out, there remains the possibility of independently performing PET and MR imaging, with software combination of the two imaging modalities to produce images with high-resolution morphologic information and lower-resolution functional information.[115]

An area of synergy between PET and MR imaging is the assessment of myocardial viability. Both imaging modalities can assess myocardial viability. Although PET has been the gold standard for many years, MR imaging is proving an attractive alternative. Delayed-enhancement MR imaging is limited, however, to a black/white pattern of signal alteration, with white representing nonviable myocardium and black representing viable myocardium. Knuesel and colleagues[116] studied tissue classification with respect to functional recovery after revascularization and showed the limitations of MR imaging to capture the variability and biologic complexity of involved segments.

A second area of synergy is the assessment of cardiac innervation. PET can image cardiac innervation using the cathecolamine analog, carbon-11 (C-11) hydroxyephedrine. This can be combined with high-resolution morphologic imaging and wall motion imaging by MR imaging. Bengel and colleagues[117] used this approach to delineate cardiac regional innervation and control mechanisms in normal subjects, in patients who had dilated cardiomyopathy, and in patients after heart transplantation.

A third area of synergy is the assessment of cardiac masses. MR imaging can be used for precise anatomic delineation of a primary or metastatic cardiac tumor, whereas FDG-PET can characterize its metabolic activity. This can be used for initial assessment of the tumor or for assessment of treatment response.

FLUORINE-18–LABELED FLUORODEOXYGLUCOSE–POSITRON EMISSION TOMOGRAPHY/CT OR FLUORINE-18–LABELED FLUORODEOXYGLUCOSE–POSITRON EMISSION TOMOGRAPHY/MR IMAGING ATHEROSCLEROSIS IMAGING IN LARGE ARTERIES

Formation of atherosclerotic plaque is a dynamic inflammatory process that involves interactions between atherogenic lipoproteins and macrophages (Fig. 9). Accumulation of cholesteryl ester in plaque macrophages leads to formation of foam cells. Foam cells are characteristically present in atherosclerotic lesions, occupying most of the plaque, leading to the progression of the pathologic process.[118] Vulnerable atherosclerotic plaque is characterized by a large lipid core, a thin fibrous cap, a preponderance of inflammatory cells, and a relative paucity of vascular smooth muscle cells, which make vessels prone to rupture.[119] Macrophage foam cells contribute extensively to the development of inflammation in plaque by secreting different inflammatory cytokines and metalloproteinases that break down the matrix proteins in the fibrous cap.[120,121] Thus, macrophages are considered an important determinant of plaque vulnerability and are a major target for imaging.

Rupture of the atherosclerotic plaque and its subsequent thrombosis or embolism, rather than the stenosis of the atherosclerotic artery itself,

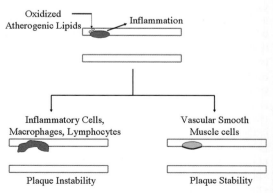

Fig. 9. Pathophysiology of atherosclerosis.

are the major determinants for serious clinical complications, such as sudden cardiac death or stroke. It is known that 70% of plaque ruptures occur in lesions that cause less than 50% stenosis.[122,123] Epidemiologic studies have shown that a large proportion of patients who have suffered from sudden cardiac events have no prior cardiovascular symptoms.[124] More importantly, it has been noted that acute coronary syndromes often result from plaque rupture at sites with no or only modest luminal narrowing on angiographic examination.[125] Angiography, the current gold standard imaging modality for assessing the arterial lumen, cannot identify inflamed plaque or nonstenotic plaques, which may be particularly prone to inflammation and rupture.[126] Thus, an ideal imaging modality should be able to identify not only the degree of stenosis but also the inflammatory status and vulnerability of a plaque. Contrast-enhanced ultrasonography with microbubbles targeted to inflammatory markers, such as P-selectin, has the potential to identify inflamed plaque in the segment of an artery being imaged. However, it suffers from the limitations of operator dependency and inability to evaluate a large body area in one setting. Several modalities are competing to address the issue of identifying the vulnerable plaques, but FDG–PET/CT or FDG–PET/MR imaging, combined functional and structural whole-body imaging modalities, likely hold the most potential for this purpose. Most of the studies so far have been performed with FDG–PET/CT.

FDG is a radiotracer that accumulates in disease sites with increased glycolysis, and it is known that activated inflammatory cells have significantly increased glycolysis. Therefore, it is generally believed that increased glucose uptake and metabolism in the plaque macrophages account for the visualization of vulnerable atherosclerosis lesion by FDG-PET imaging. Animal studies have demonstrated that FDG uptake in plaque is correlated with plaque macrophage density and inflammatory status. It was also shown that there was an approximately fivefold higher FDG uptake within an injury-induced atherosclerotic iliac artery in New Zealand white rabbits compared with uptake in the contralateral uninjured iliac artery in the same animals.[127–129] There was significant correlation between FDG uptake and macrophage density in the plaque. Also, FDG uptake correlated with vascular inflammation (macrophage density) but not with vessel wall thickness, plaque thickness, or smooth muscle cell staining. The results suggest that macrophages are responsible for the accumulation of FDG in atherosclerotic lesions.

Tahara and colleagues[130] recently determined the prevalence of inflammation in carotid artery atherosclerosis by FDG-PET in 100 consecutive human patients who underwent screening carotid artery ultrasonography for carotid atherosclerosis. FDG-PET revealed inflammation (defined as standardized uptake value [SUV] ≥ 1.6) in 12 of 41 [29%] patients who had documented carotid atherosclerosis by carotid artery ultrasonography and in 6 of 59 (10.2%) patients who did not have carotid atherosclerosis. In a pilot study of eight patients who had carotid stenosis, Rudd and colleagues used autoradiography to show that tritiated deoxyglucose accumulated in plaque macrophages when incubated with fresh carotid endarterectomy specimens in vitro from three of the eight patients. FDG uptake was higher in symptomatic lesions than in the contralateral asymptomatic lesions.[131] Recent research related to this observation in 17 patients showed a significant correlation between FDG-PET uptake by carotid plaque and macrophage staining from the corresponding histologic sections of specimens removed during endarterectomy.[132]

A prospective clinical study suggests that FDG-PET may be able to monitor drug-induced changes in plaque inflammation. The study included 43 subjects in whom FDG-PET imaging was performed for voluntary cancer screening. In this population, incidental FDG uptake was noted in the thoracic aorta or carotid arteries. Subjects then were randomly assigned to strict dietary management or to administration of simvastatin in addition to dietary management. After 3 months, FDG-PET showed significantly decreased FDG uptake in the atherosclerotic plaques in the simvastatin group, whereas no change was noted in the group with dietary management alone.[133] One of the major effects of statins is to promote plaque stability by decreasing plaque macrophage content and activity.[134] Findings suggest that FDG-PET can identify a decrease in plaque inflammation much earlier than structural changes detected by MR imaging, which was reportedly detected after 12 months of simvastatin treatment.[135] Similarly, Ogawa and colleagues[136] showed that FDG-PET detected the reduction of plaque inflammation by the anti-inflammatory drug, probucol, which is known to decrease macrophage infiltration in the plaques.

FDG uptake in large arteries detected by PET was noted as early as 1987 in patients who had vasculitis.[137] The aortic accumulation of FDG initially was interpreted as a physiologic process possibly due to blood pool activity.[138] Work from investigators at the Hospital of the University of Pennsylvania first linked FDG uptake in the great vessels to atherosclerosis. In a retrospective study, the authors found vascular FDG uptake was present in 50% of the patients.[139] Further work demonstrated that age and hypercholesterolemia were correlated consistently with FDG uptake in arteries.[140] Others confirmed these findings with one study also noting hypertension as a risk factor.[141,142] Bural and colleagues[143] recently examined the presence of arterial FDG uptake in 149 patients who had PET scans and showed that the prevalence and intensity of FDG uptake in large arteries generally increase with aging. Diffuse FDG uptake was readily detected in lower-extremity atherosclerotic arteries in diabetic patients.[144] The positive correlation between arterial FDG uptake and cardiovascular risk factors, such as age and hypercholesterolemia, suggests a promising role for FDG-PET imaging in the detection of atherosclerosis and evaluation of plaque inflammatory activity.

FDG uptake can be identified in different segments of the large arteries, including the carotid arteries, ascending aorta, aortic arch, descending thoracic aorta, and abdominal aorta and in the iliac and femoral arteries. In severe atherosclerosis, FDG uptake can be visualized in most of the arterial system. Dunphy and colleagues[145] reported that FDG uptake was more common in the aorta, compared with coronary and carotid arteries, and was most prevalent in the proximal aortic segments. More frequent FDG uptake was observed in the thoracic aorta compared with the abdominal aorta.[142,145]

There is significant disparity between FDG uptake on PET images and the presence and extent of calcification in the arteries on CT images. Congruent FDG uptake and calcification were observed in only 2% to 14% of the sites in different studies.[141,142,145] Ben-Haim and colleagues[142] described three different patterns of PET/CT findings in the vascular wall in patients: (1) PET negative and CT positive (PET−/CT+), (2) PET and CT positive (PET+/CT+), and (3) PET positive and CT negative (PET−/CT+). Recently they have further evaluated changes of these patterns over time in 50 patients who had had follow-up PET/CT studies 8 to 26 months apart. Changes in patterns over time were noted in the vascular wall abnormalities in 48% of subjects who had PET+ sites on initial scan, compared with only 4% of subjects who had PET− sites.[146] The study suggests that PET detects plaques with dynamic active changes due to an ongoing inflammatory process, whereas CT identifies chronic calcification as a manifestation of the late stage of the disease. These findings are entirely consistent with the cell biology of atherosclerosis.

Inflammation, as measured by FDG uptake, likely is transient and may forecast future complications, whereas calcification, as measured by CT, is seen in the advanced lesions, and is of debatable pathophysiologic significance.[147]

An important question regarding the role of PET in atherosclerosis imaging is whether or not vascular FDG uptake can be linked to cardiovascular events. Davies and colleagues evaluated 12 patients who had recent transient ischemic attack and severe carotid artery stenosis in the ipsilateral carotid artery who were awaiting endarterectomy of the most severely stenotic lesions. Seven of the 12 patients had high FDG uptake in the lesion, which was targeted for endarterectomy, and three of the remaining five patients had FDG uptake in the nonstenotic lesions located in the vascular territory that was considered likely to be appropriate for the presenting symptoms.[148] In another pilot study in 13 patients who had symptomatic carotid atherosclerosis, PET images revealed FDG accumulation at the site of the symptomatic plaque in all patients, with 11 (85%) exhibiting significant uptake (SUV ≥ 2.7). Six (54%) patients who had intense FDG uptake suffered from one of the primary endpoints: two died during follow-up, three had recurrent nonfatal ipsilateral ischemic stroke, and one had restenosis after stenting. FDG uptake was found significantly correlated with the degree of stenosis detected by angiography.[149] These findings suggest that FDG-PET may be able to assess the degree of inflammation in the stenotic and nonstenotic culprit lesions and potentially could be used to identify lesions that are responsible for embolic events.

Paulmier and colleagues[150] recently compared the rate of cardiovascular events in two otherwise matched groups of patients who had and who did not have detectable arterial FDG uptake. Cardiovascular events were significantly more frequent in the high-FDG uptake group than in the low-FDG uptake group. A multivariate analysis showed that the extent of arterial FDG uptake was a unique factor significantly related to the occurrence of a recent event. Conversely, calcification was a single factor related to old cardiovascular events. The investigators concluded that vascular FDG uptake may indicate a dynamic inflammatory process in the atherosclerotic plaque, which is related to increased cardiovascular event. There are limitations to this study, such as selection bias due to the retrospective nature of the research and small number of the cardiovascular events observed, which affected the statistical power. Nevertheless, this investigation is important and highlights the right direction for evaluating the role of FDG uptake as a potential risk factor and marker for cardiovascular event. A prospective study thus would provide direct evidence for such speculations.

Atherosclerosis is a systemic inflammatory disease that involves multiple vessels, and therefore, it is important and essential to quantify the degree and the extent of the disease regionally and on a larger scale in the entire body. By quantifying plaque inflammation, it may be possible to predict the natural course of the disease and the risk for plaque rupture and to monitor the effect of therapy.

SUV, a semiquantitative measure which is commonly used for assessing disease activity with PET imaging, can provide information about the severity of the inflammatory process in the arterial wall even before it is clinically symptomatic or visible by structural imaging techniques. Bural and colleagues[151] from the authors' group developed a novel quantitative method to measure the extent of atherosclerosis in the aorta by combing SUV measurements on PET with volumetric data of the aortic wall provided by CT. With this method, inner and outer wall contours of the aortic wall were manually drawn on each axial CT image and the respective wall areas in multiple samples in four aortic segments (ascending thoracic, arch, descending thoracic, and abdominal) were calculated as the net wall regions by subtracting the inner from the outer surface area. Net aortic wall areas then were multiplied by slice thickness to yield aortic wall volumes. The products of aortic wall volumes and mean SUVs over each segment were calculated for each segment and called atherosclerotic burden or atheroburden (AB) value. This approach provides the means to integrate structural and functional data into a single quantitative parameter. Aortic wall volumes, mean SUVs, and ABs in each segment were compared in three age groups spanning 6 decades in 18 patients. Significant differences in the age groups were found for segmental ABs and or the entire aorta. The age-related progression in mean SUV and volume appeared linear, whereas the progression of AB relative to age appeared exponential, suggesting a major escalation in the overall atherosclerotic process with aging that can be determined only by this approach.

In a recent study, Rudd and colleagues[152] compared two methods of artery FDG uptake measurement: the mean and maximum blood-normalized SUV, known as the target-to-background ratio (TBR). A region of interest was drawn around the artery on every slice of the coregistered transaxial PET/CT images, and a mean and maximum SUV were acquired on each slice, which was subsequently normalized to the venous blood

FDG activity. By averaging the SUVs for all slices within an arterial territory, the mean and maximum SUVs for each artery region were calculated. The investigators found that the mean and maximum TBR measurements for quantifying FDG uptake are equally reproducible, and they suggested that the mean TBR be used for tracking systemic arterial therapies, whereas the maximum TBR is optimal for detecting and monitoring local, plaque-based therapy.

Data have suggested a great potential role for FDG–PET/CT in imaging and predicting the nature of atherosclerosis in large arteries. FDG uptake in large arteries is associated with cardiovascular risk factors. FDG accumulates in plaque macrophages and uptake is correlated with plaque macrophage density and inflammatory status. Vascular FDG uptake and calcification do not overlap significantly and changes of FDG uptake are common, suggesting that FDG uptake may represent a dynamic inflammatory process. Vascular FDG uptake can be attenuated by simvastatin in patients and by anti-inflammatory drug, probucol, in rabbits. FDG uptake in arteries has been linked to cardiovascular events in some preliminary studies. With its high sensitivity and the ability for optimal quantification of the disease process, FDG–PET/CT would allow for early diagnosis and accurate evaluation of response to treatment of atherosclerosis.

FUTURE APPLICATIONS FOR POSITRON EMISSION TOMOGRAPHY IMAGING IN CARDIOVASCULAR CONDITIONS

In addition to imaging myocardial perfusion, myocardial metabolism, and atherosclerosis, PET imaging is being evaluated for certain other important cardiac conditions. Various PET radiopharmaceuticals are in development for cardiac neuronal imaging and potentially can be used to evaluate the inter-relationships between cardiac sympathetic and parasympathetic mechanisms and their interactions with metabolic mechanisms, mechanisms of neural regulation of the coronary circulation and heart rate, the role of the sympathetic nervous system in the genesis of ventricular arrhythmias, and the role of autonomic system dysfunction in the heart failure. Evaluation of cardiovascular neural regulation may provide valuable information in cardiac transplantation (which is accompanied by denervation but may show late sympathetic innervation) and in patients who have diabetic cardiomyopathy (which is associated with regional autonomic cardiac neuropathy).

The cardiac sympathetic nervous system has been assessed using PET radiopharmaceuticals, such as F18-fluorodopamine, C-11 epinephrine, C-11 metahydroxyephedrine, and C-11 phenylephrine (in human clinical trials with credible results) whereas the cardiac parasympathetic nervous system has been assessed using vesamicol-based agents such as: F18-labeled fluoroethoxybenzovesamicol.[153] The low density and focal distribution of the cardiac parasympathetic nervous system limits imaging, however, and there still is a need to identify PET tracers with optimal tracer kinetics for cardiac neuronal imaging. In addition, several PET radiotracers have been developed to image the adrenergic and muscarinic receptors in the heart. These include C-11 CGP-12177 for b1 and b2 adrenoceptors, C-11 GB67 for a1 adrenoceptors, and C-11 MQNB for M1 and M2 muscarinic receptors.[154-156] These are, in effect, PET radioligands for postsynaptic myocardial receptor proteins, which offer true postganglionic receptor imaging.

Cardiac PET also has been applied for noninvasive assessment of cardiac gene therapy. Animal experiments in rodents have shown that with a dedicated small animal PET, or microPET, noninvasive imaging of PET reporter genes combined with PET reporter probes affords determination of the location, magnitude, and time course of gene expression.[157,158] Although these experiments still need to be translated into clinical practice, the potential to noninvasively track gene therapy transfer and expression places cardiac PET imaging in the center of the molecular imaging paradigm for cardiovascular imaging.

REFERENCES

1. Bax JJ, Visser FC, van Lingen A, et al. Metabolic imaging using F18-fluorodeoxyglucose to assess myocardial viability. Int J Cardiovasc Imaging 1997;13(2):145–55, discussion 57–60.
2. Krivokapich J, Smith GT, Huang SC, et al. 13N ammonia myocardial imaging at rest and with exercise in normal volunteers. Quantification of absolute myocardial perfusion with dynamic positron emission tomography. Circulation 1989;80(5):1328–37.
3. Hutchins GD, Schwaiger M, Rosenspire KC, et al. Noninvasive quantification of regional blood flow in the human heart using N-13 ammonia and dynamic positron emission tomographic imaging. J Am Coll Cardiol 1990;15(5):1032–42.
4. Choi Y, Huang SC, Hawkins RA, et al. A simplified method for quantification of myocardial blood flow using nitrogen-13-ammonia and dynamic PET. J Nucl Med 1993;34(3):488–97.
5. Beanlands RS, Muzik O, Melon P, et al. Noninvasive quantification of regional myocardial flow reserve in patients with coronary atherosclerosis using nitrogen-13 ammonia positron emission tomography. Determination of extent of altered vascular reactivity. J Am Coll Cardiol 1995;26(6):1465–75.
6. Choi Y, Huang SC, Hawkins RA, et al. Quantification of myocardial blood flow using 13N-ammonia and PET: comparison of tracer models. J Nucl Med 1999;40(6):1045–55.
7. Schwaiger M, Ziegler SI, Bengel FM. Assessment of myocardial blood flow with positron emission tomography. In: Pohost GM, O'Rourke RA, Berman DS, editors. Imaging in cardiovascular disease. Philadelphia: Lippincott Williams and Wilkins; 2000. p. 195–212.
8. Bacharach SL, Bax JJ, Case J, et al. PET myocardial glucose metabolism and perfusion imaging: Part 1-Guidelines for data acquisition and patient preparation. J Nucl Cardiol 2003;10(5):543–56.
9. Beller GA, Bergmann SR. Myocardial perfusion imaging agents: SPECT and PET. J Nucl Cardiol 2004;11(1):71–86.
10. Sampson UK, Dorbala S, Limaye A, et al. Diagnostic accuracy of rubidium-82 myocardial perfusion imaging with hybrid positron emission tomography/computed tomography in the detection of coronary artery disease. J Am Coll Cardiol 2007;49(10):1052–8.
11. Go RT, Marwick TH, MacIntyre WJ, et al. A prospective comparison of rubidium-82 PET and thallium-201 SPECT myocardial perfusion imaging utilizing a single dipyridamole stress in the diagnosis of coronary artery disease. J Nucl Med 1990;31(12):1899–905.
12. Stewart RE, Schwaiger M, Molina E, et al. Comparison of rubidium-82 positron emission tomography and thallium-201 SPECT imaging for detection of coronary artery disease. Am J Cardiol 1991;67(16):1303–10.
13. Bateman TM, Heller GV, McGhie AI, et al. Diagnostic accuracy of rest/stress ECG-gated Rb-82 myocardial perfusion PET: comparison with ECG-gated Tc-99m sestamibi SPECT. J Nucl Cardiol 2006;13(1):24–33.
14. Nandalur KR, Dwamena BA, Choudhri AF, et al. Diagnostic performance of positron emission tomography in the detection of coronary artery disease: a meta-analysis. Acad Radiol 2008;15(4):444–51.
15. Patterson RE, Eisner RL, Horowitz SF. Comparison of cost-effectiveness and utility of exercise ECG, single photon emission computed tomography, positron emission tomography, and coronary angiography for diagnosis of coronary artery disease. Circulation 1995;91(1):54–65.
16. Schoenhagen P, Halliburton SS, Stillman AE, et al. Noninvasive imaging of coronary arteries: current and future role of multi-detector row CT. Radiology 2004;232(1):7–17.

17. Schoepf UJ, Becker CR, Ohnesorge BM, et al. CT of coronary artery disease. Radiology 2004; 232(1):18–37.

18. Leber AW, Knez A, Becker A, et al. Accuracy of multidetector spiral computed tomography in identifying and differentiating the composition of coronary atherosclerotic plaques: a comparative study with intracoronary ultrasound. J Am Coll Cardiol 2004;43(7):1241–7.

19. Di Carli M, Dorbala S, Limaye A, et al. Clinical value of hybrid PET/CT cardiac imaging: complementary roles of multi-detector CT coronary angiography and stress PET perfusion imaging. J Am Coll Cardiol 2006;47(4):115A.

20. Klocke FJ, Baird MG, Lorell BH, et al. ACC/AHA/ASNC guidelines for the clinical use of cardiac radionuclide imaging–executive summary: a report of the American College of Cardiology/American Heart association task force on practice guidelines (ACC/AHA/ASNC committee to revise the 1995 guidelines for the clinical use of cardiac radionuclide imaging). J Am Coll Cardiol 2003;42(7):1318–33.

21. Budoff MJ. Computed Tomography. In: Budoff MJ, Shinbane JS, editors. Cardiac CT imaging: diagnosis of cardiovascular disease. London: Springer-Verlag; 2006. p. 1–18.

22. Callister TQ, Raggi P, Cooil B, et al. Effect of HMG-CoA reductase inhibitors on coronary artery disease as assessed by electron-beam computed tomography. N Engl J Med 1998;339(27):1972–8.

23. O'Rourke RA, Brundage BH, Froelicher VF, et al. American College of Cardiology/American Heart Association Expert Consensus Document on electron-beam computed tomography for the diagnosis and prognosis of coronary artery disease. J Am Coll Cardiol 2000;36(1):326–40.

24. Wayhs R, Zelinger A, Raggi P. High coronary artery calcium scores pose an extremely elevated risk for hard events. J Am Coll Cardiol 2002;39(2):225–30.

25. Agatston AS, Janowitz WR, Hildner FJ, et al. Quantification of coronary artery calcium using ultrafast computed tomography. J Am Coll Cardiol 1990; 15(4):827–32.

26. Devries S, Wolfkiel C, Shah V, et al. Reproducibility of the measurement of coronary calcium with ultrafast computed tomography. Am J Cardiol 1995; 75(14):973–5.

27. Callister TQ, Cooil B, Raya SP, et al. Coronary artery disease: improved reproducibility of calcium scoring with an electron-beam CT volumetric method. Radiology 1998;208(3):807–14.

28. Rybicki FJ, Otero HJ, Steigner ML, et al. Initial evaluation of coronary images from 320-detector row computed tomography. Int J Cardiovasc Imaging 2008;24(5):535–46.

29. de Groot E, Jukema JW, van Boven AJ, et al. Effect of pravastatin on progression and regression of coronary atherosclerosis and vessel wall changes in carotid and femoral arteries: a report from the regression growth evaluation Statin study. Am J Cardiol 1995;76(9):40C–6C.

30. Desjardins B, Kazerooni EA. ECG-gated cardiac CT. AJR Am J Roentgenol 2004;182(4):993–1010.

31. Scanlon PJ, Faxon DP, Audet AM, et al. ACC/AHA guidelines for coronary angiography. A report of the American College of Cardiology/American Heart Association Task Force on practice guidelines (Committee on Coronary Angiography). Developed in collaboration with the society for cardiac angiography and interventions. J Am Coll Cardiol 1999;33(6):1756–824.

32. Smith SC Jr, Dove JT, Jacobs AK, et al. ACC/AHA guidelines for percutaneous coronary intervention (revision of the 1993 PTCA guidelines)—executive summary: a report of the American College of Cardiology/American Heart Association task force on practice guidelines (Committee to revise the 1993 guidelines for percutaneous transluminal coronary angioplasty) endorsed by the society for cardiac angiography and interventions. Circulation 2001;103(24):3019–41.

33. Goldstein JA, Gallagher MJ, O'Neill WW, et al. A randomized controlled trial of multi-slice coronary computed tomography for evaluation of acute chest pain. J Am Coll Cardiol 2007;49(8): 863–71.

34. Ehara M, Kawai M, Surmely JF, et al. Diagnostic accuracy of coronary in-stent restenosis using 64-slice computed tomography: comparison with invasive coronary angiography. J Am Coll Cardiol 2007;49(9):951–9.

35. Schiller NB, Shah PM, Crawford M, et al. Recommendations for quantitation of the left ventricle by two-dimensional echocardiography. American Society of Echocardiography Committee on standards, subcommittee on quantitation of two-dimensional echocardiograms. J Am Soc Echocardiogr 1989;2(5):358–67.

36. Dujardin KS, Enriquez-Sarano M, Rossi A, et al. Echocardiographic assessment of left ventricular remodeling: are left ventricular diameters suitable tools? J Am Coll Cardiol 1997;30(6):1534–41.

37. Helak JW, Reichek N. Quantitation of human left ventricular mass and volume by two-dimensional echocardiography: in vitro anatomic validation. Circulation 1981;63(6):1398–407.

38. Yamaoka O, Yabe T, Okada M, et al. Evaluation of left ventricular mass: comparison of ultrafast computed tomography, magnetic resonance imaging, and contrast left ventriculography. Am Heart J 1993;126(6):1372–9.

39. Zaidi H, Hasegawa B. Determination of the attenuation map in emission tomography. J Nucl Med 2003;44(2):291–315.

40. Uren NG, Crake T, Lefroy DC, et al. Reduced coronary vasodilator function in infarcted and normal myocardium after myocardial infarction. N Engl J Med 1994;331(4):222–7.

41. Yoshinaga K, Katoh C, Noriyasu K, et al. Reduction of coronary flow reserve in areas with and without ischemia on stress perfusion imaging in patients with coronary artery disease: a study using oxygen 15-labeled water PET. J Nucl Cardiol 2003;10(3): 275–83.

42. Thompson RC, McGhie AI, Moser KW, et al. Clinical utility of coronary calcium scoring after nonischemic myocardial perfusion imaging. J Nucl Cardiol 2005;12(4):392–400.

43. Berman DS, Wong ND, Gransar H, et al. Relationship between stress-induced myocardial ischemia and atherosclerosis measured by coronary calcium tomography. J Am Coll Cardiol 2004;44(4):923–30.

44. Schelbert HR. 18F-deoxyglucose and the assessment of myocardial viability. Semin Nucl Med 2002;32(1):60–9.

45. Keng FY. Clinical applications of positron emission tomography in cardiology: a review. Ann Acad Med Singap 2004;33(2):175–82.

46. Alderman EL, Fisher LD, Litwin P, et al. Results of coronary artery surgery in patients with poor left ventricular function (CASS). Circulation 1983; 68(4):785–95.

47. Emond M, Mock MB, Davis KB, et al. Long-term survival of medically treated patients in the Coronary Artery Surgery Study (CASS) Registry. Circulation 1994;90(6):2645–57.

48. Passamani E, Davis KB, Gillespie MJ, et al. A randomized trial of coronary artery bypass surgery. Survival of patients with a low ejection fraction. N Engl J Med 1985;312(26):1665–71.

49. Alderman EL, Corley SD, Fisher LD, et al. Five-year angiographic follow-up of factors associated with progression of coronary artery disease in the Coronary Artery Surgery Study (CASS). CASS Participating Investigators and Staff. J Am Coll Cardiol 1993;22(4):1141–54.

50. Mickleborough LL, Maruyama H, Takagi Y, et al. Results of revascularization in patients with severe left ventricular dysfunction. Circulation 1995;92(9 Suppl):II73–9.

51. Kaul TK, Agnihotri AK, Fields BL, et al. Coronary artery bypass grafting in patients with an ejection fraction of twenty percent or less. J Thorac Cardiovasc Surg 1996;111(5):1001–12.

52. Miller DC, Stinson EB, Alderman EL. Surgical treatment of ischemic cardiomyopathy; is it ever too late? Am J Surg 1981;141(6):688–93.

53. Luciani GB, Faggian G, Razzolini R, et al. Severe ischemic left ventricular failure: coronary operation or heart transplantation? Ann Thorac Surg 1993; 55(3):719–23.

54. Ellis SG, Fisher L, Dushman-Ellis S, et al. Comparison of coronary angioplasty with medical treatment for single- and double-vessel coronary disease with left anterior descending coronary involvement: long-term outcome based on an Emory-CASS registry study. Am Heart J 1989;118(2):208–20.

55. Shan K, Constantine G, Sivananthan M, et al. Role of cardiac magnetic resonance imaging in the assessment of myocardial viability. Circulation 2004;109(11):1328–34.

56. Tillisch J, Brunken R, Marshall R, et al. Reversibility of cardiac wall-motion abnormalities predicted by positron tomography. N Engl J Med 1986;314(14): 884–8.

57. Gropler RJ, Geltman EM, Sampathkumaran K, et al. Comparison of carbon-11-acetate with fluorine-18-fluorodeoxyglucose for delineating viable myocardium by positron emission tomography. J Am Coll Cardiol 1993;22(6):1587–97.

58. Lucignani G, Paolini G, Landoni C, et al. Presurgical identification of hibernating myocardium by combined use of technetium-99m hexakis 2-methoxyisobutylisonitrile single photon emission tomography and fluorine-18 fluoro-2-deoxy-D-glucose positron emission tomography in patients with coronary artery disease. Eur J Nucl Med 1992;19(10):874–81.

59. Tamaki N, Ohtani H, Yamashita K, et al. Metabolic activity in the areas of new fill-in after thallium-201 reinjection: comparison with positron emission tomography using fluorine-18-deoxyglucose. J Nucl Med 1991;32(4):673–8.

60. Marwick TH, MacIntyre WJ, Lafont A, et al. Metabolic responses of hibernating and infarcted myocardium to revascularization. A follow-up study of regional perfusion, function, and metabolism. Circulation 1992;85(4):1347–53.

61. Tamaki N, Yonekura Y, Yamashita K, et al. Prediction of reversible ischemia after coronary artery bypass grafting by positron emission tomography. J Cardiol 1991;21(2):193–201.

62. Tamaki N, Yonekura Y, Yamashita K, et al. Relation of change in wall motion and glucose metabolism after coronary artery bypass grafting—assessment with positron emission tomography. Jpn Circ J 1991;55(9):923–9.

63. Tamaki N, Yonekura Y, Yamashita K, et al. Positron emission tomography using fluorine-18 deoxyglucose in evaluation of coronary artery bypass grafting. Am J Cardiol 1989;64(14):860–5.

64. Tamaki N, Yonekura Y, Yamashita K, et al. Value of rest-stress myocardial positron tomography using nitrogen-13 ammonia for the preoperative prediction of reversible asynergy. J Nucl Med 1989; 30(8):1302–10.

65. vom Dahl J, Eitzman DT, al-Aouar ZR, et al. Relation of regional function, perfusion, and metabolism in

patients with advanced coronary artery disease undergoing surgical revascularization. Circulation 1994;90(5):2356–66.

66. Taegtmeyer H. Myocardial metabolism. In: Phelps ME, Mazziotta J, Schelbert HR, editors. Positron emission tomography and autoradiography: principles and applications for the brain and heart. New York: Raven Press; 1986. p. 149–95.

67. Liedtke AJ. Alterations of carbohydrate and lipid metabolism in the acutely ischemic heart. Prog Cardiovasc Dis 1981;23(5):321–36.

68. Liedtke AJ. The origins of myocardial substrate utilization from an evolutionary perspective: the enduring role of glucose in energy metabolism. J Mol Cell Cardiol 1997;29(4):1073–86.

69. Liedtke AJ, Renstrom B, Hacker TA, et al. Effects of moderate repetitive ischemia on myocardial substrate utilization. Am J Phys Am J Phys 1995; 269(1 Pt 2):H246–53.

70. Liedtke AJ, Renstrom B, Nellis SH, et al. Mechanical and metabolic functions in pig hearts after 4 days of chronic coronary stenosis. J Am Coll Cardiol 1995;26(3):815–25.

71. Vanoverschelde JL, Wijns W, Depre C, et al. Mechanisms of chronic regional postischemic dysfunction in humans. New insights from the study of noninfarcted collateral-dependent myocardium. Circulation 1993;87(5):1513–23.

72. Schelbert HR, Henze E, Phelps ME, et al. Assessment of regional myocardial ischemia by positron-emission computed tomography. Am Heart J 1982;103(4 Pt 2):588–97.

73. Schwaiger M, Fishbein MC, Block M, et al. Metabolic and ultrastructural abnormalities during ischemia in canine myocardium: noninvasive assessment by positron emission tomography. J Mol Cell Cardiol 1987;19(3):259–69.

74. Kalff V, Schwaiger M, Nguyen N, et al. The relationship between myocardial blood flow and glucose uptake in ischemic canine myocardium determined with fluorine-18-deoxyglucose. J Nucl Med 1992; 33(7):1346–53.

75. Knuuti MJ, Yki-Jarvinen H, Voipio-Pulkki LM, et al. Enhancement of myocardial [fluorine-18]fluorodeoxyglucose uptake by a nicotinic acid derivative. J Nucl Med 1994;35(6):989–98.

76. Kam BL, Valkema R, Poldermans D, et al. Feasibility and image quality of dual-isotope SPECT using 18F-FDG and (99m)Tc-tetrofosmin after acipimox administration. J Nucl Med 2003;44(2): 140–5.

77. Bax JJ, Veening MA, Visser FC, et al. Optimal metabolic conditions during fluorine-18 fluorodeoxyglucose imaging; a comparative study using different protocols. Eur J Nucl Med 1997;24(1): 35–41.

78. Martin WH, Jones RC, Delbeke D, et al. A simplified intravenous glucose loading protocol for fluorine-18 fluorodeoxyglucose cardiac single-photon emission tomography. Eur J Nucl Med 1997;24(10): 1291–7.

79. Knuuti MJ, Saraste M, Nuutila P, et al. Myocardial viability: fluorine-18-deoxyglucose positron emission tomography in prediction of wall motion recovery after revascularization. Am Heart J 1994; 127(4 Pt 1):785–96.

80. Schoder H, Campisi R, Ohtake T, et al. Blood flow-metabolism imaging with positron emission tomography in patients with diabetes mellitus for the assessment of reversible left ventricular contractile dysfunction. J Am Coll Cardiol 1999;33(5): 1328–37.

81. Baer FM, Voth E, Deutsch HJ, et al. Predictive value of low dose dobutamine transesophageal echocardiography and fluorine-18 fluorodeoxyglucose positron emission tomography for recovery of regional left ventricular function after successful revascularization. J Am Coll Cardiol 1996;28(1): 60–9.

82. Bax JJ, Cornel JH, Visser FC, et al. F18-fluorodeoxyglucose single-photon emission computed tomography predicts functional outcome of dyssynergic myocardium after surgical revascularization. J Nucl Cardiol 1997;4(4):302–8.

83. Marwick TH, Nemec JJ, Lafont A, et al. Prediction by postexercise fluoro-18 deoxyglucose positron emission tomography of improvement in exercise capacity after revascularization. Am J Cardiol 1992;69(9):854–9.

84. Di Carli MF, Asgarzadie F, Schelbert HR, et al. Quantitative relation between myocardial viability and improvement in heart failure symptoms after revascularization in patients with ischemic cardiomyopathy. Circulation 1995;92(12):3436–44.

85. Pagano D, Townend JN, Littler WA, et al. Coronary artery bypass surgery as treatment for ischemic heart failure: the predictive value of viability assessment with quantitative positron emission tomography for symptomatic and functional outcome. J Thorac Cardiovasc Surg 1998;115(4):791–9.

86. Landoni C, Lucignani G, Paolini G, et al. Assessment of CABG-related risk in patients with CAD and LVD. Contribution of PET with [18F]FDG to the assessment of myocardial viability. J Cardiovasc Surg (Torino) 1999;40(3):363–72.

87. Haas F, Haehnel CJ, Picker W, et al. Preoperative positron emission tomographic viability assessment and perioperative and postoperative risk in patients with advanced ischemic heart disease. J Am Coll Cardiol 1997;30(7):1693–700.

88. Beanlands RS, Hendry PJ, Masters RG, et al. Delay in revascularization is associated with increased mortality rate in patients with severe left ventricular

dysfunction and viable myocardium on fluorine 18-fluorodeoxyglucose positron emission tomography imaging. Circulation 1998;98(19 Suppl): II51–6.

89. Eitzman D, al-Aouar Z, Kanter HL, et al. Clinical outcome of patients with advanced coronary artery disease after viability studies with positron emission tomography. J Am Coll Cardiol 1992;20(3): 559–65.

90. Lee KS, Marwick TH, Cook SA, et al. Prognosis of patients with left ventricular dysfunction, with and without viable myocardium after myocardial infarction. Relative efficacy of medical therapy and revascularization. Circulation 1994;90(6):2687–94.

91. Di Carli MF, Maddahi J, Rokhsar S, et al. Long-term survival of patients with coronary artery disease and left ventricular dysfunction: implications for the role of myocardial viability assessment in management decisions. J Thorac Cardiovasc Surg 1998;116(6):997–1004.

92. Allman KC, Shaw LJ, Hachamovitch R, et al. Myocardial viability testing and impact of revascularization on prognosis in patients with coronary artery disease and left ventricular dysfunction: a meta-analysis. J Am Coll Cardiol 2002;39(7): 1151–8.

93. Woodard PK, Bhalla S, Javidan-Nejad C, et al. Cardiac MRI in the management of congenital heart disease in children, adolescents, and young adults. Curr Treat Options Cardiovasc Med 2008; 10(5):419–24.

94. Koskenvuo JW, Karra H, Lehtinen J, et al. Cardiac MRI: accuracy of simultaneous measurement of left and right ventricular parameters using three different sequences. Clin Physiol Funct Imaging 2007;27(6):385–93.

95. Lotz J, Meier C, Leppert A, et al. Cardiovascular flow measurement with phase-contrast MR imaging: basic facts and implementation. Radiographics 2002;22(3):651–71.

96. Desai MY, Lai S, Barmet C, et al. Reproducibility of 3D free-breathing magnetic resonance coronary vessel wall imaging. Eur Heart J 2005;26(21): 2320–4.

97. Dellegrottaglie S, Fayad ZA. Does the combination of stress perfusion and delayed-enhancement MRI improve the detection of CAD? Nat Clin Pract Cardiovasc Med 2006;3(9):472–3.

98. Jakob PM, Haase A. Basic pulse sequences for fast cardiac MR imaging. MAGMA 1998;6(2–3): 84–7.

99. Chrysikopoulos HS. Clinical MR imaging and physics: a tutorial. Berlin: Springer-Verlag; 2009.

100. Swaminathan S, Horn TD, Pellowski D, et al. Nephrogenic systemic fibrosis, gadolinium, and iron mobilization. N Engl J Med 2007;357(7):720–2.

101. Marckmann P, Skov L, Rossen K, et al. Nephrogenic systemic fibrosis: suspected causative role of gadodiamide used for contrast-enhanced magnetic resonance imaging. J Am Soc Nephrol 2006;17(9): 2359–62.

102. Nguyen TD, Spincemaille P, Cham MD, et al. Free-breathing 3D steady-state free precession coronary magnetic resonance angiography: comparison of diaphragm and cardiac fat navigators. J Magn Reson Imaging 2008;28(2):509–14.

103. Doesch C, Seeger A, Hoevelborn T, et al. Adenosine stress cardiac magnetic resonance imaging for the assessment of ischemic heart disease. Clin Res Cardiol 2008;97(12):905–12.

104. Jerosch-Herold M, Kwong RY. Optimal imaging strategies to assess coronary blood flow and risk for patients with coronary artery disease. Curr Opin Cardiol 2008;23(6):599–606.

105. Ripa RS, Nilsson JC, Wang Y, et al. Short- and long-term changes in myocardial function, morphology, edema, and infarct mass after ST-segment elevation myocardial infarction evaluated by serial magnetic resonance imaging. Am Heart J 2007; 154(5):929–36.

106. Bohl S, Wassmuth R, Abdel-Aty H, et al. Delayed enhancement cardiac magnetic resonance imaging reveals typical patterns of myocardial injury in patients with various forms of non-ischemic heart disease. Int J Cardiovasc Imaging 2008;24(6):597–607.

107. Jackson E, Bellenger N, Seddon M, et al. Ischaemic and non-ischaemic cardiomyopathies–cardiac MRI appearances with delayed enhancement. Clin Radiol 2007;62(5):395–403.

108. Hansen MW, Merchant N. MRI of hypertrophic cardiomyopathy: part I, MRI appearances. AJR Am J Roentgenol 2007;189(6):1335–43.

109. Francone M, Dymarkowski S, Kalantzi M, et al. Assessment of ventricular coupling with real-time cine MRI and its value to differentiate constrictive pericarditis from restrictive cardiomyopathy. Eur Radiol 2006;16(4):944–51.

110. Chinnaiyan KM, Leff CB, Marsalese DL. Constrictive pericarditis versus restrictive cardiomyopathy: challenges in diagnosis and management. Cardiol Rev 2004;12(6):314–20.

111. Syed IS, Feng D, Harris SR, et al. MR imaging of cardiac masses. Magn Reson Imaging Clin N Am 2008;16(2):137–64, vii.

112. Saha GB. Basics of PET imaging: physics, chemistry, and regulations. 1st edition. New York: Springer Science+Business Media, Inc; 2004.

113. Christensen NL, Hammer BE, Heil BG, et al. Positron emission tomography within a magnetic field using photomultiplier tubes and lightguides. Phys Med Biol 1995;40(4):691–7.

114. Slates RB, Farahani K, Shao Y, et al. A study of artefacts in simultaneous PET and MR imaging using a prototype MR compatible PET scanner. Phys Med Biol 1999;44(8):2015–27.

115. Woods RP, Mazziotta JC, Cherry SR. MRI-PET registration with automated algorithm. J Comput Assist Tomogr 1993;17(4):536–46.

116. Knuesel PR, Nanz D, Wyss C, et al. Characterization of dysfunctional myocardium by positron emission tomography and magnetic resonance: relation to functional outcome after revascularization. Circulation 2003;108(9):1095–100.

117. Bengel FM, Ueberfuhr P, Schiepel N, et al. Myocardial efficiency and sympathetic reinnervation after orthotopic heart transplantation: a noninvasive study with positron emission tomography. Circulation 2001;103(14):1881–6.

118. Glass CK, Witztum JL. Atherosclerosis. the road ahead. Cell 2001;104(4):503–16.

119. Virmani R, Burke AP, Farb A, et al. Pathology of the vulnerable plaque. J Am Coll Cardiol 2006;47 (8 Suppl):C13–8.

120. Robbie L, Libby P. Inflammation and atherothrombosis. Ann N Y Acad Sci 2001;947:167–79, discussion 79–80.

121. Libby P. Inflammation in atherosclerosis. Nature 2002;420(6917):868–74.

122. Ambrose JA, Tannenbaum MA, Alexopoulos D, et al. Angiographic progression of coronary artery disease and the development of myocardial infarction. J Am Coll Cardiol 1988;12(1):56–62.

123. Little WC, Constantinescu M, Applegate RJ, et al. Can coronary angiography predict the site of a subsequent myocardial infarction in patients with mild-to-moderate coronary artery disease? Circulation 1988;78(5 Pt 1):1157–66.

124. Myerburg RJ. Sudden cardiac death in persons with normal (or near normal) hearts. Am J Cardiol 1997;79(6A):3–9.

125. Fuster V, Badimon L, Badimon JJ, et al. The pathogenesis of coronary artery disease and the acute coronary syndromes (2). N Engl J Med 1992; 326(5):310–8.

126. Pasterkamp G, Schoneveld AH, van der Wal AC, et al. Relation of arterial geometry to luminal narrowing and histologic markers for plaque vulnerability: the remodeling paradox. J Am Coll Cardiol 1998;32(3):655–62.

127. Ogawa M, Ishino S, Mukai T, et al. (18)F-FDG accumulation in atherosclerotic plaques: immunohistochemical and PET imaging study. J Nucl Med 2004;45(7):1245–50.

128. Tawakol A, Migrino RQ, Hoffmann U, et al. Noninvasive in vivo measurement of vascular inflammation with F-18 fluorodeoxyglucose positron emission tomography. J Nucl Cardiol 2005;12(3):294–301.

129. Lederman RJ, Raylman RR, Fisher SJ, et al. Detection of atherosclerosis using a novel positron-sensitive probe and 18-fluorodeoxyglucose (FDG). Nucl Med Commun 2001;22(7):747–53.

130. Tahara N, Kai H, Nakaura H, et al. The prevalence of inflammation in carotid atherosclerosis: analysis with fluorodeoxyglucose-positron emission tomography. Eur Heart J 2007;28(18):2243–8.

131. Rudd JH, Warburton EA, Fryer TD, et al. Imaging atherosclerotic plaque inflammation with [18F]-fluorodeoxyglucose positron emission tomography. Circulation 2002;105(23):2708–11.

132. Tawakol A, Migrino RQ, Bashian GG, et al. In vivo 18F-fluorodeoxyglucose positron emission tomography imaging provides a noninvasive measure of carotid plaque inflammation in patients. J Am Coll Cardiol 2006;48(9):1818–24.

133. Tahara N, Kai H, Ishibashi M, et al. Simvastatin attenuates plaque inflammation: evaluation by fluorodeoxyglucose positron emission tomography. J Am Coll Cardiol 2006;48(9):1825–31.

134. Crisby M, Nordin-Fredriksson G, Shah PK, et al. Pravastatin treatment increases collagen content and decreases lipid content, inflammation, metalloproteinases, and cell death in human carotid plaques: implications for plaque stabilization. Circulation 2001;103(7):926–33.

135. Corti R, Fayad ZA, Fuster V, et al. Effects of lipid-lowering by simvastatin on human atherosclerotic lesions: a longitudinal study by high-resolution, noninvasive magnetic resonance imaging. Circulation 2001;104(3):249–52.

136. Ogawa M, Magata Y, Kato T, et al. Application of 18F-FDG PET for monitoring the therapeutic effect of antiinflammatory drugs on stabilization of vulnerable atherosclerotic plaques. J Nucl Med 2006; 47(11):1845–50.

137. Theron J, Tyler JL. Takayasu's arteritis of the aortic arch: endovascular treatment and correlation with positron emission tomography. AJNR Am J Neuroradiol 1987;8(4):621–6.

138. Mochizuki Y, Fujii H, Yasuda S, et al. FDG accumulation in aortic walls. Clin Nucl Med 2001;26(1):68–9.

139. Yun M, Yeh D, Araujo LI, et al. F-18 FDG uptake in the large arteries: a new observation. Clin Nucl Med 2001;26(4):314–9.

140. Yun M, Jang S, Cucchiara A, et al. 18F FDG uptake in the large arteries: a correlation study with the atherogenic risk factors. Semin Nucl Med 2002; 32(1):70–6.

141. Tatsumi M, Cohade C, Nakamoto Y, et al. Fluorodeoxyglucose uptake in the aortic wall at PET/CT: possible finding for active atherosclerosis. Radiology 2003;229(3):831–7.

142. Ben-Haim S, Kupzov E, Tamir A, et al. Evaluation of 18F-FDG uptake and arterial wall calcifications

using 18F-FDG PET/CT. J Nucl Med 2004;45(11): 1816–21.

143. Bural GG, Torigian DA, Chamroonrat W, et al. FDG-PET is an effective imaging modality to detect and quantify age-related atherosclerosis in large arteries. Eur J Nucl Med Mol Imaging 2008;35(3): 562–9.

144. Basu S, Zhuang H, Alavi A. Imaging of lower extremity artery atherosclerosis in diabetic foot: FDG-PET imaging and histopathological correlates. Clin Nucl Med 2007;32(7):567–8.

145. Dunphy MP, Freiman A, Larson SM, et al. Association of vascular 18F-FDG uptake with vascular calcification. J Nucl Med 2005;46(8):1278–84.

146. Ben-Haim S, Kupzov E, Tamir A, et al. Changing patterns of abnormal vascular wall F-18 fluorodeoxyglucose uptake on follow-up PET/CT studies. J Nucl Cardiol 2006;13(6):791–800.

147. Weissberg PL. Noninvasive imaging of atherosclerosis: the biology behind the pictures. J Nucl Med 2004;45(11):1794–5.

148. Davies JR, Rudd JH, Fryer TD, et al. Identification of culprit lesions after transient ischemic attack by combined 18F fluorodeoxyglucose positron-emission tomography and high-resolution magnetic resonance imaging. Stroke 2005;36(12): 2642–7.

149. Arauz A, Hoyos L, Zenteno M, et al. Carotid plaque inflammation detected by 18F-fluorodeoxyglucose-positron emission tomography. Pilot study. Clin Neurol Neurosurg 2007;109(5):409–12.

150. Paulmier B, Duet M, Khayat R, et al. Arterial wall uptake of fluorodeoxyglucose on PET imaging in stable cancer disease patients indicates higher risk for cardiovascular events. J Nucl Cardiol 2008;15(2):209–17.

151. Bural GG, Torigian DA, Chamroonrat W, et al. Quantitative assessment of the atherosclerotic burden of the aorta by combined FDG-PET and CT image analysis: a new concept. Nucl Med Biol 2006;33(8):1037–43.

152. Rudd JH, Myers KS, Bansilal S, et al. Atherosclerosis inflammation imaging with 18F-FDG PET: carotid, iliac, and femoral uptake reproducibility, quantification methods, and recommendations. J Nucl Med 2008;49(6):871–8.

153. Langer O, Halldin C. PET and SPET tracers for mapping the cardiac nervous system. Eur J Nucl Med Mol Imaging 2002;29(3):416–34.

154. Law MP, Osman S, Pike VW, et al. Evaluation of [11C]GB67, a novel radioligand for imaging myocardial alpha 1-adrenoceptors with positron emission tomography. Eur J Nucl Med 2000;27(1):7–17.

155. Delforge J, Le Guludec D, Syrota A, et al. Quantification of myocardial muscarinic receptors with PET in humans. J Nucl Med 1993;34(6):981–91.

156. Delforge J, Janier M, Syrota A, et al. Noninvasive quantification of muscarinic receptors in vivo with positron emission tomography in the dog heart. Circulation 1990;82(4):1494–504.

157. Wu JC, Inubushi M, Sundaresan G, et al. Positron emission tomography imaging of cardiac reporter gene expression in living rats. Circulation 2002; 106(2):180–3.

158. Inubushi M, Wu JC, Gambhir SS, et al. Positron-emission tomography reporter gene expression imaging in rat myocardium. Circulation 2003; 107(2):326–32.

Complementary Assessment of Abdominopelvic Disorders with PET/CT and MRI

Roland Hustinx, MD, PhD[a],*, Drew A. Torigian, MD, MA[b],
Gauthier Namur, MD[a]

KEYWORDS

- Cervical cancer • Pancreatic cancer
- Rectal cancer • Hepatic metastases
- Crohn's disease• Positron emission tomography
- PET/CT• PET/MR imaging

The advent of positron emission tomography (PET) and computed tomography (CT) devices has deeply modified the work-up of patients with many diseases, mainly in the field of oncology. PET/CT imaging is becoming a whole new specialty, and represents much more than the mere addition of CT and PET. Nuclear medicine physicians now benefit from the detailed anatomic information provided by CT, which helps to localize and better characterize sites of radiotracer uptake on PET. Radiologists are more accustomed to interpreting diagnostic-quality CT studies that are fully optimized for radiologic diagnosis; that is, with higher radiation dose and use of oral and intravenous contrast. They are now confronted with CT studies that are often obtained with a low-dose procedure and without contrast material, which is less than optimal in terms of diagnostic capabilities. Yet the combination of PET and low-dose unenhanced CT often leads to major positive changes in the diagnosis and staging of various malignancies. The diagnostic power of PET/CT is such that full diagnostic-quality CT often does not improve the diagnostic accuracy in a significant way. For example,

Kitajima and colleagues[1] performed a rigorous and very methodical comparison of contrast-enhanced CT (ceCT), 2-[18F]-fluoro-2-deoxy-D-glucose (FDG)-PET/CT, and PET/ceCT in 132 patients with suspected recurrent ovarian carcinoma. There was no significant difference in accuracy between PET/CT and PET/ceCT according to the patient-per-patient analysis, and an increase from 95.6% for PET/CT to 96.4% for PET/ceCT in terms of accuracy according to the lesion-per-lesion analysis. Similar conclusions can be reached in many other clinical situations,[2,3] although PET/ceCT has been shown to be the best option in others.[4] Nonetheless, as good as PET/CT is, it does not always provide all of the information needed by clinicians in some clinical situations to decide upon each patient's management.

Other imaging techniques, such as magnetic resonance (MR) imaging or ultrasonography (US), can offer new information that fully complements that provided by PET/CT, and in some scenarios yields a more complete picture of the true status of a patient's disease. MR imaging has several distinct advantages that are unmatched by other

[a] Division of Nuclear Medicine, University Hospital of Liège, Campus Universitaire du Sart Tilman B35, 4000 Liège, Belgium
[b] Department of Radiology, University of Pennsylvania School of Medicine, PA 19104, USA
* Corresponding author.
E-mail address: rhustinx@chu.ulg.ac.be (R. Hustinx).

PET Clin 3 (2009) 435–449
doi:10.1016/j.cpet.2009.02.002

diagnostic techniques. It provides high spatial resolution-multiplanar images without use of ionizing radiation and provides contrast resolution that is superior to that of CT, even when intravenous contrast material is not administered. This article discusses several examples of disease in which PET/CT and MR imaging offer a very potent combination of noninvasive diagnostic techniques. As the technical feasibility of PET/MR imaging has recently been demonstrated for human brain imaging,[5] these clinical situations may represent a good model for potential clinical applications of this emerging technology.

CERVICAL CARCINOMA

Cervical cancer is the third most common cancer in women worldwide and the second most common cause of cancer death in women.[6] The majority of the cases occur in developing countries, and screening has lead to a steady decrease in incidence in the Western world. Nonetheless, 11,070 new cases were expected to be diagnosed in the United States in 2008, with 3,870 expected deaths from the disease.[7] The staging of the disease follows the classification established by the International Federation of Gynecology and Obstetrics (FIGO).[8] This classification mainly relies upon clinical assessment of the local spread of the tumor (**Table 1**). Patients with very limited disease (FIGO stage IA1, invasion ≤ 3 mm in depth) may be treated with simple hysterectomy, without

lymphadenectomy. Early-stage disease (FIGO IB–IIA) may be treated with radical hysterectomy and pelvic lymphadenectomy or primary radiation therapy, with similar outcome. The latter is associated with more side effects, such as loss of ovarian function, so that it is often limited to patients with significant comorbidity that contraindicate surgery. Tumors with further local progression (up to FIGO stage IVA) are treated with a combination of chemotherapy and radiation therapy. Metastatic disease is associated with a very dire prognosis and is usually treated with palliative chemotherapy.[9] The FIGO staging system has regularly been subject to heavy criticism, in particular because it neglects the lymph node status of the disease, which is among the most important predictive factors of survival.[10] Furthermore, a purely clinical staging assessment underestimates the extent of the disease in about 24% of the patients with FIGO stage IB, when compared with surgical staging.[11] In addition, cervical cancer often strikes young patients for whom the possibility of childbearing in the future is an important issue. Consequently, surgical techniques have been developed to replace radical hysterectomy and preserve fertility potential, while maintaining similar long-term survival rates.[12] The decision to carry out such conservative approach is taken according to findings that are not integrated into the FIGO staging system, in particular the size of the tumor. Considering all of these elements, it clearly appears that imaging methods that are not

Table 1
International FIGO staging classification

Stage	Details
IA1	Invasive carcinoma, confined to cervix, diagnosed by microscopy. Stromal invasion ≤ 3mm in depth and ≤ 7 mm in horizontal spread
IA2	Invasive carcinoma, confined to cervix, diagnosed only by microscopy. Stromal invasion > 3 mm and < 5 mm in depth and ≤ 7 mm in horizontal spread
IB1	Invasive carcinoma, confined to cervix, microscopic lesion > IA2 or clinically visible lesion ≤ 4 cm in greatest dimension
IB2	Invasive carcinoma, confined to cervix, clinically visible lesion > 4 cm in greatest dimension
IIA	Tumor extension beyond cervix to vagina but not to lower third of vagina. No parametrial invasion
IIB	Tumor extension beyond cervix. Parametrial invasion but not to pelvic sidewall and not to lower third of vagina
IIIA	Tumor extension to lower third of vagina but not to pelvic sidewall
IIIB	Tumor extension to pelvic sidewall or causing hydronephrosis or non-functioning kidney
IVA	Tumor invasion into bladder or rectum
IVB	Distant metastasis

currently recommended within the FIGO frame, but that would reliably assess both the local extent of the disease and its nodal spread, would be of great value for helping the oncologic gynecologist to decide upon the best treatment scheme.

Local Staging

A systematic review was published in 2003, comparing the performances of CT and MR imaging in staging cervical carcinoma.[13] Through a review of a total of 57 articles, the investigators found that MR imaging was more sensitive than CT for detecting parametrial invasion (74% versus 55%), bladder invasion (75% versus 64%), and rectal invasion (71% versus 45%). Specificities were similar except for bladder invasion (91% versus 73%). Hricak and colleagues[14] reviewed 146 CT studies and 152 MR imaging studies in patients with invasive cervical cancer, and compared the findings with the surgical assessment. The interobserver agreement was higher with MR imaging than with CT for both tumor visualization and detection of parametrial invasion, although it was low with both techniques. The sensitivity of MR imaging for evaluating parametrial invasion was also higher than with CT, albeit not as high as previously reported: the area under the curve was 0.68 for MR imaging and 0.62 for CT. It is worth mentioning that in guidelines published this year, the European Society of Medical Oncology recommends abdominopelvic MR imaging to be preferred to CT in the initial staging, although with a low level of evidence. The diagnostic performances of PET and PET/CT for evaluating local spread have not been appropriately studied. Although the sensitivity for visualizing the primary tumor is usually greater than 90%, neither PET nor PET/CT are expected to provide any relevant and reliable information regarding parametrial invasion.[15]

Nodal Staging

A recent meta-analysis showed that FDG-PET was the most accurate imaging method for assessing the lymph node status of cervical cancer.[16] The pooled sensitivity and specificity were 74.7% and 97.6%, respectively, compared with 55.5% and 93.2% for MR imaging, and 57.5% and 92.3% for CT. In terms of likelihood ratios (LR), the positive LR was 15.3 for PET (6.4 for MR imaging) and the negative LR was 0.27 (0.5 for MR imaging). A total of 445 patients were included in eight articles regarding PET, but none of these included PET/CT imaging. However, recent studies reported similar results with PET/CT. In a series of 120 patients with FIGO stage IB or higher, Loft and

colleagues[17] found 75% sensitivity and 96% specificity for pelvic nodal staging, and 100% sensitivity and 99% specificity for para-aortic nodal staging. In a population of patients with clinical early-stage disease (FIGO IA or IB), Sironi and colleagues[18] found a sensitivity of 72% and specificity of 99.7%, with a pathologic gold standard obtained in over a thousand lymph nodes. All false-negative nodes were smaller than 5 mm in diameter. The low sensitivity of FDG-PET for detecting micrometastases was confirmed by Chou and colleagues[19] in a series 60 patients with nonbulky and MR imaging-negative nodal status. In this study, PET detected only 1 out of 10 malignant pelvic lymph nodes, with a median size of 4 mm by 3 mm. Using PET/CT instead of PET alone might have changed the results, although it is unlikely that a much higher sensitivity could be reached in such a population. Indeed, the gold standard was pathologic examination of lymph nodes obtained by intraoperative sentinel lymph node detection, a method known to enhance the overall detection of metastatic nodes, including micrometastases.[16] Nevertheless, the results of Chou and colleagues[19] represent an outlier in the literature, as PET and PET/CT have been consistently reported to be more accurate and more sensitive than MR imaging for nodal staging.[20–22]

The added value of metabolic imaging is particularly evident for detecting para-aortic nodal metastases.[23,24] Such involvement is infrequent in early stage disease, but is found in 15% to 30% of patients with stages FIGO IB2 and higher.[11] The higher the stage, the higher the likelihood of showing para-aortic nodal metastases, but even in patients with FIGO stages IB2/II, PET/CT had a 92% negative predictive value.[25] PET also proved useful in patients with a more advanced FIGO stage and positive lymph nodes on MR imaging, by either downstaging or upstaging the disease, with a positive impact on patient management in 45% of cases.[26] Delayed or dual time-point FDG-PET imaging may further improve the diagnostic performance compared with a conventional uptake time of 60 minutes, especially for distant lesions.[27,28] Currently, a prospective clinical trial is underway through the Gynecologic Oncology Group and American College of Radiology Imaging Network to assess the utility of preoperative FDG-PET/CT and ultrasmall superparamagnetic iron-oxide nanoparticle (USPIO) MR imaging before primary chemoradiation therapy to detect retroperitoneal lymph node metastases in patients with locoregionally advanced (IB2, IIA $\geq$ 4 cm, IIB-IVA) cervical carcinoma. On T2*-weighted USPIO MR images, lymph nodes are interpreted as abnormal if one or more discrete high-signal intensity focal defects are seen centrally or peripherally (excluding a fatty hilum) or if the node has diffusely high-signal intensity, which are assumed to indicate the presence of focal or diffuse micrometastatic disease to the lymph node, respectively. In addition, lymph nodes are considered as normal if low T2*-weighted signal intensity and moderate-high proton-density-weighted signal intensity relative to skeletal muscle is seen.

Prognostic Factors

As mentioned earlier, the FIGO staging system does not account for all relevant factors predicting the long-term outcome.[10] Both MR imaging and PET/CT provide valuable additional information. Uterine corpus invasion and high tumor volume as determined with MR imaging are independently associated with increased risk of local or nodal relapse.[29] As the lymph node status strongly influences survival,[30,31] the good diagnostic performances of PET and PET/CT in that setting should in all likelihood translate into prognostic significance. Few data are available, but initial results confirm this hypothesis.[32–34] Both pelvic and para-aortic PET-positive lymph nodes are strongly associated with shorter disease-free survival compared with PET-negative nodes.[34] Furthermore, the intensity of the FDG uptake by the para-aortic lymph nodes seems to be a significant predictive factor, especially when combined with the FIGO stage.[35] In a series of 70 patients, the 5-year overall survival rate was 84% in patients with FIGO stage less than or equal to II and maximum standard uptake value (SUV) less than 3.3, compared with 50% in patients with higher FIGO stages and higher SUVs.[35] At this point, however, the clinical relevance of such findings is uncertain and further studies are needed before considering use of the metabolic activity as a parameter directly influencing therapeutic planning. Two examples of MR imaging and PET/CT images in the setting of cervical cancer are shown in **Figs. 1** and **2**.

PANCREATIC CANCER
Pancreatic Adenocarcinoma

Pancreatic ductal adenocarcinoma is increasing in incidence and remains associated with a very dire prognosis. The estimated number of new diagnoses in 2008 in the United States is 37,680, with an estimated 34,290 deaths.[7] Surgery is the only curative treatment, but only a minority of patients has resectable disease at presentation. The median survival in case of locally advanced or metastatic disease does not exceed 10 months.[36] CT is the preferred modality for diagnosing

pancreatic adenocarcinoma. A meta-analysis performed in 2005 reported sensitivities of 91% for CT, 84% for MR imaging, and 76% for US in the diagnosis of pancreatic adenocarcinoma, with specificities of 85%, 82%, and 75%, respectively.[37] FDG-PET has been extensively studied in this setting, with sensitivity ranging from 85% to 100%, and specificity ranging from 67% to 99%.[38] The sensitivity is reduced by elevated blood-glucose levels, which is a common occurrence in patients with pancreatic cancer.[39] Specificity may be hampered by significant uptake in inflammatory masses, including both chronic and acute pancreatitis.[40,41] PET/CT has brought significant improvements as compared with PET alone, especially for evaluating the resectability of the lesion. The positive predictive value for cancer is high (91%–97%), whereas the negative predictive value is somewhat lower (64%–68%).[42,43] Such a low figure must be tempered by the small number of benign pancreatic lesions in the population studied (less than 25%). More importantly, PET/CT changed management in 11% to 16% of the patients, and a Swiss publication showed a favorable cost-effectiveness ratio, with an estimated $1.07 saved per patient, obtained mainly by avoiding unnecessary surgery in five cases.[43] It should be noted, however, that the methodologic approach has been criticized and that the cost-effectiveness of the study cannot be considered as fully established.[44]

More recently, Strobel and colleagues proposed the so-called "one-stop-shop" imaging for the preoperative evaluation of pancreatic cancer, combining PET and ceCT in a single imaging session. Such an approach is logical, as on the one hand ceCT clearly depicts the shape and size of the lesion as well as its relationship with adjacent structures, such as the mesenteric vasculature, whereas on the other hand, PET displays the highest sensitivity for detecting distant lesions. In their study, Strobel and colleagues found a 82% positive predictive value and a 96% negative predictive value for evaluating resectability with PET/ceCT, greater than with PET alone and unenhanced PET/CT, although the difference was not statistically significant with the latter.

MR imaging is not superior to CT and PET/CT in the diagnosis and staging of pancreatic adenocarcinoma, but is often used to solve specific problems, for example in patients with inconclusive CT results.[45] Furthermore, MR cholangiopancreatography provides excellent images of the extrahepatic biliary tract and pancreatic ducts, and is therefore a strong alternative to invasive endoscopic retrograde cholangiopancreatography, at least for diagnostic purposes.[46] Combination of

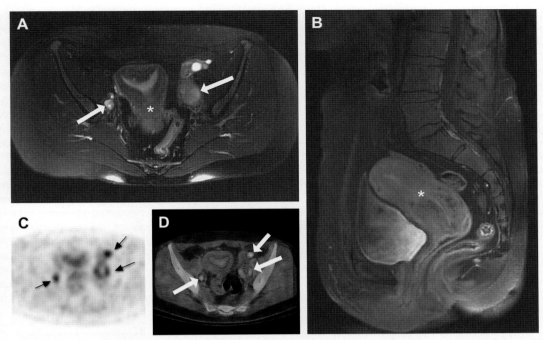

Fig. 1. Patient newly diagnosed with FIGO stage IIb squamous cell carcinoma of cervix. Axial fat-suppressed T2-weighted (*A*) and sagittal fat-suppressed contrast-enhanced T1-weighted (*B*) images show invasion of uterine corpus (*) and anterior vaginal wall, as well as bilateral iliac lymphadenopathy (*arrows*). Axial FDG-PET (*C*) and fused PET/CT images (*D*) also show hypermetabolic nodal metastases (*arrows*).

PET/CT and MR imaging could therefore constitute a powerful diagnostic and staging approach, as both MR imaging and PET characterize the pancreatic lesion, with MR imaging defining its relationship with adjacent structures, including the vasculature and pancreaticobiliary ductal system, and PET/CT identifying distant metastases, especially to the liver. The relative

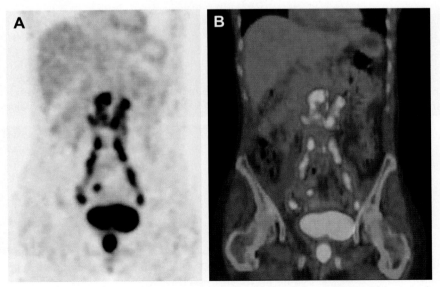

Fig. 2. Patient with nodal spread of cervical cancer. Coronal PET (*A*) and fused PET/CT (*B*) images show increased FDG uptake within bilateral iliac and para-aortic lymph node chains.

contribution of PET/CT plus MR imaging compared with PET/ceCT would be worth evaluating, as without the multiple-phase CT a lower radiation dose would be delivered and no iodinated contrast agent would be needed. **Fig. 3** shows MR imaging and PET/CT images from a patient with pancreatic cancer.

Cystic Pancreatic Lesions

Cystic pancreatic lesions are often incidental findings not related to the initial clinical indications for abdominal imaging studies performed in patients. These lesions may be malignant, such as by intraductal papillary mucinous tumors and macroscopic mucinous cystadenomas/cystadenocarcinomas, but may also be benign, such as by microcystic serous cystadenomas or pseudocysts. The diagnosis remains to be a challenge and relies upon a combination of techniques, as no single modality is able to achieve the diagnostic

certainty necessary to direct the treatment choice in all cases.[47] MR imaging and CT are generally considered to perform equally and fairly well for differentiating benign from malignant lesions.[47,48] Endoscopic ultrasonography (EUS) with fine needle aspiration is useful, as it allows for analysis of the internal cystic fluid. High content in carcinoembryonic antigen (CEA) and presence of mucin or cancer cells are all strong indicators for a mucinous tumor. Nevertheless, MR and CT images of these cystic lesions may be very difficult to interpret. MR imaging provides higher soft-tissue contrast, which may represent an advantage in this setting.[49] Two distinct studies from the same group of investigators reported excellent results in the characterization of cystic lesions with FDG-PET.[50,51] Sensitivity was 94% overall, 80% for detecting carcinomas in situ, and 95% for invasive carcinomas. All these characteristics were superior to those obtained with CT. These findings were not confirmed by Mansour and colleagues,[52]

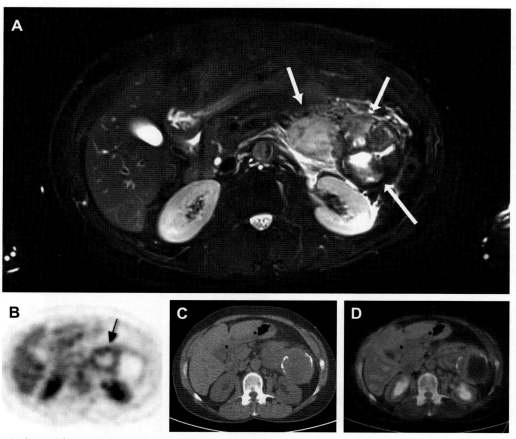

Fig. 3. Patient with pancreatic cancer. Axial fat-suppressed T2-weighted image (*A*) demonstrates bilobed heterogenous high signal intensity mass in pancreatic tail (*arrows*). Axial PET (*B*), CT (*C*), and fused PET/CT (*D*) images from FDG-PET/CT examination show mass with peripheral areas of FDG uptake (*arrows*), indicating central cystic or necrotic change.

who found a much lower sensitivity (57%) in a population of 21 patients who underwent surgery. There is no data regarding integrated PET/CT imaging in this setting, although Tann and colleagues[53] retrospectively reviewed 30 PET/CT and ceCT performed in patients with pancreatic cystic lesions. They found unusually low sensitivity (57%) and specificity (65%) for PET, using an SUV cut-off of 2.5. Nonetheless, the combined reading of the PET and ceCT data was more sensitive than either modality alone, with a specificity that remained similar to that observed with ceCT alone.

RECTAL CANCER

An estimated 40,740 new cases of rectal cancer are expected to occur in 2008 in the United States. There is no separate figure for rectal cancer mortality, but the expected number of deaths from colorectal cancer is 49,960.[7] The staging process is used to evaluate the local depth of tumor invasion (T stage), the presence and number of involved lymph nodes (N stage), and distant metastases (M stage). Early-stage disease (T1-2N0) is treated by surgery, followed by adjuvant combined radiation and chemotherapy in case of positive nodes at pathology, or locally more advanced disease (pT3). Patients with locally advanced disease (T3–T4 or N+) undergo neoadjuvant radiation therapy or combined treatment, followed by surgery. Metastatic disease will be evaluated, and synchronous or staged metastatic resection is performed whenever possible, usually following neoadjuvant chemotherapy.[54] Staging is therefore of primary importance, both at the local and distant level.

A meta-analysis comparing EUS, CT, and MR imaging for local and nodal staging of rectal cancer was published in 2004.[55] MR imaging and EUS are equally sensitive for identifying muscularis propria invasion (94%), and EUS is more specific (86% versus 69%). EUS is more sensitive (90%) than both CT (79%) and MR imaging (82%) for detecting perirectal tissue invasion, with comparable specificities (75%–78%). The sensitivity of all three techniques is similar for detecting adjacent organ invasion (70%–74%) or lymph node involvement (55%–67%). For lymph node staging, the low sensitivity is also associated with a poor specificity (74%–78%). In addition to the TNM stage, the relationship between the tumor and the circumferential resection margin (CRM) is critical, as this parameter has a major impact on the local recurrence rate. The CRM is assessed at pathology, and a tumor within 1 mm to 2 mm of the resection margin defines a positive CRM. Therefore, precise knowledge of the CRM before

surgery would be of great value. Indeed, downstaging may be achieved through preoperative chemoradiotherapy but the decision to treat is not taken lightly, given the impact on relapse rate on the one hand and the significant treatment-associated side effects on the other hand.[56] A recently published multicenter prospective study correlated the maximal extramural depth of tumor spread according to the preoperative MR imaging with the pathologic gold standard.[57] The results were quite impressive, as MR imaging and pathologic assessments were within 0.5 mm of each other. In 22 out of 295 patients (7.5%), MR imaging overestimated the extramural depth of invasion by more than 5 mm, which would have led to inappropriate management of the patients. This compares favorably with the 18% of overstaging rating observed with EUS in a recent prospective therapeutic trial.[58] In fact, a meta-analysis published in 2004 concluded that MR imaging was the only imaging modality that predicts the circumferential resection margin with reasonable accuracy.[59]

Nodal staging remains problematic, regardless of which conventional imaging technique is used. According to most initial studies, FDG-PET had a limited sensitivity for detecting regional metastatic lymph nodes from colorectal cancer, mainly because of their close spatial relationship with a bulky primary tumor. In those cases, the nodes cannot be distinguished from the tumor.[60,61] More recent studies, however, are more encouraging. Bassi and colleagues[62] found, with PET/CT, additional regional lymph nodes in 3 out of 25 patients whose conventional work-up included CT and EUS (change from N0 to N1). In a series of 83 patients with rectal cancer, PET/CT changed the stage of the disease in 26 cases (31%), including 17 changes in N stages, equally distributed between upstaging and downstaging.[63] Approximately two-thirds of the patients were evaluated with MR imaging and the remainder with EUS; all had abdominopelvic CT. Similarly, Gearhart and colleagues[64] found discordant findings with PET/CT in 14 out of 37 patients with low rectal cancer initially evaluated with CT and either MR imaging or EUS. The most common finding was detection of additional lymph nodes, half of them located in the iliac or inguinal areas. Such locations may be explained by the sample population, which included lower rectal primary tumors. It should be noted that, similar to colon cancer, PET/CT also has a high sensitivity for detecting distant metastases, including those located in the liver.[65]

In addition to contributing to the staging, PET/CT provides additional information that is useful in the subgroup of patients with locally advanced disease. As mentioned earlier, the standard of care for these patients is chemoradiotherapy. As radiation therapy is becoming increasingly conformal, the delineation of the target volume is critical to achieve the best local tumor control, while sparing normal tissue radiation damage. The metabolic volume is therefore increasingly taken into account to define the target volume. A recent study showed an average increase in the gross tumor volume of 24% when defined with PET/CT, as compared with the CT-defined gross tumor volume.[62] Furthermore, as demonstrated by several studies, the metabolic response predicts the pathologic response after chemoradiotherapy.[66–68] Methodologic issues remain to be clarified, such as how to assess the metabolic response or what the best time-frame is for imaging after completion of treatment. However, this field is involved in active investigation, and Kalff and colleagues[69] recently reported that radiation changes were not a factor limiting the capacity of PET to predict the outcome when performed within 6 weeks after completion of therapy. **Fig. 4** shows PET/CT and MR images of a patient with metastatic rectal cancer.

LIVER METASTASES

The liver is the most frequent site of hematogenous metastatic dissemination. Although virtually all cancer types may spread to the liver, colorectal cancer ranks first in the list of primary tumors, and close to 50% of colorectal cancer patients develop liver metastases, either initially or during the course of the disease. Provided that patients are carefully selected, surgery is efficient and relatively safe, as the 5-year survival rate after curative resection of liver metastases may reach 58%.[70] The conventional patient-selection criteria for resectability of colorectal metastases—that is, no more than three small metastases, ability to achieve a resection margin of at least 1 cm, and no extrahepatic disease—have been expanded in a major way. The selection criteria now rely upon technical considerations, so that all patients whose performance status is acceptable and whose metastatic lesions may technically be removed with negative margins and adequate residual hepatic volume/reserve, either through primary intent or after appropriate preparatory treatment (such as neoadjuvant chemotherapy, radiofrequency ablation, or portal vein embolization) are eligible for resectability.[70]

Two meta-analyses investigate the ability of various imaging methods for detecting liver metastases. Both found higher sensitivity for FDG-PET. The first one was published in 2002 and included studies published until 2000.[71] It concluded that

at equivalent specificity, PET was significantly more sensitive than CT and US, and marginally more sensitive than MR imaging (90% and 76%, respectively). A second meta-analysis was published in 2005 and included more recent studies, up to December 2003.[37] This study focused on liver metastases from colorectal cancer and left US out of the analysis because of its very low sensitivity for detecting small metastases. With 94.6%, PET imaging was again the most sensitive technique in the patient-per-patient analysis, compared with 64.7% for CT and 75.8% for MR imaging. Differences were smaller in the lesion-per-lesion analysis, with sensitivities of 75.9%, 63.8%, and 64.4%, respectively. It was also shown that enhancement with gadolinium (Gd) or superparamagnetic iron oxide (SPIO) improved the sensitivity of MR imaging. SPIO is taken up by the reticuloendothelial Kupffer cells in the liver, resulting in a decrease in the normal liver signal intensity on the T2-weighted images, whereas metastases to the liver do not lose signal intensity. Manganese (Mn)-based hepatobiliary MR imaging contrast agents, such as mangafodipir trisodium (MnDPDP), may also be useful to image the liver, as they are taken up by the hepatocytes, so that the signal intensity from the normal hepatocellular tissue of the liver is increased on T1-weighted images. There is no consensus as to which of these contrast agents should be preferred, although liver-specific contrast agents, either hepatobiliary or reticuloendothelial agents, appear to provide diagnostic advantages over unenhanced and Gd-enhanced MR imaging alone.[72] However, in routine clinical practice, the use of liver-specific MR imaging contrast agents remains limited, whereas the employment of Gd-based MR imaging contrast agents remains the most popular method in the majority of diagnostic imaging facilities.

Several studies investigating the added value of PET/CT have been published in the past few years. Both ceCT and FDG-PET/CT were reported to be highly sensitive in a series of 76 colorectal cancer patients with liver metastases, and PET/CT was slightly more specific, especially in patients with a history of liver surgery.[73] Others found similar sensitivities for ceCT, SPIO-MR imaging, and FDG-PET/CT for detecting liver metastases on a patient-per-patient basis.[74] FDG-PET/CT was slightly less sensitive in the lesion-per-lesion analysis, but was also more specific. Similar results were found by Kong and colleagues,[75] who performed PET/CT and MnDPDP-MR imaging in 65 patients with suspected liver involvement from colorectal cancer. Both techniques performed equally well in terms of sensitivity, with a slight

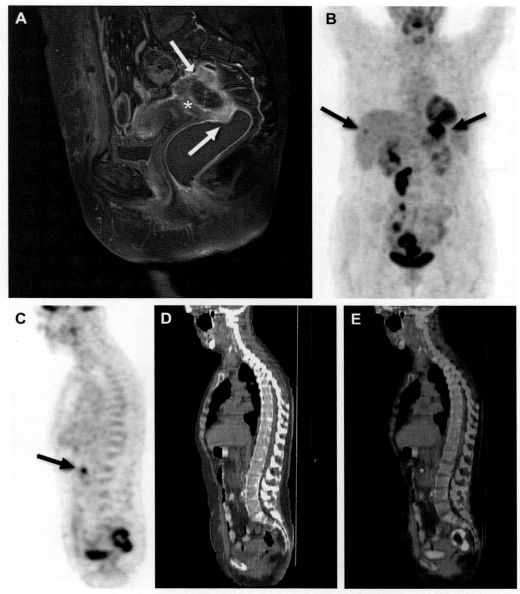

Fig. 4. Patient with upper rectal adenocarcinoma. Sagittal fat-suppressed contrast-enhanced T1-weighted image (A) reveals local spread to tumor (arrows) to posterior wall of uterus (*). Coronal (B) and sagittal (C) PET images, sagittal CT image (D), and sagittal fused PET/CT image (E) from FDG-PET/CT examination show rectal mass with FDG uptake, metastases to both lobes of liver (arrows in B), and omental implant (arrow in C) in keeping with peritoneal carcinomatosis.

advantage for MR imaging for detecting small metastases. Two recent studies emphasized an increase in diagnostic performance for PET/ceCT as compared with PET/CT.[76,77] In a study by Soyka and colleagues,[76] the main benefit was observed in patients who underwent surgical resection of liver metastases. In these patients, ceCT was needed for exact localization of lesions. In the study by Cantwell and colleagues,[77] the

sensitivity (67%) and specificity (60%) of PET/CT were both markedly lower than all of those values reported in the literature thus far. In any case, most studies reach similar conclusions: PET/CT is equally effective or superior to ceCT for detecting liver metastases, MR imaging with liver-specific contrast agents is more sensitive than PET/CT for identifying small subcentimeter lesions, and the whole-body PET/CT survey detects additional extrahepatic lesions that lead to changes in patient management in 20% to 25% of cases.[73,75] The combination of MR imaging and PET/CT therefore appears as ideally suited for optimal detection of hepatic metastases from colorectal cancer and other malignancies, and for staging of those patients, especially in the preoperative setting. **Fig. 5** illustrates PET/CT and MR images from a patient with metastatic colon cancer.

CROHN'S DISEASE

Crohn's disease (CD) is a chronic inflammatory disease of the gastrointestinal tract. Clinically, it often presents with successive periods of clinical relapse and remission. Pathologically, it is considered as a chronic active disease with a continuous inflammatory process. CD is frequently complicated by fibrotic or deeply penetrating lesions, leading to intestinal strictures and fistulas. Only a minority of patients are affected by these complications at diagnosis, although they occur in up to 50% to

60% of patients after 10 years of disease. The goal of treatment is to maintain as good a quality of life as possible by sustaining remission and avoiding complications. Monitoring the activity of the disease may be challenging, especially in patients with symptoms suggesting active disease but with biologic markers within the normal range, and in patients with clinically inactive disease but who may silently evolve toward stricturing or fistulizing complications. Blood inflammatory markers, such as C-reactive protein (CRP) serum levels may be useful, but are imperfectly correlated to inflammatory intestinal lesions.[78] Endoscopic evaluation is considered the gold standard to assess intestinal lesions, but ileocolonoscopy is invasive, unpleasant for patients, and sometimes cannot be completed because of inaccessibility of some bowel segments. Endoscopic assessment is also limited to the evaluation of mucosal lesions, while the disease may affect deeper portions of the bowel wall.

Cross-sectional imaging methods are now used in routine practice to evaluate patients with CD. CT is particularly useful for diagnosing bowel-wall

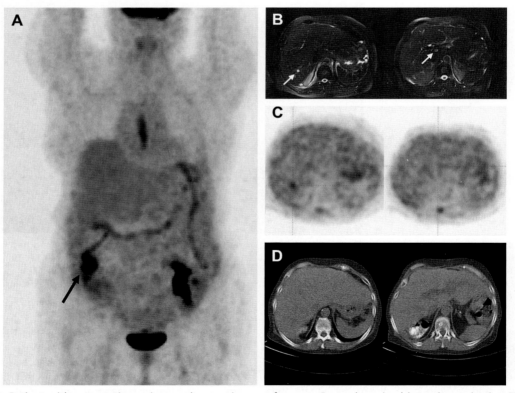

Fig. 5. Patient with metastatic mucinous adenocarcinoma of cecum. Coronal maximal intensity projection FDG-PET image (*A*) before surgery demonstrates avid FDG uptake in cecal tumor (*arrow*). Eleven months later, patient's serum CEA level increased and additional imaging was performed. Axial fat-suppressed T2-weighted images (*B*) show two subcentimeter high signal intensity metastases in liver, only one of which demonstrates increased FDG uptake on axial FDG-PET images (*C*), and neither of which is visible on low-dose unenhanced CT images (*D*).

thickening and abdominal complications of CD, and MR imaging is very useful for the evaluation of perianal CD, particularly for the delineation of fistulous and sinus tracts. CT enterography and MR enterography (MRE) are also emerging as tools to assess both disease extent and activity in small-bowel CD.[79,80] CT has come under scrutiny because of the radiation dose associated with the study. Indeed, the use of CT has significantly increased over the past 15 years, leading to cumulative effective doses higher than 75 mSv in small subgroups of high-risk patients.[81] The impact of the radiation dose is of particular concern in younger patients, and there is call among the clinical gastroenterology community for the development of procedures with limited radiation exposure.[82] Although MR imaging does not involve the use of ionizing radiation, the best images of the small bowel are obtained with MRE, which is often not as well tolerated by patients. Ongoing studies are underway to assess the value of MRE and MR colonography with oral contrast material. Clinical results are variable, but this is an area of research that is rapidly changing.[83–85]

Initial results with FDG-PET in inflammatory bowel disease were very encouraging, in particular in pediatric patients.[86,87] More recently, FDG-PET/CT was investigated by two different groups with similar results. In a pilot study including 12 patients (seven with CD and five with ulcerative colitis), Meisner and colleagues[88] found a good correlation between metabolic activity and clinical score.

In a more homogeneous and slightly larger series, Louis and colleagues[89] found significant correlations between the metabolic score on the one hand, and the clinical, biologic, and endoscopic scores on the other hand. More importantly, as the sensitivity for detecting the most severe bowel involvement was very high, FDG-PET/CT could be used as a screening test in selected CD patients. In the case of negative PET/CT results, the likelihood of active disease is very low, so that a clinical follow up might be sufficient. The positive predictive value remains imperfect and abnormal findings should be further confirmed, currently using endoscopy. The main advantage of PET/CT is its capability of performing a whole-body survey, thus investigating the entire digestive tract while maintaining a relatively low radiation dose. Further studies should investigate clinical algorithms for combining FDG-PET/CT as an initial triage tool in patients with proven CD and clinical or biologic suspicion of disease reactivation, and MR imaging as a surveillance tool. **Fig. 6** shows PET/CT images from a patient with active CD.

SUMMARY

With the selected abdominopelvic disorders described above, as well as in other disease conditions, PET/CT and MR imaging are complementary in many respects. In cervical cancer, MR imaging is the best method for defining the

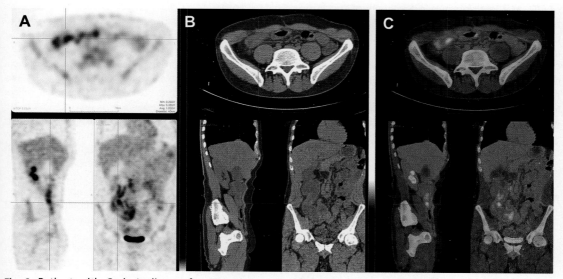

Fig. 6. Patient with Crohn's disease for 15 years, status after prior surgeries and treatment with anti-tumor necrosis factor-α agent, now with clinical exacerbation and elevated serum CRP level. Multiplanar FDG-PET (*A*), low-dose unenhanced CT (*B*), and fused FDG-PET/CT images (*C*) reveal increased FDG uptake in and wall thickening of within several locations of terminal ileum and right colon.

tumor volume and its spread to adjacent structures and organs, such as the uterine corpus, parametrium, or bladder, whereas FDG-PET/CT is the most accurate noninvasive technique for assessing the nodal status, both in the pelvic and para-aortic areas. These parameters are not integrated in the FIGO staging system, despite their critical importance as predictors of patient prognosis, and the combination of PET/CT and MR imaging is now widely viewed as a mainstay in the pretreatment assessment of cervical cancer. Pancreatic lesions are often a diagnostic challenge, and the combined information from MR imaging or EUS and PET/CT offer the highest accuracy regarding lesion characterization and tumor extent, both local and distant. Again, PET/CT and MR imaging is an extremely powerful combination, where MR imaging exquisitely defines the T stage of the tumor and PET/CT demonstrates its strength in assessment of the N and M stages of tumor. PET/CT provides value in locally advanced rectal cancers, as it contributes to definition of the target volume during radiation-treatment planning, preoperative evaluation of the response to chemoradiation, and detection of distant metastatic disease, whereas MR imaging provides excellent structural evaluation of the local extent of tumor. For the assessment of hepatic metastatic disease, MR imaging is able to delineate the presence of hepatic lesions, particularly when subcentimeter in size, whereas PET/CT provides lesional metabolic information for treatment monitoring purposes as well as improved detection of extrahepatic sites of metastatic disease. In the setting of CD, MR imaging provides details of the structural extent of bowel involvement and abdomino-pelvic complications of disease, including fistulous and sinus tract formation, whereas PET/CT provides information regarding the activity of disease, which is particularly important for treatment-monitoring purposes. Someday, PET/MR imaging may be used clinically for assessment of abdominopelvic disorders as the ultimate expression of the complementary nature of these imaging modalities.

REFERENCES

1. Kitajima K, Murakami K, Yamasaki E, et al. Performance of integrated FDG-PET/contrast-enhanced CT in the diagnosis of recurrent ovarian cancer: comparison with integrated FDG-PET/non-contrast-enhanced CT and enhanced CT. Eur J Nucl Med Mol Imaging 2008;35(8):1439–48.
2. Schaefer NG, Hany TF, Taverna C, et al. Non-Hodgkin lymphoma and Hodgkin disease: coregistered FDG PET and CT at staging and restaging–do we need contrast-enhanced CT? Radiology 2004;232(3):823–9.
3. Rodriguez-Vigil B, Gomez-Leon N, Pinilla I, et al. PET/CT in lymphoma: prospective study of enhanced full-dose PET/CT versus unenhanced low-dose PET/CT. J Nucl Med 2006;47(10):1643–8.
4. Strobel K, Heinrich S, Bhure U, et al. Contrast-enhanced 18F-FDG PET/CT: 1-stop-shop imaging for assessing the resectability of pancreatic cancer. J Nucl Med 2008;49(9):1408–13.
5. Pichler BJ, Wehrl HF, Judenhofer MS. Latest advances in molecular imaging instrumentation. J Nucl Med 2008;49(Suppl 2):5S–23S.
6. Kamangar F, Dores GM, Anderson WF. Patterns of cancer incidence, mortality, and prevalence across five continents: defining priorities to reduce cancer disparities in different geographic regions of the world. J Clin Oncol 2006;24(14):2137–50.
7. American Cancer Society. Cancer facts and figures 2008. Atlanta: American Cancer Society; 2008.
8. Benedet JL, Bender H, Jones H 3rd, et al. FIGO staging classifications and clinical practice guidelines in the management of gynecologic cancers. FIGO Committee on Gynecologic Oncology. Int J Gynaecol Obstet: The official organ of the International Federation of Gynaecology and Obstetrics 2000;70(2):209–62.
9. Whitcomb BP. Gynecologic malignancies. Surg Clin North Am 2008;88(2):301–17 vi.
10. Petignat P, Loubeyre P. Should we modify the current FIGO staging system for early-stage cervical cancer? Expert Rev Anticancer Ther 2008;8(7):1015–7.
11. Lagasse LD, Creasman WT, Shingleton HM, et al. Results and complications of operative staging in cervical cancer: experience of the Gynecologic Oncology Group. Gynecol Oncol 1980;9(1):90–8.
12. Beiner ME, Covens A. Surgery insight: radical vaginal trachelectomy as a method of fertility preservation for cervical cancer. Nat Clin Pract Oncol 2007;4(6):353–61.
13. Bipat S, Glas AS, van der Velden J, et al. Computed tomography and magnetic resonance imaging in staging of uterine cervical carcinoma: a systematic review. Gynecol oncol 2003;91(1):59–66.
14. Hricak H, Gatsonis C, Coakley FV, et al. Early invasive cervical cancer: CT and MR imaging in preoperative evaluation - ACRIN/GOG comparative study of diagnostic performance and interobserver variability. Radiology 2007;245(2):491–8.
15. Magne N, Chargari C, Vicenzi L, et al. New trends in the evaluation and treatment of cervix cancer: the role of FDG-PET. Cancer Treat Rev 2008;34(8):671–81.
16. Selman TJ, Mann C, Zamora J, et al. Diagnostic accuracy of tests for lymph node status in primary

cervical cancer: a systematic review and meta-analysis. CMAJ 2008;178(7):855–62.

17. Loft A, Berthelsen AK, Roed H, et al. The diagnostic value of PET/CT scanning in patients with cervical cancer: a prospective study. Gynecol Oncol 2007; 106(1):29–34.

18. Sironi S, Buda A, Picchio M, et al. Lymph node metastasis in patients with clinical early-stage cervical cancer: detection with integrated FDG PET/CT. Radiology 2006;238(1):272–9.

19. Chou HH, Chang TC, Yen TC, et al. Low value of [18F]-fluoro-2-deoxy-D-glucose positron emission tomography in primary staging of early-stage cervical cancer before radical hysterectomy. J Clin Oncol 2006;24(1):123–8.

20. Park W, Park YJ, Huh SJ, et al. The usefulness of MRI and PET imaging for the detection of parametrial involvement and lymph node metastasis in patients with cervical cancer. Jpn J Clin Oncol 2005;35(5):260–4.

21. Choi HJ, Roh JW, Seo SS, et al. Comparison of the accuracy of magnetic resonance imaging and positron emission tomography/computed tomography in the presurgical detection of lymph node metastases in patients with uterine cervical carcinoma: a prospective study. Cancer 2006;106(4):914–22.

22. Husain A, Akhurst T, Larson S, et al. A prospective study of the accuracy of 18Fluorodeoxyglucose positron emission tomography (18FDG PET) in identifying sites of metastasis prior to pelvic exenteration. Gynecol Oncol 2007;106(1):177–80.

23. Yeh LS, Hung YC, Shen YY, et al. Detecting para-aortic lymph nodal metastasis by positron emission tomography of 18F-fluorodeoxyglucose in advanced cervical cancer with negative magnetic resonance imaging findings. Oncol Rep 2002;9(6): 1289–92.

24. Yildirim Y, Sehirali S, Avci ME, et al. Integrated PET/CT for the evaluation of para-aortic nodal metastasis in locally advanced cervical cancer patients with negative conventional CT findings. Gynecol Oncol 2008;108(1):154–9.

25. Boughanim M, Leboulleux S, Rey A, et al. Histologic results of para-aortic lymphadenectomy in patients treated for stage IB2/II cervical cancer with negative [18F]fluorodeoxyglucose positron emission tomography scans in the para-aortic area. J Clin Oncol 2008;26(15):2558–61.

26. Chao A, Ho KC, Wang CC, et al. Positron emission tomography in evaluating the feasibility of curative intent in cervical cancer patients with limited distant lymph node metastases. Gynecol Oncol 2008; 110(2):172–8.

27. Ma SY, See LC, Lai CH, et al. Delayed (18)F-FDG PET for detection of paraaortic lymph node metastases in cervical cancer patients. J Nucl Med 2003;44(11):1775–83.

28. Yen TC, Ng KK, Ma SY, et al. Value of dual-phase 2-fluoro-2-deoxy-d-glucose positron emission tomography in cervical cancer. J Clin Oncol 2003;21(19): 3651–8.

29. Narayan K, Fisher RJ, Bernshaw D. Patterns of failure and prognostic factor analyses in locally advanced cervical cancer patients staged by magnetic resonance imaging and treated with curative intent. Int J Gynecol Cancer 2008;18(3):525–33.

30. Hsu CT, Cheng YS, Su SC. Prognosis of uterine cervical cancer with extensive lymph node metastases. Special emphasis on the value of pelvic lymphadenectomy in the surgical treatment of uterine cervical cancer. Am J Obstet Gynecol 1972;114(7): 954–62.

31. LaPolla JP, Schlaerth JB, Gaddis O, et al. The influence of surgical staging on the evaluation and treatment of patients with cervical carcinoma. Gynecol Oncol 1986;24(2):194–206.

32. Grigsby PW, Siegel BA, Dehdashti F. Lymph node staging by positron emission tomography in patients with carcinoma of the cervix. J Clin Oncol 2001; 19(17):3745–9.

33. Miller TR, Pinkus E, Dehdashti F, et al. Improved prognostic value of 18F-FDG PET using a simple visual analysis of tumor characteristics in patients with cervical cancer. J Nucl Med 2003;44(2):192–7.

34. Unger JB, Lilien DL, Caldito G, et al. The prognostic value of pretreatment 2-[18F]-fluoro-2-deoxy-D-glucose positron emission tomography scan in women with cervical cancer. Int J Gynecol Cancer 2007;17(5):1062–7.

35. Yen TC, See LC, Lai CH, et al. Standardized uptake value in para-aortic lymph nodes is a significant prognostic factor in patients with primary advanced squamous cervical cancer. Eur J Nucl Med Mol Imaging 2008;35(3):493–501.

36. Faria SC, Tamm EP, Loyer EM, et al. Diagnosis and staging of pancreatic tumors. Semin Roentgenol 2004;39(3):397–411.

37. Bipat S, Phoa SS, van Delden OM, et al. Ultrasonography, computed tomography and magnetic resonance imaging for diagnosis and determining resectability of pancreatic adenocarcinoma: a meta-analysis. J Comput Assist Tomogr 2005;29(4):438–45.

38. Delbeke D, Pinson CW. Pancreatic tumors: role of imaging in the diagnosis, staging, and treatment. J Hepatobiliary Pancreat Surg 2004;11(1):4–10.

39. Zimny M, Bares R, Fass J, et al. Fluorine-18 fluorodeoxyglucose positron emission tomography in the differential diagnosis of pancreatic carcinoma: a report of 106 cases. Eur J Nucl Med 1997;24(6): 678–82.

40. Zimny M, Buell U, Diederichs CG, et al. False-positive FDG PET in patients with pancreatic masses: an issue of proper patient selection? Eur J Nucl Med 1998;25(9):1352.

41. Shreve PD. Focal fluorine-18 fluorodeoxyglucose accumulation in inflammatory pancreatic disease. Eur J Nucl Med 1998;25(3):259–64.

42. Farma JM, Santillan AA, Melis M, et al. PET/CT fusion scan enhances CT staging in patients with pancreatic neoplasms. Ann Surg Oncol 2008; 15(9):2465–71.

43. Heinrich S, Goerres GW, Schafer M, et al. Positron emission tomography/computed tomography influences on the management of resectable pancreatic cancer and its cost-effectiveness. Ann Surg 2005; 242(2):235–43.

44. Taylor M, Warnock GL, Powell J, et al. Canadian Association of General Surgeons and American College of Surgeons evidence based reviews in surgery. 22. The use of PET/CT scanning on the management of resectable pancreatic cancer. Can J Surg 2007;50(5):400–2.

45. Sahani DV, Shah ZK, Catalano OA, et al. Radiology of pancreatic adenocarcinoma: current status of imaging. J Gastroenterol Hepatol 2008;23(1):23–33.

46. Sakai Y, Tsuyuguchi T, Tsuchiya S, et al. Diagnostic value of MRCP and indications for ERCP. Hepato-gastroenterology 2007;54(80):2212–5.

47. Katz DS, Friedel DM, Kho D, et al. Relative accuracy of CT and MRI for characterization of cystic pancreatic masses. AJR Am J Roentgenol 2007;189(3): 657–61.

48. Visser BC, Yeh BM, Qayyum A, et al. Characterization of cystic pancreatic masses: relative accuracy of CT and MRI. AJR Am J Roentgenol 2007;189(3): 648–56.

49. Balci NC, Semelka RC. Radiologic features of cystic, endocrine and other pancreatic neoplasms. Eur J Radiol 2001;38(2):113–9.

50. Sperti C, Pasquali C, Decet G, et al. F-18-fluorodeoxyglucose positron emission tomography in differentiating malignant from benign pancreatic cysts: a prospective study. J Gastrointest Surg 2005;9(1):22–8, discussion 8–9.

51. Sperti C, Bissoli S, Pasquali C, et al. 18-fluorodeoxyglucose positron emission tomography enhances computed tomography diagnosis of malignant intraductal papillary mucinous neoplasms of the pancreas. Ann Surg 2007;246(6):932–7, discussion 7–9.

52. Mansour JC, Schwartz L, Pandit-Taskar N, et al. The utility of F-18 fluorodeoxyglucose whole body PET imaging for determining malignancy in cystic lesions of the pancreas. J Gastrointest Surg 2006;10(10): 1354–60.

53. Tann M, Sandrasegaran K, Jennings SG, et al. Positron-emission tomography and computed tomography of cystic pancreatic masses. Clin Radiol 2007;62(8):745–51.

54. Nagy VM. Updating the management of rectal cancer. J Gastrointestin Liver Dis 2008;17(1): 69–74.

55. Bipat S, Glas AS, Slors FJ, et al. Rectal cancer: local staging and assessment of lymph node involvement with endoluminal US, CT, and MR imaging–a meta-analysis. Radiol 2004;232(3):773–83.

56. Nagtegaal ID, Quirke P. What is the role for the circumferential margin in the modern treatment of rectal cancer? J Clin Oncol 2008;26(2):303–12.

57. MERCURY study group. Extramural depth of tumor invasion at thin-section MR in patients with rectal cancer: results of the MERCURY study. Radiology 2007;243(1):132–9.

58. Sauer R, Becker H, Hohenberger W, et al. Preoperative versus postoperative chemoradiotherapy for rectal cancer. N Engl J Med 2004;351(17):1731–40.

59. Lahaye MJ, Engelen SM, Nelemans PJ, et al. Imaging for predicting the risk factors—the circumferential resection margin and nodal disease–of local recurrence in rectal cancer: a meta-analysis. Semin Ultrasound CT MR 2005;26(4):259–68.

60. Abdel-Nabi H, Doerr RJ, Lamonica DM, et al. Staging of primary colorectal carcinomas with fluorine-18 fluorodeoxyglucose whole-body PET: correlation with histopathologic and CT findings. Radiology 1998;206(3):755–60.

61. Kantorova I, Lipska L, Belohlavek O, et al. Routine (18)F-FDG PET preoperative staging of colorectal cancer: comparison with conventional staging and its impact on treatment decision making. J Nucl Med 2003;44(11):1784–8.

62. Bassi MC, Turri L, Sacchetti G, et al. FDG-PET/CT imaging for staging and target volume delineation in preoperative conformal radiotherapy of rectal cancer. Int J Radiat Oncol Biol Phys 2008;70(5):1423–6.

63. Davey K, Heriot AG, Mackay J, et al. The impact of 18-fluorodeoxyglucose positron emission tomography-computed tomography on the staging and management of primary rectal cancer. Dis Colon Rectum 2008;51(7):997–1003.

64. Gearhart SL, Frassica D, Rosen R, et al. Improved staging with pretreatment positron emission tomography/computed tomography in low rectal cancer. Ann Surg Oncol 2006;13(3):397–404.

65. Park IJ, Kim HC, Yu CS, et al. Efficacy of PET/CT in the accurate evaluation of primary colorectal carcinoma. Eur J Surg Oncol 2006;32(9):941–7.

66. Capirci C, Rampin L, Erba PA, et al. Sequential FDG-PET/CT reliably predicts response of locally advanced rectal cancer to neo-adjuvant chemoradiation therapy. Eur J Nucl Med Mol Imaging 2007;34(10):1583–93.

67. Cascini GL, Avallone A, Delrio P, et al. 18F-FDG PET is an early predictor of pathologic tumor response to preoperative radiochemotherapy in locally advanced rectal cancer. J Nucl Med 2006;47(8): 1241–8.

68. Konski A, Li T, Sigurdson E, et al. Use of molecular imaging to predict clinical outcome in patients with

rectal cancer after preoperative chemotherapy and radiation. Int J Radiat Oncol Biol Phys 2008, in press.

69. Kalff V, Ware R, Heriot A, et al. Radiation changes do not interfere with postchemoradiation restaging of patients with rectal cancer by FDG PET/CT before curative surgical therapy. Int J Radiat Oncol Biol Phys 2008, in press.

70. Pawlik TM, Schulick RD, Choti MA. Expanding criteria for resectability of colorectal liver metastases. Oncol 2008;13(1):51–64.

71. Kinkel K, Lu Y, Both M, et al. Detection of hepatic metastases from cancers of the gastrointestinal tract by using noninvasive imaging methods (US, CT, MR imaging, PET): a meta-analysis. Radiology 2002; 224(3):748–56.

72. Schima W, Kulinna C, Langenberger H, et al. Liver metastases of colorectal cancer: US, CT or MR? Cancer Imaging 2005;5(Spec No A):S149–56.

73. Selzner M, Hany TF, Wildbrett P, et al. Does the novel PET/CT imaging modality impact on the treatment of patients with metastatic colorectal cancer of the liver? Ann Surg 2004;240(6):1027–34, discussion 35–6.

74. Rappeport ED, Loft A, Berthelsen AK, et al. Contrast-enhanced FDG-PET/CT vs. SPIO-enhanced MRI vs. FDG-PET vs. CT in patients with liver metastases from colorectal cancer: a prospective study with intraoperative confirmation. Acta Radiol 2007;48(4): 369–78.

75. Kong G, Jackson C, Koh DM, et al. The use of (18)F-FDG PET/CT in colorectal liver metastases-comparison with CT and liver MRI. Eur J Nucl Med Mol Imaging 2008;35(7):1323–9.

76. Soyka JD, Veit-Haibach P, Strobel K, et al. Staging pathways in recurrent colorectal carcinoma: is contrast-enhanced 18F-FDG PET/CT the diagnostic tool of choice? J Nucl Med 2008;49(3):354–61.

77. Cantwell CP, Setty BN, Holalkere N, et al. Liver lesion detection and characterization in patients with colorectal cancer: a comparison of low radiation dose non-enhanced PET/CT, contrast-enhanced PET/CT, and liver MRI. J Comput Assist Tomogr 2008;32(5): 738–44.

78. Cellier C, Sahmoud T, Froguel E, et al. Correlations between clinical activity, endoscopic severity, and biological parameters in colonic or ileocolonic Crohn's disease. A prospective multicentre study of 121 cases. The Groupe d'Etudes Therapeutiques des Affections Inflammatoires Digestives. Gut 1994; 35(2):231–5.

79. Malago R, Manfredi R, Benini L, et al. Assessment of Crohn's disease activity in the small bowel with MR-enteroclysis: clinico-radiological correlations. Abdom Imaging 2008;33(6):669–75.

80. Sinha R, Nwokolo C, Murphy PD. Magnetic resonance imaging in Crohn's disease. BMJ 2008; 336(7638):273–6.

81. Desmond AN, O'Regan K, Curran C, et al. Crohn's disease: factors associated with exposure to high levels of diagnostic radiation. Gut 2008;57(11): 1524–9.

82. Peloquin JM, Pardi DS, Sandborn WJ, et al. Diagnostic ionizing radiation exposure in a population-based cohort of patients with inflammatory bowel disease. Am J Gastroenterol 2008;103(8):2015–22.

83. Kuehle CA, Langhorst J, Ladd SC, et al. Magnetic resonance colonography without bowel cleansing: a prospective cross sectional study in a screening population. Gut 2007;56(8):1079–85.

84. Florie J, Wasser MN, Arts-Cieslik K, et al. Dynamic contrast-enhanced MRI of the bowel wall for assessment of disease activity in Crohn's disease. AJR Am J Roentgenol 2006;186(5):1384–92.

85. Negaard A, Paulsen V, Sandvik L, et al. A prospective randomized comparison between two MRI studies of the small bowel in Crohn's disease, the oral contrast method and MR enteroclysis. Eur Radiol 2007;17(9):2294–301.

86. Loffler M, Weckesser M, Franzius C, et al. High diagnostic value of 18F-FDG-PET in pediatric patients with chronic inflammatory bowel disease. Ann N Y Acad Sci 2006;1072:379–85.

87. Skehan SJ, Issenman R, Mernagh J, et al. 18F-fluorodeoxyglucose positron tomography in diagnosis of paediatric inflammatory bowel disease. Lancet 1999;354(9181):836–7.

88. Meisner RS, Spier BJ, Einarsson S, et al. Pilot study using PET/CT as a novel, noninvasive assessment of disease activity in inflammatory bowel disease. Inflamm Bowel Dis 2007;13(8):993–1000.

89. Louis E, Ancion G, Colard A, et al. Noninvasive assessment of Crohn's disease intestinal lesions with (18)F-FDG PET/CT. J Nucl Med 2007;48(7): 1053–9.

Evaluation of Musculoskeletal Disorders with PET, PET/CT, and PET/MR Imaging

Karen Chen, MD*, Judy Blebea, MD, Jean-Denis Laredo, MD,
Wengen Chen, MD, PhD, Abass Alavi, MD, PhD (Hon), DSc (Hon),
Drew A. Torigian, MD, MA

KEYWORDS

- Musculoskeletal • Oncology
- Metabolic bone disease • Arthroplasty • Diabetic foot
- Positron emission tomography (PET) • PET/CT • PET/MRI

Imaging plays a major role in the diagnosis and management of musculoskeletal disorders. Conventional imaging methods, including plain film radiography, CT, and MR imaging, provide high-resolution structural information. These modalities are somewhat insensitive, however, for detecting early disease and often fail to distinguish between active and inactive lesions related to prior disease. Early diagnosis or exclusion of infection and inflammation are crucial for optimal management of patients. PET is an imaging technique that provides functional information through the distribution and uptake of positron-emitting radiotracers. Two commonly used radiotracers for PET imaging of musculoskeletal disorders are F18-fluorodeoxyglucose (FDG) and ^{18}F–sodium fluoride (^{18}F-NaF); the former is most commonly used in clinical practice. ^{18}F-NaF has great promise, however, and likely will replace conventional technetium-based compounds.

FDG originally was used to image brain function in healthy and disease states. With the advent of whole-body imaging techniques in the latter half of the 1980s, it became apparent that glucose metabolism also was elevated in malignancies and in infectious and noninfectious inflammatory processes. ^{18}F-NaF previously was used widely for skeletal imaging after its introduction in the 1960s and subsequent FDA approval in 1972[1]

but was replaced by technetium Tc 99m (^{99m}Tc) agents by the 1970s due to the wide spread of the tracer which allows generating optimal images with existing gamma cameras. With the rapid introduction of PET cameras, ^{18}F-NaF may become the skeletal imaging radiotracer of choice due to its rapid blood clearance, which results in high target-to-background ratio over a short period of time. Also, PET/CT imaging of the skeleton provides detailed structure and function correlation.

Although PET mainly has been used for assessing patients who have cancer, there are several specific clinical scenarios when PET, PET/CT, or PET/MR imaging may prove as beneficial in examining musculoskeletal disorders, including infection, diabetic foot, painful arthroplasty, metabolic bone marrow/bone disease, back pain, nonmalignant bone marrow disorders, and arthritis. In general, morphologic imaging with CT or MR imaging is limited by low sensitivity for early disease detection and lack of specificity of diagnosis in many settings in spite of providing excellent anatomic detail. In particular, CT provides excellent detail of the cortical and trabecular bone, whereas MR imaging provides excellent soft tissue contrast for the assessment of the bone marrow, muscles, tendons, ligaments, cartilaginous structures, and fat. PET is in general

Department of Radiology, Hospital of the University of Pennsylvania, 3400 Spruce Street, Philadelphia, PA 19104, USA
* Corresponding author.
E-mail address: Karen.Chen@uphs.upenn.edu (K. Chen).

PET Clin 3 (2009) 451–465
doi:10.1016/j.cpet.2009.03.003
1556-8598/09/$ – see front matter. Published by Elsevier, Inc.

much more sensitive and specific in the detection and characterization of musculoskeletal disorders but is limited by its relatively low spatial resolution. Therefore, combined morphologic imaging provided by CT or MR imaging and molecular imaging with PET by using hybrid PET/CT or PET/MR imaging scanners maximizes the strengths of both imaging approaches. PET/MR imaging, however, has not been fully developed for routine clinical use, but the prospects for its routine use are strong, based on preliminary results generated. The purpose of this article is to outline the current clinical use of PET imaging for the evaluation of musculoskeletal disorders and to touch on PET/CT and the future potential of PET/MR imaging and PET/CT/MR imaging fused data sets. Because the application of FDG-PET in musculoskeletal infections has been well described in the literature, this article focuses on the use of ^{18}F-NaF PET in musculoskeletal disorders, including the role of FDG-PET in the specific clinical settings.

TECHNICAL ASPECTS OF MUSCULOSKELETAL PET IMAGING

FDG is a glucose analogue that is transported into cells by membrane glucose transporters and becomes trapped intracellularly after being phosphorylated by hexokinase into FDG-6-phosphate. It is commonly used in cancer imaging, as it accumulates at sites of neoplasia and can be used to image infection and inflammation, as it also accumulates in activated inflammatory cells, such as lymphocytes and macrophages that have increased levels of glycolysis.[2,3]

^{18}F-NaF is a bone-specific agent, and is useful for the assessment of blood flow and new bone formation.[4,5] Currently it is not commonly used for PET imaging because of lack of reimbursement. ^{18}F-NaF seeks bone by diffusing through the capillaries into the bone extracellular fluid. Its plasma clearance is more rapid than that of ^{99m}Tc–methylene diphosponate (MDP) because of its small molecular weight and negligible protein binding, and this rapid clearance contributes to a high target-to-background ratio on PET images. At sites of rapid bone crystal turnover, it undergoes ion exchanges with apatite to form ^{18}F-fluoroapatite.[1] The amount and rapidity of radiotracer uptake, therefore, reflect relative blood flow and radiotracer delivery and osteoblast activity. It is, therefore, useful for the assessment of metabolic bone disease, bone graft viability, healing fractures, osteonecrosis, and primary and metastatic tumors.

FDG-PET imaging requires patient preparation prior to examination and requires fasting for at least 4 hours prior to examination. Serum glucose level is measured prior to FDG administration and ideally should be less than 150 mg/dL for oncologic applications, whereas for the assessment of infection and noninfectious inflammation hyperglycemia, up to 200 mg/dL does not seem to have a significant effect on the sensitivity of FDG-PET.[6] After intravenous administration of FDG, emission images are acquired 60 to 90 minutes later. An external source of radiation (typically cesium Cs 137 for PET only scanners and a low-dose CT x-ray tube for PET/CT scanners) is used during the imaging session to obtain transmission images for emission data attenuation correction purposes.

After image reconstruction, PET and CT or MR image data sets are coregistered using software and viewed on a dedicated workstation for diagnostic interpretation. For patients undergoing MR imaging (as a separate examination from PET or potentially in the future on a hybrid PET/MR imaging scanner), a thorough screening for metallic and electronic devices or objects by trained personnel prior to entry into the scanning room is imperative to prevent potential patient injury due to the effects of the powerful magnetic field. As such, the presence of orbital metallic foreign bodies (such as those from welding) and certain other non–MR imaging–compatible metallic or electronic devices (such as ferromagnetic aneurysm clips or transvenous pacemakers) are contraindications for MR imaging (and thus PET/MR imaging) examinations.[7–11] Attenuation correction of emission PET data using MR imaging data alone during PET/MR imaging is challenging and currently an area of active investigation.[12–14]

CLINICAL APPLICATIONS OF PET/CT FOR MUSCULOSKELETAL DISORDERS
Malignant Disorders

Cancer imaging is one of the main clinical indications for FDG-PET alone or as part of PET/CT (and in the future PET/MR imaging). FDG-PET provides a comprehensive quantitative assessment of the entire body, which is particularly useful in patients who have skeleton metastatic disease, lymphoma, primary musculoskeletal sarcoma, and multiple myeloma, and also may be useful to direct sites of biopsy to maximize the field from diagnostic prospects (**Figs. 1** and **2**).

Spread of lymphoma to the red bone marrow is variable but is more common with non-Hodgkin's lymphoma than with Hodgkin's lymphoma.[15–17] FDG-PET has been reported as more sensitive

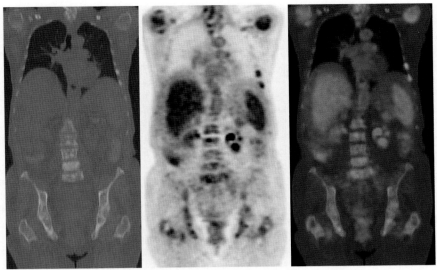

Fig. 1. Coronal CT (*left*), coronal FDG-PET (*middle*), and FDG–PET/CT (*right*) images in 70-year-old woman who had metastatic breast carcinoma demonstrate extensive multifocal sclerotic bone marrow metastases with increased FDG uptake involving lumbar spine, proximal humeri, left ribs, and pelvic bones.

and accurate than CT or MR imaging alone for overall evaluation of lymphoma spread in the entire body and is indicated for the staging, monitoring, and restaging of lymphoma.[18,19] With regards to evaluation of lymphomatous involvement of the red bone marrow, meta-analysis of 587 patients demonstrated a 54% sensitivity and 92% specificity of FDG-PET for bone marrow lesions. Sensitivity varied with the subtype and grade of the lymphoma and was greater in high grade

(73%) than in low-grade (30%) lymphomas. Cases of positive PET findings but negative marrow biopsy results often indicated missed bone marrow sampling by the initial bone marrow biopsy with subsequent confirmation with rebiopsy or follow-up imaging.[20] In a study by Schaefer and colleagues[21] of 50 consecutive patients who had Hodgkin's lymphoma or aggressive non-Hodgkin's lymphoma, however, additional FDG–PET/CT information regarding uni- or multifocal bone

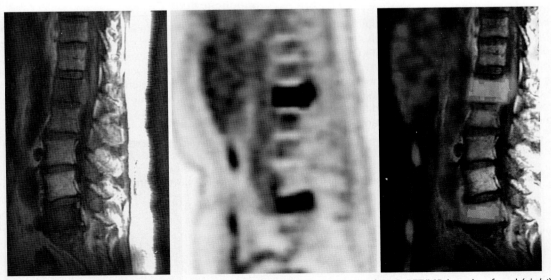

Fig. 2. Sagittal T1-weighted MR (*left*), sagittal FDG-PET (*middle*), and sagittal FDG–PET/MR imaging fused (*right*) images of patient who had metastatic disease to lumbar spine. PET image shows metabolically active tumor whereas MR image shows abnormal signal intensity in L1 and L5 vertebral bodies providing accurate anatomic localization.

involvement resulted in lymphoma upstaging in 21 (42%) patients compared with the combined information provided by CT and bone marrow biopsy. Overall, results suggest that FDG–PET/CT outperforms FDG-PET alone and CT alone in the staging of patients who have lymphoma and that data on the diagnostic performance of whole-body MR imaging for this application are lacking, justifying the need for future well-designed prospective studies.[22]

PET/CT can improve the accuracy of preoperative staging of soft tissue and bone sarcomas. FDG uptake in tumor correlates with histologic grade, and the improved anatomic localization from PET/CT (83%) provides more accurate staging than PET alone (70%) and conventional imaging (77%).[23,24] In a series of 117 patients who had various sarcomas, PET/CT decreased overstaging and changed tumor diagnosis from unresectable to resectable in 2% of patients.[24] FDG-PET in conjunction with MR imaging also is useful for evaluating therapeutic response in the setting of musculoskeletal sarcoma.[25]

Osseous involvement is one of the criteria of the Durie and Salmon classification of myeloma for treatment.[26] In the management of solitary plasmacytoma, it is paramount to confirm that the lesion actually is solitary. Traditionally, osseous lesions are detected using whole-body plain film radiography, but radiographs often underestimate disease burden in the bone marrow, especially when there is early disease.[27] The staging system then was updated to include FDG-PET or MR imaging of the spine.[28] A study comparing imaging modalities reported that FDG-PET detects focal bone marrow disease better than bone scintigraphy or MR imaging but was suboptimal for detection of diffuse disease (**Fig. 3**).[29] When combined with bone scintigraphy, FDG-PET modified the clinical management of more patients than bone scintigraphy and MR imaging, suggesting a complementary role of bone scintigraphy and PET in the staging of patients who had multiple myeloma.

18F-NaF PET/CT can be used for the evaluation of skeleton metastases in a fashion similar to bone scintigraphy. In particular, 18F-NaF PET/CT is more likely to detect skeletal metastases of tumors that typically have low FDG avidity, such as thyroid cancer and renal cell cancer (**Fig. 4**).[30] When used to evaluate high-risk prostate cancer patients, 18F-NaF PET/CT was reported more sensitive than planar or single photon emission CT (SPECT) bone scintigraphy or 18F-NaF PET alone, with sensitivities of 100%, 70%, and 92%, respectively. 18F-NaF PET/CT also was more specific, with specificities of 100%, 82%, and 62%, respectively.[31]

18F-NaF is not specific for malignant tumors as it also can accumulate in benign osseous abnormalities. Although it has a higher sensitivity than bone scintigraphy in the evaluation of malignancy, this sensitivity is counterbalanced by a high rate of false-positive results.[32] Therefore, for this clinical application, 18F-NaF PET requires correlation, such as CT or MR imaging, to improve it specificity, which in the future will be provided by the hybrid PET/CT or PET/MR imaging scanners. One study that compared 18F-NaF PET/CT to PET alone showed an increase in specificity of the former for lesions (97% versus 72%, respectively) and for patients (88% versus 56%, respectively).[30]

Metabolic Bone Disease

Diseases affecting the structure of bone, such as Paget's disease, osteoporosis, and renal osteodystrophy, often are associated with changes in bone turnover. As such, serial evaluation and quantification of regional disease activity by 18F-NaF PET may be useful to assess bone

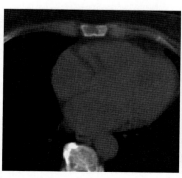 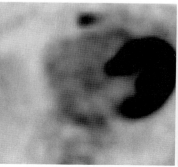 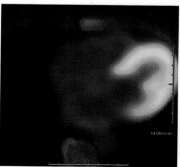

Fig. 3. Axial CT (*left*), FDG-PET (*middle*), and PET/CT (*right*) images in 68-year-old woman who had multiple myeloma demonstrate FDG avid lytic lesion involving right aspect of sternum.

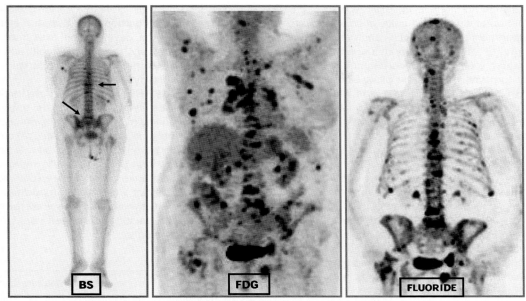

Fig. 4. Coronal ^{99m}Tc-MDP planar scintigraphic image (*left*) shows metastatic involvement of thoracic and lumbar spine. Coronal FDG-PET (*middle*) and ^{18}F-fluoride PET (*right*) images demonstrate greater number of osseous metastases. Note lack of soft tissue uptake on ^{18}F-fluoride PET image, further increasing sensitivity for detection of osseous lesions adjacent to sites of physiologic or pathophysiologic FDG uptake. BS, ^{99m}Tc bone scan. (*Reprinted from* Langsteger W, Heinisch M, Fogelman I. The role of fluorodeoxyglucose, 18F-dihydroxyphenylalanine, 18F-choline, and 18F-fluoride in bone imaging with emphasis on prostate and breast. Semin Nucl Med 2006;36(1):73–92; with permission.)

turnover and changes due to therapeutic response.[33-36] Although ^{99m}Tc bone scintigraphy allows for qualitative assessment of disease activity, ^{18}F-NaF PET provides tomographic images with high spatial resolution and allows accurate quantification, which may not be achievable with SPECT. Based on reports in the literature, by using ^{18}F-NaF, a response to therapy can be detected in as short as 1 month after therapeutic intervention.[37]

Methods of quantifying disease activity in Paget's disease initially were described with dynamic ^{18}F-NaF PET. Scans were performed by first obtaining a 15-minute transmission scan for attenuation correction followed by a dynamic 60-minute emission scan.[37] Arterial plasma activity was measured from counts obtained from the aorta on PET images or from direct arterial access. The dynamic scan combined with arterial plasma activity allowed for calculation of clearance of radiotracer from plasma to the bone tissue, transport of fluoride ions between extravascular bone compartment to plasma, and plasma clearance of fluoride to bone mineral.

Subsequent studies have demonstrated that maximum standardized uptake value (SUV), a much simpler measurement than calculating tracer clearance and transport into different

plasma and bone components, correlates well with net uptake of fluoride to bone mineral and thus osteoblastic disease activity.[34] Response to treatment, manifesting as a decrease in osteoblastic activity, correlated with decreasing maximum SUV, indicating that maximum SUV can be used as a means to assess disease activity. This approach allows for simplification of the PET examination by eliminating the need for dynamic image acquisition and arterial access.

With the metabolic diseases, such as Paget's disease, increases in the resorption and formation of bone have been reported.[38] Current treatment of Paget's disease relies on the blockage of bone remodeling through administration of bisphosphonates.[39] Thus, serial ^{18}F-NaF PET scans can be used to assess response to therapy[40] and to follow-up patients over time after therapy has been completed.[36] Similar to Paget's disease, fibrous dysplasia also may benefit from ^{18}F-NaF PET assessment of response to bisphophonate therapy.

In a study of renal osteodystrophy, Messa and colleagues[36] evaluated 11 patients by using ^{18}F-NaF PET and demonstrated that the calculated rate constant of net incorporation of ^{18}F-NaF into bone correlated well with serum alkaline phosphatase, a marker of bone turnover and serum parathyroid hormone level. This result was similar to that obtained through calculation with a three-compartment model or Patlak analysis. Moreover, the rate of ^{18}F-NaF incorporation into bone also correlated well with histomorphometric indices of bone turnover in iliac crest biopsies. The indices were higher in patients who had high-turnover renal osteodystrophy compared to those in patients who had low bone-turnover diseases or in healthy subjects.

[18]F-NaF PET may be useful in evaluating osteoporosis in postmenopausal women. Postmenopausal women have been found to demonstrate increased bone turnover compared to their premenopausal counterparts.[41,42] Blake and colleagues evaluated 69 postmenopausal women using ^{18}F-NaF PET and showed a statistically significant difference in bone turnover between patients treated with hormone replacement and untreated women. These findings suggest that ^{18}F-NaF PET could be used to monitor changes in bone turnover in patients undergoing treatment for osteoporosis.[43]

Back Pain in Adolescence

SPECT imaging has been important for the evaluation of back pain in athletically active youths, particularly for evaluation of spondylolysis. Given the high sensitivity of ^{18}F-NaF PET for bone remodeling, PET may demonstrate osseous stress changes prior to the development of a fracture (**Fig. 5**).[44] Alternatively, lack of abnormal uptake indicates an old fracture, which is no longer remodeling. In a study of 15 patients who had back pain, ^{18}F-NaF PET/CT demonstrated treatable abnormalities in 10 patients.[44] In another study of 94 patients who had back pain using ^{18}F-NaF PET only, a possible source of back pain was revealed in 55%, similar to the rate with bone scintigraphy with SPECT but with improved resolution and shortened imaging time. Total radiation dose was similar with the two modalities.[45] The negative predictive value (NPV) was strong, and symptoms of back pain resolved spontaneously without intervention.

Bone Viability

[18]F-NaF PET also can be used to measure bone blood flow and to assess the extent of viable bone in the femoral heads. This is useful particularly in the setting of trauma or reconstructive surgery. Schiepers and colleagues[46] demonstrated that a decrease in blood flow or decreased ^{18}F-NaF influx predicted the eventual need for joint arthroplasty. In the setting of a joint replacement, ^{18}F-NaF shows normal uptake in the bone

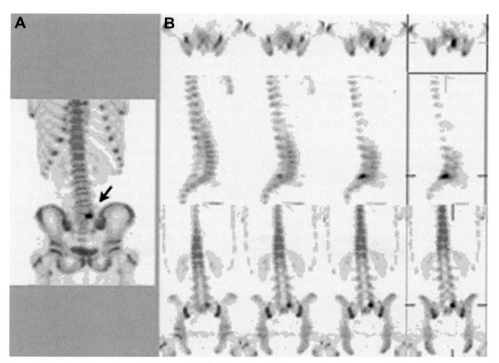

Fig. 5. Coronal planar (*A*) and multiplanar (*B*) ^{18}F-fluoride PET images in 12-year-old female gymnast who had lower back pain shows increased focal uptake in left posterior element of L5 vertebra in keeping with stress reaction (*arrow*).

underlying the resurfacing prosthesis.[47] Bone graft material sometimes is used to aid in stabilization of joint prostheses. Two studies investigated the uptake of ^{18}F-NaF in bone graft used in hip arthroplasties. The uptake in the allograft was similar to the adjacent cortical bone immediately after surgery but decreased compared to adjacent cortical bone on late follow-up (9 months to 5 years), indicating normal bony incorporation.[48,49]

Bone Marrow Imaging

Changes in marrow composition and imaging appearance occur with age. In infants, marrow is predominantly red and hematopoietic. With age, there is progressive replacement of red hematopoietic marrow with yellow fatty marrow. This marrow conversion process is almost total (red to yellow marrow) in the appendicular skeleton and partial (with a decrease in the ratio of red to yellow marrow) in the axial skeleton. In the appendicular skeleton, the conversion begins in the distal phalanges and proceeds in a centripetal fashion. In long bones, the conversion begins in the epiphysis and diaphysis and progresses proximally and distally with faster conversion in the distal bone.[50]

An understanding of the age- and gender-specific differences in marrow is essential to providing an accurate diagnosis of benign and malignant skeleton disorders. Pathologic conditions can alter marrow composition by replacing normal marrow, although a variety of nonmalignant conditions that increase erythrocyte demand also can alter marrow composition. Some of these conditions include long-distance running, living in a high-altitude location, and smoking. These changes in the bone marrow are seen more commonly in women than men and manifest as an increase in red marrow within the distal metaphyseal region of the humeri or femora or in the metaphyseal region of the proximal tibiae. Chronic anemia, myelofibrosis, and malignant infiltration of the bone marrow result in additional demands for hematopoiesis, also leading to reconversion of yellow to red marrow. Red marrow reconversion in the long bones begins in the metaphyses, following a reverse pattern of the physiologic conversion of red to yellow marrow.

Although FDG is not a bone marrow specific tracer, it can be used to examine the red marrow activity and detect bone marrow involvement by benign or malignant processes. In contrast to traditional bone marrow imaging agents, which rely on the absence or decrease of physiologic uptake in sites of disease, FDG demonstrates increased uptake in lesions based on increases in metabolic activity, which is the main advantage of FDG as a bone marrow tracer for the detection of metabolically active lesions. In contrast, traditional bone marrow agents show decreased uptake in sites of metabolically active and inactive disease.

The main pitfall of using FDG-PET to image the bone marrow occurs in the setting of granulocyte colony-stimulating factor therapy, which results in physiologically hypermetabolic bone marrow. In this setting, the increased FDG uptake in the bone marrow can simulate diffuse metastatic disease (**Fig. 6**). Furthermore, the increased

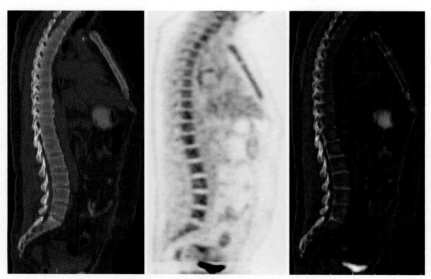

Fig. 6. Sagittal CT (*left*), FDG-PET (*middle*), and FDG–PET/CT (*right*) images in 52-year-old man treated with chemotherapy for colon carcinoma. Note diffuse increased FDG uptake throughout bone marrow of spine and sternum without corresponding CT abnormality, in keeping with post-treatment bone marrow stimulation.

background uptake can make it difficult to assess treatment response of focal marrow metastases. The metabolic rate of the bone marrow rapidly decreases 3 to 5 days after the cessation of granulocyte colony-stimulating factor therapy. Although FDG uptake can remain higher than at baseline for up to 4 weeks, a 5-day delay after cessation of therapy prior to performing FDG-PET is adequate for the bone marrow to return toward baseline levels of metabolic activity, allowing for the accurate delineation of focal marrow lesions and assessment of treatment response.[51]

Pain Related to Prior Arthroplasty

Pain is not an uncommon symptom after joint replacement. The most common cause of joint replacement failure is aseptic loosening. In a few patients, pain is caused by infection, creating a critical clinical challenge in distinguishing patients who have aseptic loosening from those who have prosthetic or periprosthetic infection.[52] The current mainstays for diagnostic imaging of patients who have pain related to arthroplasty are plain film radiography, CT, planar scintigraphy, and sometimes MR imaging. Plain film radiography is limited because the appearance of prosthetic or periprosthetic infection is not different from that of loosening or granulomatous disease. Images of CT and MR imaging frequently have poor image quality due to artifacts from the metallic hardware, making the assessment for infection difficult if not impossible. Functional imaging with three-phase ^{99m}Tc-labeled bone seeking agent scintigraphy, gallium citrate GA 67 (^{67}Ga) scintigraphy, or a combination of indium In 111 (^{111}In) leukocyte and ^{99m}Tc–sulfur colloid bone marrow scintigraphy is of limited value because of the nontomographic nature of images generated. Overall, these techniques have low accuracy and are time consuming, particularly

for ^{111}In-leukocyte and ^{99m}Tc–sulfur colloid scintigraphy.[53] Data have shown, however, that FDG-PET has a potential role in detecting infection in hip prostheses and to a lesser extent in knee prostheses. FDG-PET imaging with use of an external radioactive source for creation of transmission images (rather than PET/CT) is highly sensitive for detection of infection, is not affected by artifacts caused by the metallic components of the prosthesis that is seen with CT or MR imaging, and provides higher-resolution images than those of conventional nuclear medicine techniques.

In a study of 113 patients who had 127 hip prostheses and pain, results of images with FDG-PET were compared with those of the standard of preoperative tests, intraoperative findings, histopathology, and clinical findings for the diagnosis of periprosthetic infection. PET findings were suggestive of septic loosening if increased uptake was observed at the stem-prosthesis interface (**Fig. 7**), whereas uptake adjacent to the neck of the prosthesis was interpreted as a nonspecific reaction (**Fig. 8**). Of 35 positive studies, 28 were confirmed as infected. Of 92 negative studies, 87 were proved aseptic. Overall, the sensitivity, specificity, positive predictive value (PPV), and NPV of FDG-PET were 85%, 93%, 80%, and 95%, respectively, compared to the performance characteristics of ^{99m}Tc–sulfur colloid and ^{111}In–white blood cell (WBC) scintigraphy, which were substantially lower (**Fig. 9**).[54] Therefore, FDG-PET seems promising for accurate diagnosis of infection in the setting of the painful hip after arthroplasty.

The authors' group reported that in a study involving 38 hip prostheses and 36 knee prostheses, the sensitivity, specificity, and accuracy of FDG-PET for detecting infection were 90%, 89.3%, and 89.5%, respectively, for hip prostheses, and 90.9%, 72.0%, and 77.8%, respectively, for knee prostheses (**Fig. 10**).[55] In an

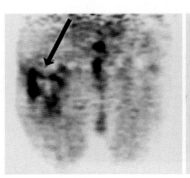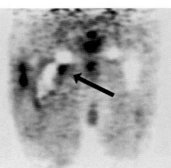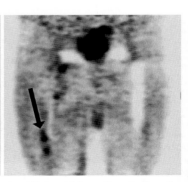

Fig. 7. Coronal FDG-PET images in patient who had right hip pain and prior bilateral hip arthroplasties show intense FDG uptake surrounding proximal and distal femoral components in keeping with infection (*arrows*).

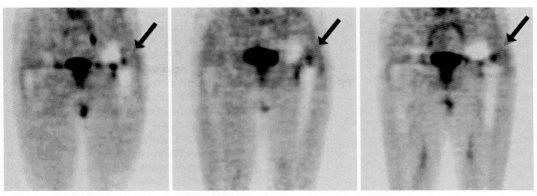

Fig. 8. Coronal FDG-PET images performed at 3 (*left*), 6 (*middle*), and 12 (*right*) months after left hip replacement show no significant change in increased FDG uptake (*arrows*) surrounding neck of hip prosthesis consistent with nonspecific reactive change.

attempt to compare the accuracy of FDG-PET with combined ^{99m}Tc–sulfur colloid bone marrow imaging and ^{111}In-WBC scintigraphy for the diagnosis of periprosthetic infection, Pill and colleagues[56] prospectively enrolled 89 patients who had 92 painful hip prostheses. These patients were given the option of undergoing combined FDG-PET and ^{99m}Tc–sulfur colloid bone marrow imaging/^{111}In-WBC scintigraphy or FDG-PET alone. FDG-PET correctly diagnosed 20 of 21 infected cases (sensitivity of 95.2%) and excluded infection in 66 of the 71 aseptic hips (specificity of 93%) with a PPV of 80% (20/25) and a NPV of 98.5% (66/67). Combined ^{99m}Tc–sulfur colloid bone marrow imaging/^{111}In-WBC scintigraphy correctly identified 5 of 10 infected cases (sensitivity of 50%) and excluded this complication in 39 of 41 aseptic cases (specificity of 95.1%) corresponding to a PPV and NPV of 41.7% (5/12) and 88.6% (39/44), respectively. Based on these results, the investigators concluded that FDG-PET is a promising diagnostic tool for distinguishing septic from aseptic painful hip prostheses.

Chacko and colleagues[57] studied the location and intensity of FDG uptake in 41 total hip prostheses from 32 patients with complete clinical follow-up data. Twelve had periprosthetic infection and 11 displayed moderately increased FDG uptake along the interface between the bone and prosthesis. In contrast, FDG-PET of patients who had loosening of the hip prosthesis without infection revealed intense uptake around the femoral head or neck components of prostheses with SUVs as high as 7. The investigators concluded that the amount of increased FDG uptake is less important than the location of increased FDG uptake when this technique is used to diagnose periprosthetic infection in patients who have undergone prior hip arthroplasty. By adopting the standard criterion of presence of FDG uptake between the bone and prosthesis at the level of the mid shaft portion of the prosthesis, the accuracy of FDG-PET is substantially enhanced.

It is likely that FDG-PET will play a pivotal role in the evaluation of complicated lower-limb prostheses, especially after the criteria for infection

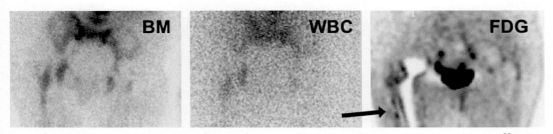

Fig. 9. A 73-year-old woman who had right hip pain 14 years after right hip arthroplasty. Coronal ^{99m}Tc-MDP planar scintigraphic image (*left*) and coronal ^{111}In-WBC planar scintigraphic image (*middle*) show mildly increased uptake surrounding proximal femoral component of right hip prosthesis. Coronal FDG-PET image (*right*) demonstrates increased FDG uptake surrounding lateral aspect of proximal femoral component in keeping with periprosthetic infection (*arrow*). BM, ^{99m}Tc bone scan.

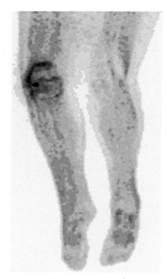

Fig. 10. A 58-year-old woman who had painful left knee prosthesis. Coronal FDG-PET maximal intensity projection image from posterior projection reveals diffusely increased FDG uptake surrounding left knee prosthesis interface on both sides of joint space in keeping with infection.

and aseptic loosening are fully defined by well-designed prospective studies. A recent meta-analysis has indicated that the FDG-PET sensitivity in identifying hip prosthesis infections was 82.8% and the specificity 87.3%. PET based on FDG could be a valid option if further research is able to specify uptake patterns that are specific for septic and aseptic loosening.[58]

Osteomyelitis

Acute osteomyelitis is commonly diagnosed by a combination of physical examination, laboratory findings, and imaging studies, including three-phase bone scintigraphy and MR imaging. Therefore, only a few studies regarding the role of FDG-PET in this clinical setting have been reported compared to that of chronic osteomyelitis. The main advantage of FDG-PET over other nuclear medicine techniques is its high spatial and contrast resolution, enabling it to distinguish between soft tissue infection and osteomyelitis.

Several groups have shown that FDG–PET/CT is accurate in differentiating between osteomyelitis and soft tissue involvement by infection (**Fig. 11**). In particular, preliminary data comparing FDG-PET, MR imaging, and plain film radiography for evaluation of osteomyelitis in the diabetic foot by Nawaz and colleagues[59] showed a sensitivity, specificity, PPV, and NPV for FDG-PET of 78%, 93%, 78%, and 93%, respectively, whereas MR imaging and plain film radiography showed a sensitivity, specificity, PPV, and NPV of 95%, 78%, 56%, and 98% and 57%, 85%, 57%, and 85%, respectively.

de Winter and colleagues[60] investigated the role of FDG-PET in detecting chronic musculoskeletal infection in an unselected patient population. Among 60 patients who had a suspected infection, 29 had an area of increased uptake, and infection was confirmed in 25 by histopathologicl studies or microbiologic culture. In 35 patients, no area of increased uptake was seen, and none of these patients was shown to have infection. The overall sensitivity, specificity, and accuracy were 100%, 88%, and 93%, respectively. Among four false-positive results, the investigators report that two most likely were related to the effects of recent surgery. FDG-PET was especially useful in detecting uptake in the axial skeleton, an area for which WBC scanning is of limited value. The researchers concluded that FDG-PET is highly accurate as

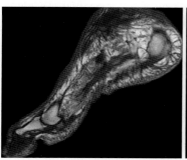
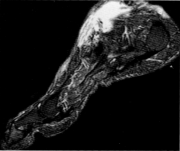
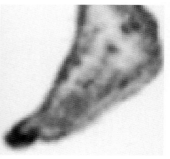

Fig. 11. A 50-year-old diabetic man. Sagittal T1-weighted (*left*) and fat-suppressed T2-weighted (*middle*) images through foot show decreased T1-weighted and increased T2-weighted signal intensity within distal phalanx of great toe with cortical destruction seen as loss of very low signal intensity osseous margin on T1-weighted images. Sagittal FDG-PET image (*right*) shows intense FDG uptake in same location. These findings are in keeping with osteomyelitis.

a single technique for the evaluation of chronic osteomyelitis. Another prospective study, by Meller and colleagues,[61] of 30 patients who had suspected active chronic osteomyelitis concluded that FDG-PET is superior to ^{111}In-WBC imaging in the diagnosis of chronic osteomyelitis in the central skeleton. FDG-PET accurately detects spinal osteomyelitis and could potentially replace ^{67}Ga for this purpose.

A recent meta-analysis showed that FDG-PET not only is the most sensitive imaging modality for detecting chronic osteomyelitis but also has a greater specificity than radiolabeled WBC scintigraphy, bone scintigraphy, or MR imaging.[62] In this meta-analysis, the pooled sensitivity demonstrated that FDG-PET was the most sensitive technique, with a sensitivity of 96% compared to 82% for bone scintigraphy, 61% for radiolabeled WBC scintigraphy, 78% for combined bone and radiolabeled WBC scintigraphy, and 84% for MR imaging. The pooled specificity demonstrated that bone scintigraphy had the lowest specificity, with a specificity of 25% compared with 60% for MR imaging, 77% for radiolabeled WBC scintigraphy, 84% for combined bone and radiolabeled WBC scintigraphy, and 91% for FDG-PET.

It is expected that FDG-PET imaging will be used routinely in the near future to determine the presence or the absence of an infectious focus, to monitor response to antimicrobial treatment, and to determine when treatment can safely be discontinued.

Diabetic Foot Complications

Differentiation between osteomyelitis and Charcot's neuroarthropathy in the diabetic patient population is a clinical and radiologic challenge. Use of MR imaging to distinguish between Charcot's neuroarthropathy and osteomyelitis sometimes can be difficult given that signal abnormalities in the bone and bone marrow frequently are nonspecific in etiology.

In a small study, Höpfner and colleagues compared FDG-PET with a dedicated full-ring PET scanner, FDG-PET with a coincidence camera, and MR imaging. The full-ring PET scanner accurately diagnosed Charcot's arthropathy in all 39 patients who had surgically proved Charcot's arthropathy for a sensitivity of 100%. The coincidence PET camera was 77% sensitive and MR imaging showed a sensitivity of 79%.[63]

Data from the authors' group[64] showed that in four groups, total 63 patients, a low degree of diffuse FDG uptake was observed in Charcot joints **(Fig. 12)**, which were clearly distinguishable from normal joints. The maximum SUV in Charcot joints varied from 0.7 to 2.4, whereas that of midfoot of normal control subjects and of patients who had an uncomplicated diabetic foot ranged from 0.2 to 0.7 and from 0.2 to 0.8, respectively. The maximum SUV of sites of osteomyelitis as a complication of the diabetic foot ranged from 2.9 to 6.2. Overall, the sensitivity and accuracy of FDG-PET in the diagnosis of Charcot's neuroarthropathy were 100% and 93.8%, respectively, and for MR imaging the values were 76.9% and 75.0%, respectively. These results indicate the usefulness of FDG-PET in the setting of the diabetic foot to reliably differentiate Charcot's neuroarthropathy from osteomyelitis. In summary, FDG-PET can differentiate between Charcot's neuroarthropathy, osteomyelitis, and soft tissue infection in the diabetic foot.

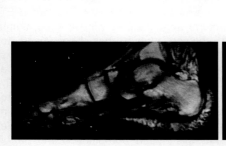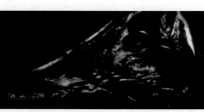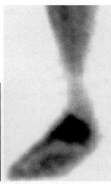

Fig. 12. A 57-year-old diabetic woman. Sagittal T1-weighted (*left*) and fat-suppressed T2-weighted (*middle*) images of foot demonstrate fragmentation and disorganization of joints of midfoot with reactive high T2-weighted signal intensity bone marrow. Sagittal FDG-PET maximal intensity projection image (*right*) of foot demonstrates mild FDG uptake in corresponding location. These findings are in keeping with Charcot's neuroarthropathy.

Arthritis

The most common form of inflammatory arthritis is rheumatoid arthritis, affecting 1% of the population.[65] It is characterized by chronic autoimmune inflammation with leukocyte infiltrate and proliferation of the synovial membrane, which result in destruction of bone and cartilage. As FDG accumulates in activated leukocytes, FDG-PET potentially can directly reveal the inflammatory process before the secondary changes of hyperemia or erosions are seen on bone scintigraphy and plain film radiography, respectively.[66,67] The clinical usefulness of FDG-PET for evaluation of the inflammatory arthritides currently is under investigation, but there is promising data that suggest a correlation of imaging results with clinical findings.

In a small series of patients who had clinically active inflammatory arthritis, FDG-PET positivity was correlated to clinical findings of pain, tenderness, and swelling.[68] The positivity rate of PET (69%) was similar to those of MR imaging (69%) and ultrasonography (75%) at baseline. In addition, there was a strong correlation between an elevated SUV and increased synovial thickness measured at MR imaging or ultrasonography on baseline studies. Decreases in SUV after treatment correlated with decreases in synovial enhancement, serum C-reactive protein levels, and serum metalloproteinase-3 levels but not with synovial thickness on MR imaging.[69,70]

A recent study evaluated the role of FDG–PET/CT in assessing the inflammatory activity of the rheumatoid synovium.[71] The extent and area of synovial inflammation were well delineated with this imaging approach, which was found more informative than conventional radiographic techniques. The degree of FDG uptake as an indication of the severity of the inflammatory process may become an important source of information in other rheumatologic conditions, such as osteoarthritis. In a recent study, the authors examined patients who had osteoarthritis and painful knee joints. Of the 18 knees that were reported to be painful, 78% had knee joint space maximum SUVs that exceeded the average maximum SUV of control knee joints, and 83% had synovial maximum SUVs that exceeded the average maximum SUV of control knees. The difference between the two groups was found significant for joint space and synovial uptake of FDG. The authors concluded that pain in the joint due to inflammation is associated with increased metabolic activity as seen on FDG-PET.[72]

FUTURE PROSPECTS

Increasingly, disorders involving the entire musculoskeletal system can be assessed by PET methodologies. Although FDG will be of great value in the assessment of inflammatory and infectious processes, ^{18}F-NaF PET may replace planar scintigraphy or SPECT imaging using single gamma-emitter radiopharmaceuticals for the evaluation of osseous abnormalities. This will be of great importance particularly in examination of the axial skeleton where a large volume of tissue is projected onto a single projection image.

Other novel radiotracers may play a role for examining specific pathologic states. Among these are those to assess bone marrow diseases due to variable pathologic states. ^{18}F-fluorothymidine (FLT), a radiolabeled thymidine analogue that reflects cellular proliferation, may be of value in differentiating proliferative marrow from hematologic malignancies, such as leukemia and multiple myeloma.[73,74] In addition, FLT may aid in determining early response to chemotherapy in the setting of hematologic malignancy, as cytotoxic chemotherapy will affect cell division earlier and to a greater extent than glucose metabolism.[75] Other radiotracers, including copper 60 diacetyl-bis (N^4-methylthiosemicarbazone), 2-(2-nitroimidazol-1H-yl)-N-(3-^{18}F-fluoropropyl-acetamide), and [2-(2-nitro-1H-imidazol-1-yl)-N-(2.2,3,3,3-pentafluoropropyl-acetamide)], diffuse into normally oxygenated and deoxygenated tissues but are retained in substantially higher concentration in hypoxic tissues.[76,77] These hypoxia agents may play a future role in optimal understanding of diseases that cause ischemia in the marrow space, such as sickle cell anemia.

Likewise, PET/CT will be a useful adjunct for most of the clinical applications of this modality in the axial and appendicular skeleton. Because of the poor sensitivity of CT in the detection of bone marrow abnormalities in certain disorders, however, correlative assessment between PET and structural abnormalities will be suboptimal. PET/MR imaging already has been used to depict the exact location of meniscal tears with associated synovitis.[78] Therefore, the authors believe that the introduction of PET/MR imaging will add a major dimension to research and clinical applications of PET in a variety of musculoskeletal disorders. We expect that this hybrid combination will be of critical value for the assessment of musculoskeletal abnormalities associated with bone marrow and soft tissue abnormalities.

SUMMARY

FDG-PET has an established role in the evaluation of hip periprosthetic infection and musculoskeletal malignancies. Determination of its role in the management of inflammatory arthritis and diabetic foot complications is ongoing. The reintroduction of ^{18}F-NaF as a PET radiotracer may advantageously replace ^{99m}Tc-MDP for some nononcologic applications, including treatment monitoring of Paget's disease and fibrous dysplasia. The combination of CT or MR imaging with PET imaging synergistically maximizes the diagnostic potential of a combined structural-functional imaging approach for the detection, characterization, and monitoring of myriad musculoskeletal disorders.

REFERENCES

1. Grant FD, Fahey FH, Packard AB, et al. Skeletal PET with 18F-fluoride: applying new technology to an old tracer. J Nucl Med 2008;49(1):68–78.

2. Bleeker-Rovers CP, de Kleijn EM, Corstens FH, et al. Clinical value of FDG PET in patients with fever of unknown origin and patients suspected of focal infection or inflammation. Eur J Nucl Med Mol Imaging 2004;31(1):29–37.

3. Zhuang H, Yu JQ, Alavi A. Applications of fluorodeoxyglucose-PET imaging in the detection of infection and inflammation and other benign disorders. Radiol Clin North Am 2005;43(1):121–34.

4. Blau M, Ganatra R, Bender MA. 18 F-fluoride for bone imaging. Semin Nucl Med 1972;2(1):31–7.

5. Hawkins RA, Choi Y, Huang SC, et al. Evaluation of the skeletal kinetics of fluorine-18-fluoride ion with PET. J Nucl Med 1992;33(5):633–42.

6. Zhuang HM, Cortes-Blanco A, Pourdehnad M, et al. Do high glucose levels have differential effect on FDG uptake in inflammatory and malignant disorders? Nucl Med Commun 2001;22(10):1123–8.

7. Kelly WM, Paglen PG, Pearson JA, et al. Ferromagnetism of intraocular foreign body causes unilateral blindness after MR study. AJNR Am J Neuroradiol 1986;7(2):243–5.

8. Klucznik RP, Carrier DA, Pyka R, et al. Placement of a ferromagnetic intracerebral aneurysm clip in a magnetic field with a fatal outcome. Radiology 1993;187(3):855–6.

9. Boutin RD, Briggs JE, Williamson MR. Injuries associated with MR imaging: survey of safety records and methods used to screen patients for metallic foreign bodies before imaging. AJR Am J Roentgenol 1994; 162(1):189–94.

10. Kulshrestha M, Misson G. Magnetic resonance imaging and the dangers of orbital foreign bodies. Br J Ophthalmol 1995;79(12):1149.

11. Shinbane JS, Colletti PM, Shellock FG. MR in patients with pacemakers and ICDs: Defining the issues. J Cardiovasc Magn Reson 2007;9(1):5–13.

12. Hofmann M, Pichler B, Scholkopf B, et al. Towards quantitative PET/MRI: a review of MR-based attenuation correction techniques. Eur J Nucl Med Mol Imaging 2009;36(Suppl 1):S93–104.

13. Hofmann M, Steinke F, Scheel V, et al. MRI-based attenuation correction for PET/MRI: a novel approach combining pattern recognition and atlas registration. J Nucl Med 2008;49(11):1875–83.

14. Beyer T, Weigert M, Quick HH, et al. MR-based attenuation correction for torso-PET/MR imaging: pitfalls in mapping MR to CT data. Eur J Nucl Med Mol Imaging 2008;35(6):1142–6.

15. Foucar K, McKenna RW, Frizzera G, et al. Bone marrow and blood involvement by lymphoma in relationship to the Lukes–Collins classification. Cancer 1982;49(5):888–97.

16. Lambertenghi-Deliliers G, Annaloro C, Soligo D, et al. Incidence and histological features of bone marrow involvement in malignant lymphomas. Ann Hematol 1992;65(2):61–5.

17. McKenna RW, Hernandez JA. Bone marrow in malignant lymphoma. Hematol Oncol Clin North Am 1988;2(4):617–35.

18. Fletcher JW, Djulbegovic B, Soares HP, et al. Recommendations on the use of 18F-FDG PET in oncology. J Nucl Med 2008;49(3):480–508.

19. Isohashi K, Tatsumi M, Higuchi I, et al. 18F-FDG-PET in patients with malignant lymphoma having long-term follow-up: staging and restaging, and evaluation of treatment response and recurrence. Ann Nucl Med 2008;22(9):795–802.

20. Pakos EE, Fotopoulos AD, Ioannidis JP. 18F-FDG PET for evaluation of bone marrow infiltration in staging of lymphoma: a meta-analysis. J Nucl Med 2005;46(6):958–63.

21. Schaefer NG, Strobel K, Taverna C, et al. Bone involvement in patients with lymphoma: the role of FDG-PET/CT. Eur J Nucl Med Mol Imaging 2007; 34(1):60–7.

22. Kwee TC, Kwee RM, Nievelstein RA. Imaging in staging of malignant lymphoma: a systematic review. Blood 2008;111(2):504–16.

23. Bastiaannet E, Groen H, Jager PL, et al. The value of FDG-PET in the detection, grading and response to therapy of soft tissue and bone sarcomas; a systematic review and meta-analysis. Cancer Treat Rev 2004;30(1):83–101.

24. Tateishi U, Yamaguchi U, Seki K, et al. Bone and soft-tissue sarcoma: preoperative staging with fluorine 18 fluorodeoxyglucose PET/CT and conventional imaging. Radiology 2007;245(3):839–47.

25. Bredella MA, Caputo GR, Steinbach LS. Value of FDG positron emission tomography in conjunction with MR imaging for evaluating therapy response

in patients with musculoskeletal sarcomas. AJR Am J Roentgenol 2002;179(5):1145–50.

26. Durie BG, Salmon SE. A clinical staging system for multiple myeloma. Correlation of measured myeloma cell mass with presenting clinical features, response to treatment, and survival. Cancer 1975; 36(3):842–54.

27. Durie BG, Waxman AD, D'Agnolo A, et al. Whole-body (18)F-FDG PET identifies high-risk myeloma. J Nucl Med 2002;43(11):1457–63.

28. Durie BG, Kyle RA, Belch A, et al. Myeloma management guidelines: a consensus report from the Scientific Advisors of the International Myeloma Foundation. Hematol J 2003;4(6):379–98.

29. Fonti R, Salvatore B, Quarantelli M, et al. 18F-FDG PET/CT, 99mTc-MIBI, and MRI in evaluation of patients with multiple myeloma. J Nucl Med 2008.

30. Langsteger W, Heinisch M, Fogelman I. The role of fluorodeoxyglucose, 18F-dihydroxyphenylalanine, 18F-choline, and 18F-fluoride in bone imaging with emphasis on prostate and breast. Semin Nucl Med 2006;36(1):73–92.

31. Even-Sapir E, Metser U, Mishani E, et al. The detection of bone metastases in patients with high-risk prostate cancer: 99mTc-MDP Planar bone scintigraphy, single- and multi-field-of-view SPECT, 18F-fluoride PET, and 18F-fluoride PET/CT. J Nucl Med 2006;47(2):287–97.

32. Even-Sapir E, Metser U, Flusser G, et al. Assessment of malignant skeletal disease: initial experience with 18F-fluoride PET/CT and comparison between 18F-fluoride PET and 18F-fluoride PET/CT. J Nucl Med 2004;45(2):272–8.

33. Patel S, Pearson D, Hosking DJ. Quantitative bone scintigraphy in the management of monostotic Paget's disease of bone. Arthritis Rheum 1995; 38(10):1506–12.

34. Installe J, Nzeusseu A, Bol A, et al. (18)F-fluoride PET for monitoring therapeutic response in Paget's disease of bone. J Nucl Med 2005;46(10):1650–8.

35. Frost ML, Cook GJ, Blake GM, et al. A prospective study of risedronate on regional bone metabolism and blood flow at the lumbar spine measured by 18F-fluoride positron emission tomography. J Bone Miner Res 2003;18(12):2215–22.

36. Messa C, Goodman WG, Hoh CK, et al. Bone metabolic activity measured with positron emission tomography and [18F]fluoride ion in renal osteodystrophy: correlation with bone histomorphometry. J Clin Endocrinol Metab 1993;77(4):949–55.

37. Cook GJ, Blake GM, Marsden PK, et al. Quantification of skeletal kinetic indices in Paget's disease using dynamic 18F-fluoride positron emission tomography. J Bone Miner Res 2002; 17(5):854–9.

38. Meunier PJ, Coindre JM, Edouard CM, et al. Bone histomorphometry in Paget's disease. Quantitative and dynamic analysis of pagetic and nonpagetic bone tissue. Arthritis Rheum 1980;23(10):1095–103.

39. Devogelaer JP. Modern therapy for Paget's disease of bone: focus on bisphosphonates. Treat Endocrinol 2002;1(4):241–57.

40. Cook GJ, Lodge MA, Blake GM, et al. Differences in skeletal kinetics between vertebral and humeral bone measured by 18F-fluoride positron emission tomography in postmenopausal women. J Bone Miner Res 2000;15(4):763–9.

41. Fogelman I, Bessent R. Age-related alterations in skeletal metabolism—24-hr whole-body retention of diphosphonate in 250 normal subjects: concise communication. J Nucl Med 1982;23(4):296–300.

42. Thomsen K, Johansen J, Nilas L, et al. Whole body retention of 99mTc-diphosphonate. Relation to biochemical indices of bone turnover and to total body calcium. Eur J Nucl Med 1987;13(1):32–5.

43. Blake GM, Park-Holohan SJ, Fogelman I. Quantitative studies of bone in postmenopausal women using (18)F-fluoride and (99m)Tc-methylene diphosphonate. J Nucl Med 2002;43(3):338–45.

44. Ovadia D, Metser U, Lievshitz G, et al. Back pain in adolescents: assessment with integrated 18F-fluoride positron-emission tomography-computed tomography. J Pediatr Orthop 2007;27(1):90–3.

45. Lim R, Fahey FH, Drubach LA, et al. Early experience with fluorine-18 sodium fluoride bone PET in young patients with back pain. J Pediatr Orthop 2007;27(3):277–82.

46. Schiepers C, Broos P, Miserez M, et al. Measurement of skeletal flow with positron emission tomography and 18F-fluoride in femoral head osteonecrosis. Arch Orthop Trauma Surg 1998; 118(3):131–5.

47. Forrest N, Welch A, Murray AD, et al. Femoral head viability after Birmingham resurfacing hip arthroplasty: assessment with use of [18F] fluoride positron emission tomography. J Bone Joint Surg Am 2006;88(Suppl 3):84–9.

48. Piert M, Winter E, Becker GA, et al. Allogenic bone graft viability after hip revision arthroplasty assessed by dynamic [18F]fluoride ion positron emission tomography. Eur J Nucl Med 1999;26(6):615–24.

49. Sorensen J, Ullmark G, Langstrom B, et al. Rapid bone and blood flow formation in impacted morselized allografts: positron emission tomography (PET) studies on allografts in 5 femoral component revisions of total hip arthroplasty. Acta Orthop Scand 2003;74(6):633–43.

50. Piney A. The anatomy of the bone marrow with special reference to the distribution of the red marrow. Br Med J 1922;28:792–5.

51. Blebea JS, Houseni M, Torigian DA, et al. Structural and functional imaging of normal bone marrow and evaluation of its age-related changes. Semin Nucl Med 2007;37(3):185–94.

52. Furnes O, Lie SA, Espehaug B, et al. Hip disease and the prognosis of total hip replacements. A review of 53,698 primary total hip replacements reported to the Norwegian Arthroplasty Register 1987-99. J Bone Joint Surg Br 2001;83(4):579–86.

53. Zhuang H, Yang H, Alavi A. Critical role of 18F-labeled fluorodeoxyglucose PET in the management of patients with arthroplasty. Radiol Clin North Am 2007;45(4):711–8, vii.

54. Chryssikos T, Parvizi J, Ghanem E, et al. FDG-PET imaging can diagnose periprosthetic infection of the hip. Clin Orthop Relat Res 2008;466(6):1338–42.

55. Zhuang H, Duarte PS, Pourdehnad M, et al. The promising role of 18F-FDG PET in detecting infected lower limb prosthesis implants. J Nucl Med 2001; 42(1):44–8.

56. Pill SG, Parvizi J, Tang PH, et al. Comparison of fluorodeoxyglucose positron emission tomography and (111)indium-white blood cell imaging in the diagnosis of periprosthetic infection of the hip. J Arthroplasty 2006;21(6 Suppl 2):91–7.

57. Chacko TK, Zhuang H, Stevenson K, et al. The importance of the location of fluorodeoxyglucose uptake in periprosthetic infection in painful hip prostheses. Nucl Med Commun 2002;23(9):851–5.

58. Zoccali C, Teori G, Salducca N. The role of FDG-PET in distinguishing between septic and aseptic loosening in hip prosthesis: a review of literature. Int Orthop 2009;33(1):1–5.

59. Nawaz A, Torigian D, Zhuang H, et al. Diagnostic performance of FDG-PET, MRI, and plain film radiography (PFR) in the diagnosis of acute osteomyelitis in the diabetic foot. J Nucl Med 2008;49(Suppl 1):134P.

60. de Winter F, van de Wiele C, Vogelaers D, et al. Fluorine-18 fluorodeoxyglucose-position emission tomography: a highly accurate imaging modality for the diagnosis of chronic musculoskeletal infections. J Bone Joint Surg Am 2001;83-A(5):651–60.

61. Meller J, Koster G, Liersch T, et al. Chronic bacterial osteomyelitis: prospective comparison of (18)F-FDG imaging with a dual-head coincidence camera and (111)In-labelled autologous leucocyte scintigraphy. Eur J Nucl Med Mol Imaging 2002;29(1):53–60.

62. Termaat MF, Raijmakers PG, Scholten HJ, et al. The accuracy of diagnostic imaging for the assessment of chronic osteomyelitis: a systematic review and meta-analysis. J Bone Joint Surg Am 2005;87(11): 2464–71.

63. Höpfner S, Krolak C, Kessler S, et al. Preoperative imaging of Charcot neuroarthropathy in diabetic patients: comparison of ring PET, hybrid PET, and magnetic resonance imaging. Foot Ankle Int 2004; 25(12):890–5.

64. Basu S, Chryssikos T, Houseni M, et al. Potential role of FDG PET in the setting of diabetic neuro-osteoarthropathy: can it differentiate uncomplicated Charcot's neuroarthropathy from osteomyelitis and

soft-tissue infection? Nucl Med Commun 2007; 28(6):465–72.

65. Scott DL, Symmons DP, Coulton BL, et al. Long-term outcome of treating rheumatoid arthritis: results after 20 years. Lancet 1987;1(8542):1108–11.

66. Polisson RP, Schoenberg OI, Fischman A, et al. Use of magnetic resonance imaging and positron emission tomography in the assessment of synovial volume and glucose metabolism in patients with rheumatoid arthritis. Arthritis Rheum 1995;38(6):819–25.

67. Palmer WE, Rosenthal DI, Schoenberg OI, et al. Quantification of inflammation in the wrist with gadolinium-enhanced MR imaging and PET with 2-[F-18]-fluoro-2-deoxy-D-glucose. Radiology 1995;196(3):647–55.

68. Elzinga EH, van der Laken CJ, Comans EF, et al. 2-Deoxy-2-[F-18]fluoro-D-glucose joint uptake on positron emission tomography images: rheumatoid arthritis versus osteoarthritis. Mol Imaging Biol 2007;9(6):357–60.

69. Beckers C, Jeukens X, Ribbens C, et al. (18)F-FDG PET imaging of rheumatoid knee synovitis correlates with dynamic magnetic resonance and sonographic assessments as well as with the serum level of metalloproteinase-3. Eur J Nucl Med Mol Imaging 2006; 33(3):275–80.

70. Beckers C, Ribbens C, Andre B, et al. Assessment of disease activity in rheumatoid arthritis with (18)F-FDG PET. J Nucl Med 2004;45(6):956–64.

71. Ju JH, Kang KY, Kim IJ, et al. Visualization and localization of rheumatoid knee synovitis with FDG-PET/CT images. Clin Rheumatol 2008;27(Suppl 2):S39–41.

72. Parsons M, Torigian D, Alavi A. Metabolic activity in the painful knee joint as measured on FDG-PET. J Nucl Med 2008;49(Suppl 1):270P.

73. Barthel H, Cleij MC, Collingridge DR, et al. 3′-deoxy-3′-[18F]fluorothymidine as a new marker for monitoring tumor response to antiproliferative therapy in vivo with positron emission tomography. Cancer Res 2003;63(13):3791–8.

74. Buck AK, Schirrmeister H, Hetzel M, et al. 3-deoxy-3-[(18)F]fluorothymidine-positron emission tomography for noninvasive assessment of proliferation in pulmonary nodules. Cancer Res 2002;62(12):3331–4.

75. Dittmann H, Dohmen BM, Paulsen F, et al. [18F]FLT PET for diagnosis and staging of thoracic tumours. Eur J Nucl Med Mol Imaging 2003;30(10):1407–12.

76. Evans SM, Kachur AV, Shiue CY, et al. Noninvasive detection of tumor hypoxia using the 2-nitroimidazole [18F]EF1. J Nucl Med 2000;41(2):327–36.

77. Dolbier WR Jr, Li AR, Koch CJ, et al. [18F]-EF5, a marker for PET detection of hypoxia: synthesis of precursor and a new fluorination procedure. Appl Radiat Isot 2001;54(1):73–80.

78. El-Haddad G, Kumar R, Pamplona R, et al. PET/MRI depicts the exact location of meniscal tear associated with synovitis. Eur J Nucl Med Mol Imaging 2006;33(4):507–8.

Index

Note: Page numbers of article titles are in **boldface** type.

PET Clin 3 (2009) 467–472
doi:10.1016/S1556-8598(09)00044-3
1556-8598/09/$ – see front matter © 2009 Elsevier Inc. All rights reserved.

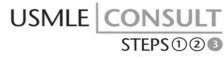